Cognitive Neuroscience of Human System

Work and Everyday Life

Human Factors and Ergonomics Series

Cognitive Neuroscience of Human Systems

Work and Everyday Life

Chris Forsythe
Huafei Liao
Michael Trumbo
Rogelio E. Cardona-Rivera

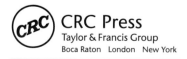

CRC Press
Taylor & Francis Group
Boca Raton   London   New York

CRC Press is an imprint of the
Taylor & Francis Group, an **informa** business

CRC Press
Taylor & Francis Group
6000 Broken Sound Parkway NW, Suite 300
Boca Raton, FL 33487-2742

First issued in paperback 2017

© 2014 by Taylor & Francis Group, LLC
CRC Press is an imprint of Taylor & Francis Group, an Informa business

No claim to original U.S. Government works

Version Date: 20150123

ISBN 13: 978-1-4665-7057-3 (hbk)
ISBN 13: 978-1-138-07337-1 (pbk)

Visit the Taylor & Francis Web site at
http://www.taylorandfrancis.com

and the CRC Press Web site at
http://www.crcpress.com

Contents

Authors

Chris Forsythe is a distinguished member of the technical staff at Sandia National Laboratories, in Albuquerque, New Mexico. He has a PhD in experimental psychology and an MS in biopsychology from the University of Memphis. His primary expertise lies in the application of technology to improve human performance. He has worked in diverse areas that include human–machine transactions, high consequence systems, cyber, automotive systems, training, and neurotechnology. His research interests encompass individual differences in the neurophysiology of human performance, advanced training technologies development, and human–machine systems integration. He regularly conducts seminars on the application of brain science to everyday life for audiences that extend from professional conference attendees to elementary school–age children and works extensively with youth to promote their interest in science and technology.

Huafei (Harry) Liao is a senior technical staff member in the Risk and Reliability Analysis Department of Sandia National Laboratories, Albuquerque, New Mexico. He has many years of experience with human performance modeling in the nuclear industry, and his work currently focuses on human factors and human reliability in complex systems and high-risk environments. He holds a BS and MS in control theories and control engineering from Tsinghua University, Beijing, China, and a PhD in human factors and ergonomics from Purdue University.

Michael C.S. Trumbo is a doctoral candidate in the Cognition, Brain, and Behavior program within the University of New Mexico Psychology Department, where he is further affiliated with the Psychology Clinical Neuroscience Center. Additionally, Michael conducts research on human performance at Sandia National Laboratories and through The Mind Research Network and Lovelace Biomedical and Environmental Research Institute. Research interests center on facilitation of human performance in both clinical and healthy populations in a variety of professional and educational realms, with a particular emphasis on the use of electrical brain stimulation in order to achieve this.

Rogelio E. Cardona-Rivera is a PhD student in computer science at North Carolina State University and is advised by Dr. R. Michael Young in the Liquid Narrative Research Group. Rogelio's thesis work is at the intersection of artificial intelligence, cognitive science, narratology, and game design and focuses on creating a cognitive model of the player's understanding of an unfolding story in an interactive narrative through the use of narrative affordances. Rogelio completed an MS in computer science at North Carolina State University and a BS in computer engineering at the University of Puerto Rico at Mayagüez. He has held internship positions at Sandia National Laboratories, Apple, The MIT/Lincoln Laboratory, and Goldman Sachs. Rogelio is a Department of Energy Computational Science graduate fellow and a GEM fellow.

1

Introduction

What do most people know about their brains? Do they know as much as they know about their favorite sports teams or their favorite celebrities? Can they describe the operations of their brains with the precision that they list the ingredients and steps in a favorite recipe or explain the nuances of playing a popular electronic game? Do they track their brains with the regularity that they follow the weather, the price of gas, or how much money they have in their wallets? Yet, all that we experience, all that we know, and all that we do is a direct, inseparable product of our brains.

For most of us, our brains serve as the conduit through which we experience life, but nothing more. We may have thoughtfully devised programs for exercising our bodies, and on any given day, we may know our weight within a couple of pounds, but we pay scant attention to the state of our brains, how we may be affecting them, how we may be affecting the brains of others, and how our own brains are being affected during the course of everyday life.

In the following chapters, our primary objective is to summarize current brain science, but most importantly, highlight and explain the practical, everyday application of brain science. Today, there may be no field that produces a larger volume of scientific papers, books, and other publications than brain science, or *neuroscience*. However, with little exception, these publications are esoteric and beyond the reach of those without the requisite academic training (i.e., generally, an advanced degree in neuroscience or a similar field). This occurs despite recognition in diverse fields ranging from education to engineering to marketing that brain science is highly relevant to these domains. Our goal is to make brain science accessible to a wide array of professions and to do so in a manner that allows readers to readily apply brain science to their own professional endeavors.

We will discuss current perspectives on brain science, as well as many recent research findings. Particular emphasis will be placed on factors that affect performance and behavior, including common vulnerabilities contributing to errors, misinterpretations, and lapses in judgment, as well as factors that affect our social interactions and allow us to work more or less effectively as teams, groups, and organizations. Special care will be taken to not present countless facts that would soon be forgotten. For example, basic brain function will be described without detailed descriptions of the related anatomical structures, given our belief that few readers will possess a thorough knowledge of neuroanatomy. Most of the material that would typically be covered in a college course concerning brain science will not be discussed here. This is because the bulk of current knowledge about the brain, while interesting, cannot be easily translated into insights and principles that may be readily applied to everyday activities. For instance, numerous research programs are working toward an understanding of how the cells of the brain operate, and interact with one another, at the smallest measurable scale (i.e., nanoscale, or one millionth of a meter). While important to many endeavors (e.g., engineering new drugs that have highly specific effects on the brain), there is little insight that can be gleamed from this knowledge to help individuals understand why people do what they do, or how to achieve more effective outcomes.

In the forthcoming chapters, the discussion will often extend beyond the science of the brain to encompass research and theories that might be best described as behavior science. There are many insights arising from the broad study of human behavior, for which many of the neural underpinnings are not well understood. Today, the traditional behavior sciences, which include psychology, sociology, anthropology, economics, and political science, are increasingly influenced by brain science. This is partly due to the growing availability of equipment to study brain function, such as the electroencephalogram (EEG), and neural imaging such as functional magnetic resonance imaging (fMRI). Additionally, there is a natural tendency for scientists to look to deeper and deeper levels, in this case the functioning of the brain, to uncover causes for the phenomena they study.

A convergence of brain science and behavior science is an inevitable outcome and the two have a reciprocal interest in embracing one another. As noted, brain science provides insight into the fundamental mechanisms of observable behavior. In kind, behavior science speaks to the mechanisms by which the environment has shaped modern humans and, particularly, our brains. As with any animal species, our brains are the product of our specific adaptations to cope with various challenges and to capitalize on opportunities afforded by the environments in which we evolved. In the same way that various species have developed complex courtship and mating rituals involving sometimes tightly choreographed sequences of behavior and response, the human brain has been shaped through evolution to respond in a specific manner to certain events within the environment.

A later chapter will discuss the ultimatum game, which is a research paradigm in which experimental test subjects are offered real, spendable money with no strings attached, yet they regularly turn it down due to the social situation created within the context of the game (Sanfey et al., 2003). This is not a matter of delayed reinforcement where one sacrifices a small, immediate reward in favor of a later, larger award. Instead, the money is there for the taking; nothing is required of them, but they routinely say, "no thanks." Why would a test subject, most likely a college student, turn down the experimenters' money? This can happen if the situation is one that triggers disgust or anger that outweighs rational considerations. While humans are not as hardwired as other animal species, there are many curious behavioral tendencies that may be triggered by placing humans within certain situations.

The unconscious has long been a prominent idea used to explain human behavior within psychology (Westen, 1999). By unconscious, we mean that there are factors that shape our psychological experience and behavior that we are not aware of (e.g., subtle emotional reactions, forgotten memories). The notion of the unconscious fell into disfavor due to the twentieth-century dismissal of the fanciful propositions of Sigmund Freud and other early psychologists. However, the basic idea that our behavior is heavily influenced, and sometimes determined, by operations of the brain for which we do not have conscious awareness has undergone a modern revival due to the realization of neuroscientists that the overwhelming majority of what the brain does occurs at an unconscious level (Eagleman, 2011).

In a forthcoming chapter, there will be discussion of research showing that by using brain imaging, the decisions an experimental test subject will make can be predicted 7–10 s before the subject is consciously aware of his or her decision (Soon et al., 2008). In other words, the experimenter looking at the brain scan knows what the subject is going to do 7–10 s before the subject knows what he or she is going to do. Accepting the importance of unconscious brain processes, one can better understand human behavior that seems irrational, counterproductive, and even self-destructive (e.g., overeating and other self-destructive indulgences). Specifically, our behavior is regularly driven by operations of the brain that we are not consciously aware of; these brain operations are the product of the unique solutions that humans adopted to survive and flourish during the history of our species. Through the convergence of brain science and behavior science, the scientific understanding of brain operations is advancing and with this understanding, principles and insights arise that may be applied in everyday life to appreciate our own behavior, counteract our vulnerabilities, and more effectively engage in social interactions.

So that there is no confusion, the subject of this book is not human evolution or evolutionary psychology, and human evolution is not a component in much of the reasoning presented for understanding the brain and behavior, or applying this understanding to everyday activities. Imagine that one is asked to explain the automobile and why it has come to take its modern form. Some consideration of roadways and how they have influenced and shaped certain facets of automobile design would be expected. Similarly, some consideration of human evolution should naturally be expected in discussing the operations of the human brain. Furthermore, setting aside the historical context, it should not be forgotten that all operations of the brain occur within the context of an individual's environmental surroundings and human behavior involves a continual interplay between a person and his or her environment, including other people, occurring at both conscious and unconscious levels.

We believe that a broader awareness and consideration of the brain from the perspective of how knowledge, principles, and practices may be applied to improve everyday life is a natural step, even a culmination, of several trends. In a thought-provoking 2011 Technology, Entertainment, Design (TED) talk, journalist David Brooks (2011) discussed the predominance of rationalism in Western thought and its misleading influence on common beliefs concerning human behavior. It is generally assumed that people will behave in a rational manner and our institutions are organized on the basis of this belief. When we contemplate other's behavior, we assume that they will behave logically, given the rules and constraints that society has put in place, and we fault them, and often punish them, when their behavior does not adhere to the expectations of rationality. Furthermore, we value logical thought, and encourage and promote those who show an aptitude and a propensity for logical modes of thinking. However, humans often behave in a manner that may be thought of as irrational (e.g., fearing activities for which there is little risk while ignoring the real risks associated with other activities, or investing vast amounts of time and effort in activities for which there are little or no rewards). Moreover, while rational thought has been at the core of many human engineering and technical accomplishments, it has not served nearly as well in formulating our institutions. Soviet communism offers a sterling example. Its engineers never imagined the magnitude of corruption that would emerge, and become institutionalized, in a system that relied on everyone sacrificing for the greater good of the state.

A growing recognition of the irrational side of human behavior, often referred to as "human nature," has begun to reshape the field of economics (Tuckett, 2011). With financial investment, everyone knows that the logical strategy is to buy low and sell high. Yet, professional investors regularly disavow this most basic principle. The propensity to follow the crowd and do what everyone else is doing is so strong that software has been put in place to slow the tide, even put on the brakes, when the crowd has developed too much momentum.

David Tuckett (2011), an economist at the University College of London, describes the situation in the financial industry, where the information available to investors is essentially limitless, yet investors can never be certain of what will happen. Institutions expect that individual investors will always generate a positive return through their investment decisions, and a string of losses can quickly cause an investor to lose his or her job. The system sustains an illusion that individual investors, as well as the market as a whole, behave rationally. However, investors often merely watch what other investors are doing, and then they do the same. Tuckett notes that for the individual investor, "if I'm doing what everyone else is doing, I may lose money, but at least I won't get fired." However, investors will rarely acknowledge the extent to which their decisions are being influenced by others, but instead they will assert, and most likely believe, stories that explain their behavior in rational terms.

These ideas concerning how the operations of the brain can predispose people to seemingly irrational behavior can be seen in current trends within marketing. Before launching multimillion-dollar advertisement campaigns, many companies are now turning to organizations that specialize in "neuromarketing" to test prospective commercials (Sands Research, 2012). In these tests, high-density EEG is used to image the activity in the brain of sample viewers as they watch a commercial. The resulting images of the viewers' brains help to identify what facets of a commercial evoke the strongest responses and, particularly, where emotional responses are evoked and how strong those emotional responses are. Sands Research Inc. has been a pioneer in this area and has made numerous striking illustrations of their techniques public through videos posted to their website and to YouTube.

Another related trend is evident in the public's interest in personal health and fitness. While physical fitness garners the bulk of the attention, there is increasing discussion of "cognitive health" and a variety of businesses and other organizations offer products and services advertised to enhance cognitive performance (SharpBrains, 2012). The range of products spans nutritional supplements to energy drinks to brain-training exercises and games to educational products. In this vein, pharmaceuticals, such as Ritalin, are being used regularly in colleges and other educational settings to achieve on-demand enhancements in cognitive performance (White et al., 2006). Interestingly, it was reported that the number of professional baseball players self-reporting their use of Ritalin and similar pharmaceuticals prescribed to treat attention deficit hyperactive disorder (ADHD) has increased significantly, in parallel with the nonmedical use of these drugs to boost scholastic performance (Schmidt, 2009). In another development, due to the increasing use of biometric monitoring devices during physical exercise (e.g., heart rate monitors), a variety of biometric monitoring devices have been introduced for tracking brain activity, with the initial emphasis on measuring and improving the quality of sleep. These developments point to an overall trend in which large sectors of the population are now asking how they might improve their brain function and are turning to various supplements, products, and activities to accomplish this.

Finally, throughout human history—whether harnessing fire, inventing the printing press, or developing the Internet—it has been technological innovation that has expanded the bounds of human capability. Yet, as technology, and the way of life that has resulted from technology, has grown increasingly complex, our achievable limits are no longer determined by technology, but instead by human cognitive and physical capacities, in concert with our abilities to cope with the ensuing stresses. There is a broadening appreciation that we have reflexively turned to technology as the solution to our problems, but time and time again, often following great expenditures of money, time, and other resources, it is realized that there is a human dimension to our problems that cannot be ignored.

Today, with the Internet, despite massive investments in technologies for cybersecurity, the human remains the weakest link and the enabling factor for the rampant growth of criminal organizations devoted to cybercrime (Kraemer et al., 2009). No historical precedent exists for the economic commitment that the United States has made to technology as a basis for achieving military might, yet progress in the Iraq and Afghan conflicts only came after embracing a counterinsurgency policy that emphasized the need to form relationships with local authorities and populations (Metz, 2007). The transformations in professional and everyday life resulting from the ready availability of inexpensive, easy-to-use personal computers are a direct product of innovations, specifically the graphical user interface, that have minimized the specialized knowledge required to use a computer. Today, consumers expect products to be designed so that they are easy to use, and they will complain, abandon, and reject products that are hard to learn and use.

Technology has pushed us to our limits and further technological advances can only occur through thorough consideration and incorporation of the human dimension in the design of products and the management of organizations. This reality necessitates greater knowledge of and attention to how humans operate so that technologies and technological systems may be synergized with the humans that use them and are affected by them. Consequently, we believe that an understanding of the brain and how its operations shape our capabilities and experiences will become critical to effectively designing, implementing, managing, and sustaining technological systems. This sentiment is not new. It has been captured in the aspirations of the augmented cognition community and its founder USN Captain (ret.) Dylan Schmorrow (Forsythe et al., 2005) and in the thinking of Raja Parasuraman, a professor at George Mason University, in advancing neuro-ergonomics as a field of study and professional practice (Parasuraman and Rizzo, 2005).

In the following chapters, a variety of topics from brain science and their relevance to everyday activities are discussed. Little attention is focused on presenting and sorting out alternative theories. Instead, the chapters focus on the science, describing the findings and the scientific studies producing these findings. Emphasis is then placed on explaining how these findings relate to everyday life and how they might be integrated into one's professional endeavors. The ultimate goal is to provide usable knowledge that may be readily applied to day-to-day activities to achieve more effective outcomes based on a fundamental understanding of how the operations of the human brain produce behavior and modulate performance.

Acknowledgments

Sandia National Laboratories is a multiprogram laboratory managed and operated by Sandia Corporation, a wholly owned subsidiary of Lockheed Martin Corporation, for the US Department of Energy's National Nuclear Security Administration under contract DE-AC04-94AL85000.

References

Brooks, D. (2011). The social animal. *TED Ideas Worth Spreading*, Retrieved June 8, 2012, http://www.ted.com/talks/david_brooks_the_social_animal.html.

Eagleman, D. (2011). *Incognito: The Secret Lives of the Brain*. New York: Pantheon.

Forsythe, C., Kruse, A. and Schmorrow, D. (2005). Augmented cognition. In C. Forsythe, T.E. Goldsmith, and M.L. Bernard (eds), *Cognitive Systems: Cognitive Models in Systems Design*, pp. 99–134. Mahwah, NJ: Lawrence Erlbaum.

Kraemer, S., Carayon, P. and Clem, J. (2009). Human and organizational factors in computer and information security: Pathways to vulnerabilities. *Computers and Security, 28*(7), 509–520.

Metz, S. (2007). *Learning from Iraq: Counter-Insurgency in American Strategy*. Carlisle, PA: Strategic Studies Institute.

Parasuraman, R. and Rizzo, M. (2005). *Neuroergonomics: The Brain at Work*. Oxford: Oxford University Press.

Sands Research. (2012). *Sands Research*, Retrieved June 8, 2012, http://www.sandsresearch.com/default.aspx.

Sanfey, A.G., Rilling, J.K., Aronson, J.A., Nystrom, L.E. and Cohen, J.D. (2003). The neural basis of economic decision-making in the ultimatum game. *Science, 300*(5626), 1755–1758.

Schmidt, M.S. (2009). What is ADHD—And why are so many Major League Baseball players getting this diagnosis? *New York Times*, December 1.

SharpBrains. (2012). Market research tracking brain fitness innovation: News, research, tech, trends, *SharpBrains*, Retrieved June 8, 2012, http://www.sharpbrains.com/.

Soon, C.S., Brass, M., Heinze, H.J. and Haynes, J.D. (2008). Unconscious determinants of free decisions in the human brain. *Nature Neuroscience, 11*, 543–545.

Tuckett, D. (2011). *Minding the Markets: An Emotional Finance View of Financial Instability*. New York: Palgrave Macmillan.

Westen, D. (1999). The scientific status of unconscious processes: Is Freud really dead? *Journal of the American Psychoanalytic Association, 47*(4), 1061–1106.

White, B.P., Becker-Blease, K.A. and Grace-Bishop, K. (2006). Stimulant medication use, misuse and abuse in an undergraduate and graduate student sample. *Journal of American College Health, 54*(5), 261–268.

2

A Few Basics

This chapter offers background information that will be useful in considering the topics discussed in subsequent chapters. This background information consists of essential facts concerning the mechanics of the brain and the techniques that are used to measure brain function, as well as perspectives for appreciating the relevance of scientific research in cognitive neuroscience to everyday situations.

Neurons: A Basic Unit of the Brain

The brain consists of many different cell types, but scientists have primarily focused their attention on a type of cell known as a *neuron*. This is not unreasonable since neurons are unique among all the cells within the body. In particular, neurons have a specialized capacity to conduct electrical current, but perhaps more importantly, they form complex networks of interconnecting cells that interact with one another in ways that scientists do not fully understand.

When a neuron fires, there is an exchange of molecules across the cell walls separating the inside and outside of the neuron that produces an electrical charge. Beginning near one end of the neuron, this exchange of electrically charged molecules travels like a wave transmitting an electrical current the length of the neuron. The initial transfer of electrically charged molecules across the neuron's cell walls is a passive process that does not require energy. However, after a neuron has fired, the cellular machinery that restores the neuron to its previous state so that it is ready to fire again is active and requires considerable energy (Byrne and Roberts, 2004).

Within the brain, neurons form extremely complex networks. A given neuron may receive input from thousands of other neurons and send output to just as many. However, the connections between neurons are generally not physical connections. Instead, there are fluid-filled gaps between one neuron and the next. When a neuron fires, specialized molecules known as *neurotransmitters* are released into the gap separating one neuron from the next. The neurotransmitter molecules may bind to points on the next neuron known as *receptors*. When a neurotransmitter binds to the receptors of a neuron it may either make that neuron more likely to fire (i.e., *excitatory*) or make it less likely to fire (i.e., *inhibitory*). When enough excitatory neurotransmitters have bound to the receptors of a nearby neuron, a threshold is surpassed and the neuron fires. As occurred with the previous neuron, a wave of electrical energy travels the length of this next neuron, and then, when the wave of electrical current reaches the end of the neuron, the neuron releases its neurotransmitters, which may then bind to the receptors of subsequent neurons.

In this brief description, I have skimmed over enough details to fill a series of books. What is important to know is that the operations of the brain involve countless electrochemical events occurring across an immensely complex web of interconnecting neurons. This is important because when we discuss measurement of the electrical activity of the brain, we should remember that the resulting signals represent the combination of countless electrochemical events involving thousands, if not millions, of individual neurons. Additionally, as will be discussed in a later chapter, the introduction of electrical or magnetic energy and certain chemical compounds (e.g., caffeine and other psychoactive substances) offers mechanisms by which the activity of the brain may be manipulated.

Furthermore, it is important to remember that the molecular machinery that gives neurons their unique capacity to transmit electrical current consumes energy. Actually, relative to other parts of the body, the brain consumes an enormous amount of energy (Mink et al., 1981). While representing only 2% of the total body weight, the brain receives 15% of the blood from the heart, and accounts for 20% of the total oxygen consumption and 25% of the total glucose consumption (i.e., blood sugar). This is important because another primary means of measuring brain activity involves recording the energy expenditure of the brain, as occurs with functional magnetic resonance imaging (fMRI). Additionally, whether by altering the availability of blood, oxygen, or glucose, the operations of the brain may be manipulated through mechanisms that affect the ability of neurons to burn energy (Kennedy and Scholey, 2000; Scholey et al., 1999).

Neurons Live in a Protected Fluid Environment

Neurons and the other cells that make up the brain live within a fluid medium (Byrne and Roberts, 2004). The cells of the brain extract substances from their fluid surroundings. These substances serve as fuel to drive the cellular machinery, and materials for sustaining cell structure and manufacturing various molecules essential to neuronal and general cellular functions. Likewise, waste from cellular operations is discharged into this fluid medium for elimination. This ongoing fluid exchange between the cells of the brain and the surrounding fluid medium is a vital facet of brain function.

The fluid environment in which the cells of the brain are submersed is pervaded by capillaries, which provide the interface between the fluid medium of the brain and the circulatory system. However, there is a special protective barrier known as the *blood–brain barrier* that blocks many substances that would otherwise pass from the circulatory system into the fluid environment of the brain (Byrne and Roberts, 2004). Of particular importance, this barrier prevents bacteria and other infectious agents from gaining access to brain cells. In fact, a major challenge in the development of drugs targeting the brain involves engineering molecules so that they can penetrate the blood–brain barrier.

Recognition of the fluid properties of the brain is important to understanding what happens when we consume various substances with behavioral or psychological effects, also known as *psychoactive* substances. One of the most widely used psychoactive substances is caffeine. When we ingest coffee, tea, soft drinks, or other beverages that contain caffeine, the caffeine molecules pass from the digestive tract into the circulatory system, which then transports them throughout the body, including the capillaries feeding the cells of the brain. The caffeine molecules pass through the blood–brain barrier and diffuse throughout the fluid medium of the brain. Within the brain, the caffeine molecules adhere to and block a specific type of receptor embedded in the walls of many neurons, that is, adenosine receptors (Fisone et al., 2004). By blocking these receptors, caffeine prevents the inhibitory effects that would otherwise occur through stimulation of these receptors. In other words, caffeine operates not by stimulating the neurons of the brain, but instead by blocking normal processes that would inhibit neuronal activity.

Over time, the body breaks down the caffeine molecules and they are gradually eliminated. However, this takes time. If one consumes a typical dose of caffeine (e.g., the 200 mg that might be found in a cup of coffee) in 4–6 h, half of those caffeine molecules will be either eliminated or rendered inert, that is, no longer effective (Hammami et al., 2010). Then, 4–6 h later, half of the remaining caffeine will be eliminated, and so on. It may be said that caffeine has a half-life of 4–6 h, assuming a normal capacity to break down and eliminate it from the body. As the concentration of caffeine in the bloodstream is reduced, so too is its concentration in the fluid medium of the brain, with a lessening of its stimulus effects on the brain.

The preceding paragraphs have discussed two key points. First, the fluid environment of the brain allows diffusion throughout the brain of substances that affect brain functioning, with the magnitude of their effects depending on their concentration. While the previous example concerned caffeine, the same holds true for nutrients derived from foods, fluids such as water or alcohol, substances manufactured by the body (e.g., hormones), gases such as oxygen, and substances suspended in gases (e.g., nicotine) that enter the circulatory system through the lungs. Second, assuming the normal breakdown and elimination of substances by the body, their concentration diminishes over time, consistent with their half-life, with a corresponding reduction in their capacity to affect brain function.

Given that the availability of nutrients and other substances vital for brain function depends on the flow of blood to the brain, this presents a mechanism for affecting the operations of the brain. There is certainly a negative effect when blood flow to the brain is diminished, such as the light-headedness that follows after standing up too quickly from a reclining posi-tion. More severely, the brief interruption of blood flow that occurs with a stroke can be deadly. But does an increase in blood flow to the brain improve brain function? The increased circulation that occurs with light exercise has been shown to enhance cognitive function for immediate activities, as well as providing longer-range benefits (Cotman and Berchtold, 2002). But merely increasing blood flow may not be sufficient. Substances that cause dilation (i.e., expansion) of the capillaries increase blood flow, yet it is unclear whether such substances produce any benefits to cognitive function (Fisher et al., 2006; Jaiswal et al., 1991; Kennedy et al., 2010; Moser et al., 2004).

The fluid exchange that occurs with increased circulation is important. Consider oxygen, which in combination with various metabolites is essen-tial to fueling the operation of brain cells. When blood reaches the brain, it has already been infused with oxygen from the lungs. Oxygen molecules are extracted and used by the brain cells. This leaves deoxygenated blood, which reenters the circulatory system. Thus, by increasing circulation, and in the process increasing the turnover of oxygenated and deoxygenated blood, brain cells are provided with ideal conditions for their functioning. To conclude this discussion, it is important to note that a primary mechanism for measuring brain activity involves the measurement of blood flow, and particularly the relative differences in oxygenated and deoxygenated blood. The measurement of the relative concentration of oxygenated and deoxygen-ated blood is the basis for two of the most common techniques for measur-ing brain function (i.e., fMRI and functional near-infrared imaging [fNIR]), although sonography techniques have also been used to directly measure the velocity of blood flow within the arteries of the brain (Stroobant and Vingerhoets, 2000).

The Brain Sustains a Homeostatic Balance

Modest enhancements to brain function may be achieved through steps that provide the brain with more fuel, or manipulate the cellular machinery, as occurs with caffeine. However, as most of us are well aware, the effects, and particularly the positive effects, of caffeine and other substances seem to diminish more quickly than their concentration. Often, the sensation that one experiences after a cup of coffee or a caffeine-rich energy drink is an immediate period of increased alertness, focus, and energy; an enhanced capacity for mental and physical work; and a more positive disposition. Then, after an hour or so, these effects have subsided and perhaps, even reversed. Yet, the concentration of caffeine in the bloodstream remains high, as is apparent from the difficulty one experiences in trying to relax and fall asleep.

With many of the measures taken to affect brain function, over time there is a diminished effect and, eventually, there may be a reversal of the effects. As with other complex biological systems, the brain seeks to sustain a homeostatic balance and efforts to alter brain function perturb this balance. Various mechanisms, many of which are poorly understood, adjust the operation of the cellular machinery of the brain to correct for perturbations and restore a homeostatic state. These adjustments involve various feedback mechanisms that can be somewhat imprecise and, due to this imprecision, may overshoot such that one does not only experience a diminished effect over time, but one experiences the opposite of the intended effect. This has been referred to as the *rebound effect* (Julien, 2001). Furthermore, while substances such as caffeine may temporarily enhance some cellular processes, other processes that are unaffected by caffeine (e.g., the molecular production of substances that are vital to brain functions) may not keep up and, eventually, fall behind. The net effect is that a temporary acceleration is followed by an extended slowdown until the cells of the brain have had a chance to reconstitute. Thus, it is important to remember that actions taken to affect the brain, and in particular those that involve the cellular machinery of the brain, often produce an opposite effect.

Yet, it is also important to recognize that the processes described here are predictable. Furthermore, at least with caffeine, despite the rebound effect, its consumption can help to make us more effective in a range of activities if it is consumed in a strategic manner (Lieberman et al., 2002). For example, research has shown caffeine-based performance enhancement for endurance exercises (Costill et al., 1978); auditory vigilance and visual reaction time (Lieberman et al., 1987); simple and choice reaction time, incidental verbal memory and visuospatial reasoning (Jarvis, 1993); and logical reasoning and semantic memory (Smith et al., 1992). However, caffeine does not seem to offer a benefit for brief intense exercise (Greer et al., 1998). Many frequent consumers of caffeine use it in a manner that is poorly calibrated to their actual needs and can often be counterproductive. For many, caffeine use begins first thing in the morning with one or more cups of coffee to get the brain going and then a few, perhaps several, more cups during the day to sustain alertness. Over time, the brain adapts to the constant caffeine intake and becomes increasingly tolerant such that larger quantities are required to produce the same effect (Evans and Griffiths, 1992). Thus, due to these adaptations, for many, caffeine consumption is primarily driven by a desire to avoid its withdrawal effects and the associated mental doldrums, not realizing the modest enhancements that are achievable when caffeine is used in a more strategic manner. This propensity for the brain to adapt in ways that sustain its homeostatic balance is important because it renders various approaches that produce short-term benefits ineffective as long-term mechanisms for achieving higher levels of cognitive function.

It is worth noting that these same adaptive mechanisms serve to sustain our cognitive capacities in conditions that would otherwise produce diminished capacities. For instance, moving from low to high altitude, there is a reduction in the concentration of oxygen in the blood, which leaves the brain unable to maintain normal levels of metabolic function, with accompanying declines in cognitive function (Kramer et al., 1993). Given continued exposure to high altitude, adaptations occur within the brain that result in the increased efficiency of metabolic functions (Hochachka et al., 1993), with this adaptation being specific to key regions of the brain (Hochachka et al., 1999). Thus, given a reduction in fuel, the brain adapts by increasing the efficiency with which it uses fuel. Unlike a piece of machinery or electronic equipment, the brain is a biological system that is designed to operate within a given range. Furthermore, being a biological system, the brain is both adaptive and self-corrective. Consequently, actions taken to affect brain function will invariably produce a homeostatic correction. Importantly, while sometimes inconvenient, this should not be thought of as a bug, but rather as reflecting the brain's inherent capacity to cope effectively with a broad range of experiences.

A Choke in the Desert Southwest

It was the mid-1990s and the basketball program of a small university in the southeastern United States had experienced a series of successful seasons. Twice within the past 4 years, they had gotten within one game of making the Final Four of the national championship tournament, meaning that they would have played in the semifinals of the national championship. These were significant accomplishments for a little-known school from an impoverished region. This season, the team had played well, at one point being one errant shot from a victory that would have earned them the ranking of the top team in the country. They were extremely talented, with three players who would go on to have professional careers in the National Basketball Association. They were not among the elite teams in the championship tournament, but given a little luck, they had a legitimate chance of winning the national championship.

They had been one of eight teams assigned to the Western Regional games of the national championship tournament in Albuquerque, New Mexico. Albuquerque is a city in the desert southwest of the United States and sits at an elevation of over 5000 ft. Consequently, the air is dry and deprived of oxygen. This presents a challenge for many visitors, and hospital emergency rooms regularly admit tourists suffering from dehydration and altitude sickness. The team had never played in Albuquerque and its players and coaches had little experience with high-altitude, desert conditions.

In the first-round game of the tournament, the team was matched against one of the weaker teams from the East Coast of the United States. For most analysts, the game was viewed as a warm-up for the tougher competition that they would face in forthcoming games. School was in session and the coaches were concerned with the players missing classes; therefore, they delayed their travel until the night before their opening game. They arrived late and everyone went to his or her hotel and slept late the next morning, before catching a bus to the arena a couple of hours prior to the game.

The first few minutes of the game were unspectacular as both teams sought to overcome the uneasiness that comes from playing in an unfamiliar arena. However, once their opponent overcame this uneasiness and began to execute their game play, the complexion of the game quickly became apparent. Instead of running their usual offense, which emphasized plays engineered to produce shot opportunities near the basket, they took a series of long-range, three-point shots. Ordinarily, this would have merely called for a defensive adjustment. However, despite their efforts, these adjustments were unsuccessful. The players became winded from the lack of oxygen, and this was compounded by their inability to adjust from a cognitive perspective. As the opposing team ran various plays, they were consistently lagging behind, comprehending plays a fraction of a second too late to respond. They were a smart team and could sense what their opponent was doing, but not quickly enough. Since their offense often benefited from playing aggressive defense, they soon found that they could neither stop their opponent nor mount an effective offense of their own. By halftime, their opponent had an insurmountable lead and the eventual outcome was lopsided, leaving the team to return home early, frustrated and embarrassed by their performance.

Two factors accounted for the cognitive deficits experienced by the players. Due to their late arrival and sleeping in the next morning, the players had not consumed enough liquids and were dehydrated, with their dehydration exacerbated by the physical demands of the game. Their liquid intake, which would normally have been sufficient, was not enough for the dry, desert conditions. Secondly, the players were accustomed to playing at sea level, or near sea level, and they struggled to perform given the thin, mountain air. Together, these factors produced cognitive deficits that might not have shown in other everyday situations. However, in the fast-paced game of basketball where decisions made in a few milliseconds determine a team's success or failure, the cognitive deficits were quite apparent. It was perhaps the most disappointing loss experienced in the long history of the school's basketball program and led to the dismissal of the coach and most of his staff, followed by several lackluster seasons.

Our Brains Are Continually Being Shaped

I like to say that there are five things that we must feed our brains. Most people can easily list the first three: (1) food, including nutrients, vitamins, and minerals; (2) fluids, and particularly water; and (3) oxygen. The fourth is sleep. We are all familiar with the mental sluggishness that follows a sleepless night. Likewise, we are all familiar with the satisfying sensation when we later allow ourselves to be overcome by our hunger for sleep. While there remains uncertainty regarding the exact benefits of sleep to the brain, the deleterious effects of sleep deprivation on brain function show that there is a definite need for regular, uninterrupted periods of sleep (Vassalli and Dijk, 2009).

Fifth, we must feed our brains with experiences. This is illustrated most dramatically with critical periods of development during which certain brain functions do not develop if there is insufficient exposure to certain environmental stimulation. Landmark studies with cats showed that when lenses were affixed to the eyes of kittens that prevented them from seeing certain geometric orientations (e.g., vertically or horizontally oriented features of their environments), their visual system was later incapable of seeing these orientations (Hubel and Wiesel, 1970). For example, kittens denied exposure to vertical features would later run into chair legs, behaving as if their brain had failed to process the corresponding visual information. With humans, critical periods in language development have been well documented. It is much easier to learn a second or third language if one is exposed to that language as a child, than if one waits until adolescence or adulthood (Snow and Hoefnagel-Hohle, 1978). In fact, research suggests that second and third (i.e., nonnative) languages learned during childhood are organized in the brain similarly to one's native language, whereas after the critical period for language development has passed, there is a different, somewhat more superficial organization of nonnative languages within the brain (Perani and Abutalebi, 2005).

While critical periods demonstrate the influence of early experience on the organization of certain functions within the brain, one might mistakenly assume that once the brain has matured, it is unchanging, and for many decades, this was the conventional wisdom within neuroscience. However, there has been a growing appreciation that the brain is not static and is modified by experience (Pascual-Leone et al., 2005). Initial evidence of the brain's malleability came from studies demonstrating its reorganization following major injuries (e.g., Merzenich et al., 1984). Within our brains, there is a map in which different brain regions correspond to different parts of the body (Buonomano and Merzenich, 1998). Physically stimulating parts of the body triggers activity in the region of the brain that maps to that body part. It was observed in monkeys that following the loss of a finger, there was a reorganization of the brain so that the area corresponding to the missing finger began to respond to stimulation of the adjacent fingers (Merzenich et al., 1984). These findings, although the product of unusual events, suggested that the mature brain is capable of some degree of reorganization and is more malleable than previously thought.

A growing number of research studies have asked whether extended practice with a given activity produces measurable changes in the brain. For instance, a widely reported study looked at London taxi drivers who are renowned for their detailed knowledge of the roadways in and around the city (Maguire et al., 2000). There is an area deep within the brain known as the hippocampus, with a subsection of this region (i.e., the posterior hippocampus) critical to our knowledge of the spatial layout of the world and our ability to navigate between places. The researchers found that the posterior region of the hippocampus was much larger in the taxi drivers as compared with a control group with the more limited experience of most Londoners navigating from place to place. Furthermore, the size of the posterior hippocampus was correlated with how long an individual had worked as a taxi driver. A subsequent study considered whether the key factor was the demands associated with navigation or merely the experience of regularly being on the road going from place to place (Maguire et al., 2006). Comparing taxi drivers with bus drivers who must follow constrained routes, the researchers found that the posterior hippocampus was larger in the taxi drivers, with the correlation between years of experience and the volume of the posterior hippocampus only present for the taxi drivers.

One might ask if individuals who are naturally endowed with a more extensive hippocampus are somehow drawn to the profession of taxi driver such that the differences were preexisting and not attributable to the experience of being a taxi driver. Controlled experimental studies with animals that compared the structure and function of the brain before and after certain experiences (e.g., learning to use sound cues to navigate a maze) have also shown differences in brain organization associated with specific experiences (Bao et al., 2004). Furthermore, a number of other studies considering the effects of extended practice for activities such as meditation (Tang et al., 2012), musical training (Schlaug et al., 2009), and reading Braille (Hamilton and Pascual-Leone, 1998) have similarly reported differences in the relative volume and organization of regions of the brain associated with these activities. More recent research has shown measurable changes in the brain attributable to comparatively little practice or experience with activities. For instance, in a study by researchers at the Mind Research Network in Albuquerque, New Mexico, using adolescent girls, relative to a control group, measurable differences in the thickness of the outer layers of the brain were found when comparing brain imaging measurements taken before and after having had 3 months of regular experience playing the computer game Tetris (Haier et al., 2009). As shown in Figure 2.1, these differences were found for areas of the brain that are generally associated with complex, coordinated movements and the integration of input entering the brain from different sensory

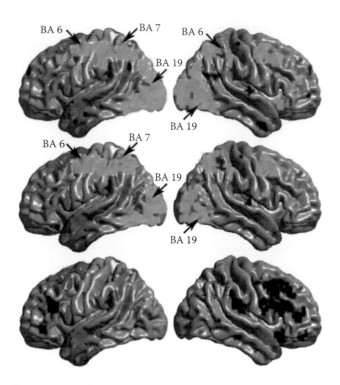

FIGURE 2.1   (See color insert)
Areas in *red* indicate regions in which there is increased cortical thickness following practice playing the game Tetris. Areas in *green* exhibit increased activation and areas in *blue* exhibit decreased activation while playing the game. The top panel represents baseline recordings, the middle panel represents recordings at follow-up, and the bottom panel represents the follow-up recordings minus the baseline recordings. (From Haier, R.J., Karama, S., Leyba, L., and Jung, R.E., *BMC Research Notes*, 2, 174, 2009. With permission.)

channels (e.g., sight, sound, and touch). fMRI measurements revealed that functional differences were also apparent, as evidenced by differential levels of brain activation; however, areas showing functional differences were distinct from areas for which there were structural differences. Similarly, in a study reported by Tang et al. (2012), subjects receiving only 11 h of a specific type of meditation training (i.e., integrative body–mind training) showed differences in the efficiency and density of the neural connections within areas of the brain associated with executive control, compared with a control group that had received equivalent training in relaxation techniques.

Generally, the trend within brain science is that as the precision with which the brain can be measured increases, we find that briefer exposure to experiences produces measurable changes in the organization and function of the brain. This is consistent with behavioral research, as well as our own personal experiences. Particularly, with learning and memory, brief exposure to events is sufficient to produce memories for seemingly unimportant details that persist for surprisingly long durations. For example, if presented with a random series of words and given no explicit instructions to try and remember the words and no subsequent opportunities to study the words, an individual can state with remarkable accuracy whether he or she had been presented with specific words from the list a week or more later (Rabinowitz and Graesser, 1976). This would suggest that, at the least, there must have been changes at a functional level within the brain such that some representation of the experience of seeing the words persisted during the intervening period of time. Similarly, a single experience in which we hear a song or eat a certain food within a given context is sufficient to forever associate that song or food with that context. What cannot be stated with certainty is the nature or extent to which the brain changes in response to specific experiences; however, experiences, even incidental, seemingly unimportant experiences, obviously have the capacity to leave an enduring impression on our brains.

While the basic structure and the fundamental circuits of the brain develop early in life and remain intact throughout life, brain science suggests that the functional organization and, to a lesser extent, the structural organization of the brain are in continual flux. The situation is not unlike that of the body. The fundamental structure and function of the body remains intact over the course of our lives (e.g., barring injury, we have 2 arms and 10 fingers that operate in a certain way). Yet, there is a continuous turnover at the cellular level and decisions we make concerning the foods and other substances that we consume, the exercise and activities in which we engage, and the conditions to which we expose our bodies continually shape the ultimate physical and functional makeup of our bodies. Similarly, the functional and, to a lesser extent, the structural makeup of our brains are being continuously shaped by the actions in which we engage and the sensory experiences to which we expose our brains. Thus, it is important to remember that, like a piece of clay that can be molded to form various shapes, our brains are malleable and whether through intentional or incidental experiences, our brains are continuously being shaped.

Many Functions May Be Localized to Specific Regions of the Brain

Modern neuroscience benefits from a growing number of techniques for measuring the activity of the brain. This is a relatively recent development, particularly brain imaging techniques such as fMRI. For much of the history of neuroscience, a primary source of knowledge regarding the brain was the study of the effects of brain damage (i.e., brain lesions). Whether the product of injury, cancerous tumors, or other causes, lesions have provided an opportunity to observe the operations of the brain when certain regions have ceased to function normally.

An early key finding was that certain operations of the brain are localized to specific regions of the brain. For instance, pioneering research by the nineteenth-century physician Paul Broca showed that damage to a region on the left side of the brain, toward the front, caused impairments in the ability to produce speech (Dronkers et al., 2007). These patients could still comprehend speech, but they experienced severe difficulties generating speech, whether verbal or written, despite no impairments associated with the muscles, tongue, or any other part of the speech apparatus. This finding indicated that for most of us, the neural circuits responsible for generating speech are localized within this particular region of the brain. Since Broca's observations concerning the localization of speech deficits, an immense literature has accumulated documenting the dysfunctions observed with damage to different regions of the brain. Today, it is common practice for neuropsychologists to administer a series of behavioral tests as a means to pinpoint the location of their patient's injuries. Furthermore, with the proliferation of brain imaging equipment and techniques, study of the localization of different functions within the brain now regularly involves nonpatient populations with normally functioning brains.

An entire career could be consumed by studying the mapping of different operations of the brain to the various regions of the brain, and the variations across individuals. The reason that this is important in applying brain science to everyday life does not involve knowing how different functions are distributed throughout the brain. Instead, localization implies a segregation of operations such that the neural circuits within a given region are uniquely designed to perform a specific operation. Where such segregation and specialization of neural circuits occur, it implies a fundamental operation of the brain. Imagine that you have just purchased a new cell phone. If you want to get the most out of this cell phone, you should read through the owner's manual and become familiar with all its functions. You might even rearrange the icons for specific functions so that you do not forget that certain operations are available to you. In the same way that our ability to make the most of electronic or other products (e.g., software products) requires that we know their various functions, our ability to get the most out of people and their brains in everyday situations hinges on some appreciation of the brain's basic operations.

We need to appreciate what brains do naturally, as opposed to those things that are doable but are not natural. For example, there are neural circuits within the brain that are specialized for the recognition of faces and it might be said that facial recognition is a basic operation of the brain (Nelson, 2001). In contrast, brains are capable of learning and recognizing similarly complex patterns of numbers, but this takes significant effort or the use of an aid, whether internal (e.g., pneumonic) or external (e.g., cheat sheet). In general, when tasks rely on operations that correspond to operations for which the brain has specialized neural circuits, these tasks are going to be easier, whereas tasks that require operations for which the brain does not have specialized circuits will be harder and may require some type of aid. The localization of functions to different regions of the brain and the specialization of the constituent neural circuits for these operations reveal the basic operations of our brain, and are a clue to what is going to be hard and what is going to be easy.

Furthermore, by understanding the specialized operations of the brain, there is an opportunity to develop designs that are tailored to maximally engage the innate capacities of the brain. For example, considerable research has focused on a region near the center of the brain that seems to be most sensitive to conditions in which one recognizes that one has committed an error (Carter et al., 1998). Studies show increased activity across the neural circuits in this area (i.e., anterior cingulate cortex) that corresponds to sensing that one has made a mistake. Furthermore, where knowledge of an error is based on some type of feedback (e.g., error message), the level of brain activation tends to vary with regard to how surprising it is for the individual to learn that he or she has made a mistake (Yasuda et al., 2004). Thus, unexpected negative feedback produces more activation than feedback that is less surprising. This research indicates that a basic operation of the brain is to detect when we have committed an error, as well as to differentiate errors on the basis of how unexpected or surprising they are. Knowing about this basic operation of the brain, one might speculate on how best to deliver feedback. Specifically, continuous negative feedback can be ineffective because a person eventually becomes sensitized and no longer responds. However, carefully timed negative feedback can get a person's attention in that it is surprising and causes the person to stop and rethink how he or she is approaching a task. This example illustrates how an understanding of the operations of the functional circuits of the brain can be applied to achieve more effective system and product designs.

Everyday Activities Involve Integrated Functions Dispersed throughout the Brain

While there is localization of functions to specific regions of the brain, it is important to remember that at any given time, there is extensive activity involving many different regions throughout the brain. Images depicting the activity of the brain, such as those based on fMRI, may pinpoint specific regions that are active while performing a laboratory task. However, the activity of the brain is not limited to those regions. These images are created using statistical techniques that compare the brain activity measured while performing a task with the activity seen during a baseline condition, such as sitting quietly. The activity depicted in these images reflects variations from the baseline condition, or where there is the greatest elevation in brain activity. Thus, what we are really seeing is the differential engagement of brain regions, or which regions become somewhat more active than their neighboring regions.

Also, one must keep in mind that most images of the brain are the product of carefully controlled experiments that are designed so that the person is focused on a single distinct task. To see how the brain appears during everyday activities, I recommend looking at the videos posted on YouTube by Sands Research (2014). This is a company that specializes in neuromarketing. Its clients consist of major corporations that are developing advertising campaigns and want to know how consumers will respond to different messages. In several videos, you see a television commercial and next to it are images depicting the activity of the brain that are measured using high-density electroencephalogram (EEG) as a test subject watched the commercial. During some points in the commercial, the activity of the brain is somewhat restricted, often centered on the areas specialized for visual processes. At other times, the activity spreads rapidly across the brain, encompassing almost the entire brain. It is particularly interesting to observe the ebb and flow of brain activity that occurs in response to the changing events within the commercial. It is apparent that the activity of the brain during everyday activities is highly dynamic, with activity emanating from different areas, extending and receding, enveloping surrounding regions, and sometimes being overtaken by waves of activity originating from other areas.

Given that there is localization of certain functions, yet the everyday activity of the brain involves the simultaneous activation and dynamic interplay of different brain regions, how might one best think about how the brain operates during everyday life? The neurons of the brain are organized into complex circuits, with circuits specialized for performing certain operations. The operations performed by each neural circuit are somewhat like computer programs. There are many different types of operations. For instance, in the visual system, there are circuits specialized for detecting objects oriented at a specific angle or objects of a specific color or objects moving in a specific direction. One may think of the brain as a massive collection of circuits that are designed to perform many different specialized operations. During everyday life, various circuits are active at any given time, with the involvement and the combination of circuits differing in response to ongoing demands. The product is a highly dynamic, yet well-integrated organization of diverse functions.

However, our mental experience generally involves the seamless integration of different operations. Imagine the experience on a windy day in which there is the sensation of a breeze blowing across the skin, and the sight and sound of leaves rustling, and these are combined with our ongoing stream of thoughts, which may involve reminiscence of other similarly windy days. Each facet of this experience involves different operations occurring within distinct yet integrated circuits spread throughout the brain. However, it is all combined to produce a single unified experience. In short, the brain is capable of doing a lot of different things, all at the same time, but remarkably, it puts it all together to form the coherent, seamless whole that makes up our everyday experience of the world.

The Brain Is a Complex System, Yet Is Only One Component in a Larger System of Systems

The brain is the master controller for the body. In moving about and interacting with the world around us, the body is a slave to the brain much as a remote-controlled car is a slave to its controller. It is the brain that enables the range of behavior that makes humans interesting as an animal species, including the capacity to learn and to adapt behavior in responding to changing circumstances. For these reasons, I believe that there is a predilection to see the brain as distinct from the rest of the body, and somewhat removed from our basic biological functions.

Earlier in my career, without ever realizing it, my thinking about the brain and behavior very much reflected the perspective that the brain was a master controller for the body, sitting on top of the body, issuing commands and observing their outcomes. This view changed after I had the opportunity to visit Russia and become acquainted with several researchers at Saint Petersburg State University. At some point during our discussions, I began to recognize that they had a somewhat different set of core beliefs, or model, for thinking about the brain and behavior. In particular, their model emphasized that the brain was just one of many components that make up the body, but most importantly, it worked in concert with other systems of the body, interacting with the other systems of the body in varied ways. To some extent, their perspective diminished the role of the brain, seeing the brain as one of many important parts that is neither independent of the other parts nor dominant to the other parts. This perspective differed significantly from that predominant in brain science as it was taught in the United States and Western Europe, and suggested lines of scientific inquiry that many Western scientists might find peculiar.

How does a perspective that emphasizes that the brain is just one system in a complex system of systems affect the way that we think about the brain? Foremost, attention turns to the interactions between the brain and other systems. It suggests that the functioning of the brain is affected by other systems of the body. There are some obvious examples. For instance, the brain requires fuel. This implies an interaction between the brain and the circulatory system, with the functioning of the brain modulated in response to the ability of the heart and its associated plumbing to supply an ample volume of nutrient-enriched, oxygenated blood.

The nutrients fueling the brain are derived from the foods we ingest, suggesting an interaction whereby the functioning of the brain depends on the capacity of the digestive system to extract essential substances and transfer them to the bloodstream. One might think that the interactions between the brain and the digestive system only involve nutrition. However, in a series of studies, researchers at University College Cork and McMaster University showed that the bacterial content of the gut could alter brain processes (Bravo et al., 2011). They fed mice a diet that had been supplemented with a harmless species of bacteria. After 6 weeks, the animals were subjected to tests in which they were allowed to explore spaces that included a narrow elevated walkway and an open area that offered no cover from potential predators. Ordinarily, mice are scared of these settings and will actively avoid them. Instead, the mice explored the elevated walkway and open space, showing comparatively few signs of anxiety or fear. Additionally, when placed in water, which produces a severe stress response in mice, the animals that had received the bacteria showed lower levels of stress hormones. Later, when the researchers cut the vagus nerve, which transmits neural signals between the stomach and the brain, the behavior of the animals returned to normal. It appeared that the presence of the bacteria within the stomach produced activation of the vagus nerve such that there was a relaxing effect on the brain. Additionally, when researchers studied the brains of the animals treated with the bacteria, they found measurable differences in the density of a specific receptor that has a dampening effect on brain activity (i.e., GABAergic receptors), when compared with mice that had not received the bacteria.

Oxygen also fuels the operations of the brain. The interaction between the brain and the respiratory system is familiar. The common advice when someone is upset or generally needs to relax, is to take a deep breath. Likewise, with many meditation practices, breathing is used as a basis for consciously modulating brain activity, and in some cases, inducing altered states of consciousness. Some specialized military and law enforcement personnel are taught techniques in which specific patterns of breathing are used to enhance mental readiness for critical activities (Stetz et al., 2007), with similar practices incorporated into the I Chin Ching training associated with the centuries-old martial art of Shaolin Kung Fu (Shahar, 2008).

The circulatory, digestive, and respiratory systems are only three systems within the body that interact with the brain. The interactions between the brain and the reproductive system are certainly appreciated (Geher and Miller, 2008), and there has been discussion of interactions between the brain and the immune system (Ader et al., 1990). The ways in which the brain is influenced by other bodily systems are poorly understood, and generally such interactions are not a popular topic of experimental research. Consequently, there are likely many everyday behaviors that unknowingly serve to affect the operation of the brain, as well as unrecognized opportunities for enhancing brain function.

No Two Brains Work Exactly the Same

We all know that people think differently. We all recognize that individuals have varying levels of aptitude for different activities and will often approach problems very differently. In fact, we often celebrate these differences, both in ourselves as well as in others. However, individual differences have been a difficult topic for the brain and behavioral sciences. The primary objective within these sciences has been to elucidate basic principles that are common to everyone. Within these sciences, individual differences represent noise that clouds the detection of commonalities. As previously noted, brain imaging techniques generally rely on averaging data across many different test subjects to identify the patterns of activity that are common to almost everyone. Likewise, the behavioral sciences are built on statistical techniques where variability in the data attributable to different individuals is quantified and subtracted from the calculation. Thus, behavioral science is largely the study of the average person and tells us very little about the differences between people, much less specific individuals.

In contrast, Michael Miller and colleagues at the University of California at Santa Barbara have reported studies that explicitly consider individual differences (Miller et al., 2002). These studies used a common experimental procedure within cognitive psychology where test subjects were given a series of unrelated words and were asked to try and remember them. Later, a second series of words were presented that consisted of some words that appeared in the original list and others that were not presented earlier in the study. After each word, the subjects were asked to indicate if they believed that the word was "old," meaning it was in the original list, or "new," meaning it was not in the original list. When the researchers compared the brain images recorded from subjects, they found that there was substantial variability in the predominant patterns of brain activity (see figure 2 in Miller et al., 2002). Different subjects had used different strategies to help them remember the words and these different strategies had produced different patterns of activity in their brains. For example, subjects may have repeated the word in their head, which would have engaged areas associated with the vocalization of speech, or they may have constructed a sentence containing the word, which would have engaged areas involved in language production, or they may have visualized the word, which would have engaged areas associated with visual processes.

Whether laboratory studies such as that reported by Miller and colleagues or the various tasks we encounter during everyday life, different people possess different aptitudes and experiences, and based on their individual aptitudes and experiences, they will employ different strategies to accomplish a task. It is important to remember that when we see people going about the same task in different ways, this may reflect more than mere preferences. Instead, there may be inherent neurologically based differences that cause an individual to gravitate to one strategy and not another. A preference implies arbitrariness, or that the person could have just as easily chosen an alternative strategy, and malleability such that given the will to do so, one could easily shift to a different strategy. Thus, thinking of behavior variability in terms of mere preferences instead of inherent predilections, one may feel little obligation to accommodate individual differences and the associated tendency to adopt different strategies in accomplishing one's objectives.

Where individual differences are the product of inherent variability in the organization of the brain, it may not be fair to ask someone to adopt a different strategy, or impose a different strategy on the person. A different strategy may come at the cost of additional effort, and the sense that activities do not feel natural. Handedness offers a good illustration. Whether one is right handed or left handed results from the basic organization of the brain and while one can learn to use one's alternate hand, it comes at a cost and may never feel quite right (Hugdahl and Westerhausen, 2010). While handedness is a particularly salient manifestation of differential brain organization, it represents one dimension along which the brains of different individuals may differ with there being numerous other dimensions that are reflected in individual biases toward specific strategies for accomplishing common tasks.

Our genes provide the basic instructions for creating neural circuits that are designed to perform specific operations and a general architecture for assembling these circuits into a functional brain. However, there is a lot of room for variability in the exact make up of each individual brain, with each of us being more or less endowed with each of the specialized operations that make up a functional brain. It is much like our physical bodies, where genetics offers the instructions for creating different body parts (i.e., hands, arms, legs, noses) and the general architecture for assembling these body parts to construct a functional human body. However, some have relatively longer or shorter arms and legs, or somewhat different shaped noses, and so on. It is similar with brains. In the same way that we all have our own individual appearance, we each have our own individual brain.

Our Best Measures Do Not Tell Us
Exactly How the Brain Works

There have been several decades of research in which scientists have used various measures to study the workings of the brain. Measures such as fMRI have appeared in many publications and most of us have seen images illustrating the differential activation of regions of the brain associated with various activities. However, when we say that we have measured brain activation, what exactly is meant by the term *activation*? Each of the popular techniques for measuring brain activity operates somewhat differently, providing various perspectives on the brain's functioning. The following sections briefly summarize each of these common measurement techniques and how they operate.

EEG

This is the oldest and most common technique for measuring brain activity. The cost of EEG measurement is low enough that university laboratories can easily afford the equipment and simple versions of EEG are now found in readily available commercial products. For instance, the Emotiv headset uses brain activation as an alternative means for controlling computer games and EEG units are now available that allow one to monitor the quality of one's sleep.

With EEG, electrodes are placed on the scalp that are capable of detecting the miniscule (i.e., millivolt scale) electrical currents associated with the activity of the neurons of the brain. In actuality, the electrodes detect the electrical potential between the area of the scalp immediately underneath the electrode and a reference electrode placed at a spot that is electrically inert (e.g., the earlobe). With EEG, it is important to remember that the currents being measured reflect the product of thousands, if not millions of neurons. In many respects, looking at maps illustrating the differential activation of the brain based on EEG measurement is like looking at a satellite image of the earth. It depicts the general layout, but does not provide any detail. Although, it should be noted that EEG does provide very good detail regarding the timing of brain activity, thereby allowing scientists to observe events occurring in the millisecond timescale.

fMRI

Perhaps the second most common technique for brain measurement is fMRI. Today, most hospitals and many university laboratories have facilities for fMRI measurement. This involves large, specialized equipment requiring trained staff to operate it, as well as specially designed facilities. Images depicting a large dome-like structure that surrounds the upper body of a person who is lying on his or her back are generally fMRI systems.

Within the dome-like structure, a large magnet creates an extremely powerful magnetic field, and associated sensors are capable of measuring minor fluctuations within the magnetic field. As discussed previously, blood supplies the cells of the brain with oxygen. When blood cells are carrying oxygen, they exhibit different magnetic properties than when oxygen is absent. The fMRI senses the proportion of blood carrying oxygen (i.e., oxygenated) relative to blood without oxygen (i.e., deoxygenated). Thus, with fMRI, brain activity is not measured directly, as with EEG, but indirectly. Specifically, since the operation of neurons requires oxygen, it is assumed that there is increased oxygen consumption where neurons are active. In contrast, where neurons are relatively quiet, there should be relatively less oxygen consumption.

fMRI allows measurement in the scale of millimeters pinpointing detailed differences in the activation of brain regions. However, it is a relatively slow process by which measurable differences in the proportion of oxygenated and deoxygenated blood appear in response to differential activation of brain regions. It is generally assumed that the activation observed using fMRI lags the actual activity of the brain cells by a few seconds. Consequently, while fMRI shows where activity occurs, being at such a gross timescale relative to the operations of the brain, fMRI says less about the timing of brain processes.

fNIR

Whereas fMRI requires large equipment and specialized facilities, fNIR operates on the same principle, but without many of the same constraints as fMRI. As with fMRI, fNIR infers the activity of the brain cells based on differences in the proportion of oxygenated and deoxygenated blood. However, fNIR is based on different properties of oxygenated and deoxygenated blood. Specifically, when infrared light is directed at blood cells, some of the light is absorbed by the blood cells and some is reflected. Oxygenated blood absorbs shorter wavelength light (i.e., preferentially in the 660 nm range), while deoxygenated blood absorbs longer wavelength light (i.e., preferentially in the 940 nm range). With fNIR, an infrared light, which readily passes through skin and bone, is directed at the scalp, and adjacent sensors detect the proportion of light that is reflected back after having bounced off the blood cells within the brain.

fNIR offers practical advantages over fMRI, given that the sensors are generally embedded within a small plate that is placed on the scalp, and there are no requirements for specialized facilities. However, fNIR does not offer nearly as detailed images as fMRI. Furthermore, fNIR measurements are limited to activity at the surface of the brain given that infrared light does not penetrate to deeper levels. Yet, fNIR does offer a much faster timescale than fMRI, on the order of 50 ms as opposed to 1–2 s. Nonetheless, as with fMRI, fNIR senses a by-product of brain activity (i.e., relative oxygen consumption), as opposed to directly measuring the activity of the brain.

Positron Emission Tomography (PET)

Unlike the techniques discussed previously that may be employed for either research or clinical purposes, PET is used almost exclusively in clinical settings. With PET, a radioactive substance, known as a tracer, is injected into the blood. The tracer combines a radioactive isotope with other molecules that naturally bind to specific molecules or features of the brain cells. Consequently, as the tracer diffuses throughout the brain with the circulating blood, it tends to concentrate in areas that are rich in the biological processes targeted by the tracer. For example, one common tracer closely resembles glucose, a sugar that is a primary source of fuel for neurons, and concentrates in active regions of the brain where there is disproportionate glucose utilization. The radioactive emissions from the tracer then provide the basis for obtaining an image that depicts the differential concentration of the tracer throughout the brain.

Magnetoencephalography (MEG)

As neurons transmit electrical currents, corresponding magnetic fields are created around the neurons. MEG uses sensors that are capable of detecting these weak magnetic fields as a means of measuring the electrical activity of the brain. As with fMRI, a large dome is placed over the head of the test subject, and measurements occur in a specialized facility. However, unlike fMRI, which measures the proportion of oxygenated and deoxygenated blood, MEG directly measures the magnetic fields generated through the activity of the neurons.

Each of the techniques described here for measuring the activity of the brain has proven useful in advancing our knowledge of how the brain operates. However, none of these techniques directly measures the activity of the brain cells, with the arguable exception of MEG. Instead, each is an indirect measure that provides data that scientists then use to try and infer what is really happening. I am reminded of the parable of Nastrudin. In this story, several people come across an old man on his hands and knees frantically searching under a streetlight. When they ask the old man if they can be of assistance, he replies that he has lost his house key. The passersby join the old man taking to their hands and knees and begin looking for the key. After a while, someone asks if the old man can remember where he was when he lost his key and the old man answers that he was in his home. "Why, then, are you looking here under the streetlight," asked one of the passersby, and the old man replied, "because the light is better here." Scientists use the measures we have because they are the only techniques available to illuminate the workings of the brain, yet everyone knows that we are not directly observing its operations, but using the best data we have to infer its operations.

Acknowledgments

Sandia National Laboratories is a multiprogram laboratory managed and operated by Sandia Corporation, a wholly owned subsidiary of Lockheed Martin Corporation, for the US Department of Energy's National Nuclear Security Administration under contract DE-AC04-94AL85000.

References

Ader, R., Felten, D. and Cohen, N. (1990). Interactions between the brain and immune system. *Annual Review of Pharmacology and Toxicology, 30*, 561–602.

Bao, S., Chang, E.F., Woods, J. and Merzenich, M.M. (2004). Temporal plasticity in the primary auditory cortex induced by operant perceptual learning. *Nature Neuroscience, 7*, 974–981.

Bravo, J.A., Forsythe, P., Chew, M.V., Escaravage, E., Savignac, H.M., Dinan, T.G., Bienenstock, J. and Cryan, J.F. (2011). Ingestion of *Lactobacillus* strain regulates emotional behavior and central GABA receptor expression in a mouse via the vagus nerve. *Proceedings of the National Academy of Sciences, 108*(38), 16050–16055.

Buonomano, D.V. and Merzenich, M.M. (1998). Cortical plasticity: From synapses to maps. *Annual Review of Neuroscience, 21*, 149–186.

Byrne, J.H. and Roberts, J.L. (2004). *From Molecules to Networks: An Introduction to Cellular and Molecular Neuroscience*, New York: Elsevier.

Carter, C.S., Braver, T.S., Barch, D.M., Botvinick, M.M., Noll, D. and Cohen, J.D. (1998). Anterior cingulate cortex, error detection, and the online monitoring of performance. *Science, 280*(5364), 747–749.

Costill, D.L., Dalsky, G.P. and Fink, W.J. (1978). Effects of caffeine ingestion on metabolism and exercise performance. *Medicine and Science in Sports, 10*(3), 155–158.

Cotman, C.W. and Berchtold, N.C. (2002). Exercise: A behavioral intervention to enhance brain health and plasticity. *Trends in Neurosciences, 25*(6), 295–301.

Dronkers, N.F., Plaisant, O., Iba-Zizen, M.T. and Cabanic, E.A. (2007). Paul Broca's historic cases: High resolution MR imaging of the brains of Leborne and Lelong. *Brain, 130*(5), 1432–1441.

Evans, S.M. and Griffiths, R.R. (1992). Caffeine tolerance and choice in humans. *Psychopharmacology, 108*(1–2), 51–59.

Fisher, N.D.L., Sorond, F.A. and Hollenberg, N.K. (2006). Cocoa flavanals and brain perfusion. *Journal of Cardiovascular Pharmacology, 47*, S210–S214.

Fisone, G., Borgkvist, A. and Usielle, A. (2004). Caffeine as a psychomotor stimulant: Mechanisms of action. *Cellular and Molecular Life Science, 61*(7–8), 857–872.

Geher, G. and Miller, G. (2008). *Mating Intelligence: Sex, Relationships and the Mind's Reproductive System*, New York: Lawrence Erlbaum.

Greer, F., McLean, C. and Graham, T.E. (1998). Caffeine, performance and metabolism during repeated Wingate exercise tests. *Journal of Applied Physiology, 85*(4), 1502–1508.

Haier, R.J., Karama, S., Leyba, L. and Jung, R.E. (2009). MRI assessment of cortical thickness and functional activity changes in adolescent girls following three months of practice on a visual-spatial task. *BMC Research Notes, 2*, 174.

Hamilton, R.H. and Pascual-Leone, A. (1998). Cortical plasticity associated with Braille learning. *Trends in Cognitive Sciences, 2*(5), 168–174.

Hammami, M.M., Al-Gaai, E.A., Alvi, S. and Hammami, M.B. (2010). Interaction between drug and placebo effects: A cross-over balanced placebo design trial. *Trials, 11*(110), 1–10.

Hochachka, P.W., Clark, C.M., Brown, W.D., Stanley, C., Stone, C.K., Nickles, J., Zhu, G.G., Allen, P.S. and Holden, J.E. (1993). The brain at high altitude: Hypometabolism as a defense against chronic hypoxia. *Journal of Cerebral Blood Flow and Metabolism, 14*, 671–679.

Hochachka, P.W., Clark, C.M., Matheson, G.O., Brown, W.D., Stone, C.K., Nickles, J. and Holden, J.E. (1999). Effects on regional brain metabolism of high-altitude hypoxia: A study of six U.S. marines. *Regulatory and Integrative Physiology*, *277*(1), R314–R319.

Hubel, D.H. and Wiesel, T.N. (1970). The period of susceptibility to the physiological effects of unilateral eye-closure in kittens. *Journal of Physiology*, *206*(2), 419–436.

Hugdahl, K. and Westerhausen, R. (2010). *The Two Halves of the Brain: Information Processing in the Cerebral Hemispheres*, Cambridge, MA: MIT Press.

Jaiswal, A.K., Upadhyay, S.N. and Bhattacharya, S.K. (1991). Effect of dihydroergotoxine, a cerebral vasodilator, on cognitive deficits induced by parental undernutrition and environmental impoverishment in young rats. *Indian Journal of Experimental Biology*, *29*(6), 532–537.

Jarvis, M.J. (1993). Does caffeine intake enhance absolute levels of cognitive performance? *Psychopharmacology*, *110*(1–2), 45–52.

Julien, R.M. (2001). *A Primer of Drug Action: A Concise Nontechnical Guide to the Actions, Uses and Side Effects of Psychoactive Drugs*, New York: Macmillan.

Kennedy, D.O. and Scholey, A.B. (2000). Glucose administration, heart rate and cognitive performance: Effects of increasing mental effort. *Psychopharmacology*, *149*(1), 63–71.

Kennedy, D.O., Wightman, E.L., Reay, J.L., Lietz, G., Okello, E.J., Wilde, A. and Kaskell, C.F. (2010). Effects of resveratrol on cerebral blood flow variables and cognitive performance in humans: A double blind, placebo-controlled, crossover investigation. *American Journal of Clinical Nutrition*, *91*(6), 1590–1597.

Kramer, A.F., Coyne, J.T. and Strayer, D.L. (1993). Cognitive function at high altitude. *Human Factors*, *35*(2), 329–344.

Lieberman, H.R., Tharion, W.J., Shukitt-Hale, B., Speckman, K.L. and Tulley, R. (2002). Effects of caffeine, sleep loss, and stress on cognitive performance and mood during US Navy SEAL training. *Psychopharmacology*, *164*(3), 250–261.

Lieberman, H.R., Wurtman, R.J., Emde, G.G., Roberts, C. and Coviella, L.G. (1987). The effects of low doses of caffeine on human performance and mood. *Psychopharmacology*, *92*(3), 308–312.

Maguire, E.A., Gadian, D.G., Johnsrude, I.S., Good, C.D., Ashburner, J., Frackowiack, R.S.J. and Frith, C.D. (2000). Navigation-related structural change in the hippocampi of taxi drivers. *Proceedings of the National Academy of Sciences*, *97*(8), 4398–4403.

Maguire, E.A., Woollett, K. and Spiers, H.J. (2006). London taxi drivers and bus drivers: A structural MRI and neuropsychological analysis. *Hippocampus*, *16*(12), 1091–1101.

Merzenich, M.M., Nelson, R.J., Stryker, M.P., Cynader, M.S., Schoppmann, A. and Zook, J.M. (1984). Somatosensory cortical map changes following digit amputation in adult monkeys. *Journal of Comparative Neurology*, *224*(4), 591–605.

Miller, M.B., Van Horn, J.D., Wolford, G.L., Handy, T.C., Valsangkar-Smyth, M., Inati, S., Grafton, S. and Gazzaniga, M.S. (2002). Extensive individual differences in brain activations associated with episodic retrieval are reliable over time. *Journal of Cognitive Neuroscience*, *14*(8), 1200–1214.

Mink, J.W., Blumenschine, R.J. and Adams, D.B. (1981). Ratio of central nervous system to body metabolism in vertebrates: Its constancy and functional basis. *American Journal of Physiology*, *241*(3), 203–212.

Moser, D.J., Hoft, K.F., Robinson, R.G., Paulsen, J.S., Benjamin, M.L., Schultz, S.K. and Haynes, W.G. (2004). Blood vessel function and cognition in elderly patients with atherosclerosis. *Stroke*, *35*(11), 369–372.

Nelson, C.A. (2001). The development and neural bases of face recognition. *Infant and Child Development*, *10*, 3–18.

Pascual-Leone, A., Amedi, A., Fregni, F. and Merabet, L.B. (2005). The plastic human brain cortex. *Annual Review of Neuroscience*, *28*, 377–401.

Perani, D. and Abutalebi, J. (2005). The neural basis of first and second language processing. *Current Opinion in Neurobiology*, *15*(2), 202–206.

Rabinowitz, R.J. and Graesser, A.C.I. (1976). Word recognition as a function of retrieval processes. *Bulletin of Psychonomic Society*, *7*, 75–77.

Sands Research. (2014). Sands Research—Pioneers in Marketing, Accessed January 15, 2014, http://www.sandsresearch.com/.

Schlaug, G., Forgeard, M., Zhu, L., Norton, A. and Winner, E. (2009). Training-induced neuroplasticity in young children. *Annals of the New York Academy of Sciences*, *1169*, 205–208.

Scholey, A.B., Moss, M.C., Neave, N. and Wesnes, K. (1999). Cognitive performance, hyperoxia and heart rate following oxygen administration in healthy young adults. *Physiology and Behavior*, *67*(5), 783–789.

Shahar, M. (2008). *The Shaolin Monastery: History, Religion and the Chinese Martial Arts*, Honolulu, HI: University of Hawaii Press.

Smith, A.P., Kendrick, A.M. and Maben, A.L. (1992). Effects of breakfast and caffeine on performance and mood in late morning and after lunch. *Neuropsychobiology*, *26*(4), 198–204.

Snow, C.E. and Hoefnagel-Hohle, M. (1978). The critical period for language acquisition: Evidence from second language learning. *Child Development*, *49*(4), 1114–1128.

Stetz, M.C., Thomas, M.L., Russo, M.B., Stetz, T.A., Wildzunas, R.M., McDonald, J.J., Wiederhold, B.K. and Romano, J.A. (2007). Stress, mental health and cognition. A brief review of relationships and countermeasures. *Aviation, Space and Environmental Medicine*, *78*(1), B252–B260.

Stroobant, N. and Vingerhoets, G. (2000). Transcranial Doppler ultrasonography monitoring of cerebral hemodynamics during performance of cognitive tasks: A review. *Neuropsychology Review*, *10*(4), 213–231.

Tang, Y.Y., Lu, Q., Yang, Y. and Posner, M.I. (2012). Mechanisms of white matter changes induced by meditation. *Proceedings of the National Academy of Sciences*, *109*(26), 10570–10574.

Vassalli, A. and Dijk, D.J. (2009). Sleep function: Current questions and new approaches. *European Journal of Neuroscience*, *29*(9), 1830–1841.

Yasuda, A., Sato, A., Miyawaki, K., Kumano, H. and Kuboki, T. (2004). Error-related negativity reflects detection of negative reward prediction error. *Neuroreport*, *15*(16), 2561–2565.

3

Conscious Awareness

This chapter is the first in a series of chapters devoted to specific topics. We begin with a discussion of conscious awareness. This topic is fundamental to how we think about the roles of humans within systems. Often implicitly, our systems' designs assume that humans are consciously aware of their actions and are operating in a knowing manner, cognizant of what they are doing and why they are doing it. We exhibit a bias to assume conscious awareness in interpreting the actions of others, and with our own actions, as well. It is unsatisfying to think that a person might have no explanation for an erroneous action. Likewise, it is hard to accept that the logic on which we base our beliefs might often reflect an after-the-fact rationalization. This is understandable given that we experience life through the medium of conscious awareness and have limited access to those processes and knowledge that exist outside our conscious awareness. In filling our roles as designers, engineers, analysts, managers, or otherwise, there is value in recognizing the extent to which our assumptions regarding conscious awareness shape our thinking and often make us vulnerable to certain biases, as well as the influence of others.

One of the major trends within brain science over the past decade has been a growing recognition of how little we are aware of the operations of our brains, and that the overwhelming majority of what happens within our heads occurs at the largely inaccessible level we think of as the unconscious (Custers and Aarts, 2010; Vedantam, 2010).

Unlike other parts of the body that are richly endowed with sensory receptors, we have no practical mechanisms that allow us to sense and experience stimuli arising from the tissues that make up our brains. The surface of the body is covered with tactile (i.e., touch) sensors. The muscles and joints possess sensors that are responsive to their motion and relative position. Pain sensors occur throughout the body, providing unpleasant sensations when they are exposed to destructive or noxious stimuli. In contrast, our primary sense of the brain comes through conscious self-reflection. Yet, this reflection tells us little about the operations of the brain. It mostly offers a glimpse of our memory as occurs when we visualize things we have seen, or recollect something that we have heard or felt, or construct scenes within our heads. In general, we lack a direct sense of our brains, with our conscious experience and self-reflection a product of the operations of our brains, as opposed to a direct sensory experience of our brains.

The distinction between the conscious mind and the unconscious brain is important because it is central to the ways that we think about ourselves and others. Our conscious minds create the sense that we have control over our actions and, to a large extent, our thoughts, and we generally approach the world as if this is the case. Likewise, we assume the same with others, and assign responsibility to them for their actions and thoughts. When we interact with others, we experience it as an interaction between two conscious minds, with each participant in the interaction being responsible for what he or she says, thinks, and does. Similarly, when we observe the actions of others, we assume that they are consciously aware of what they are doing and their actions are intentional and deliberate. These are deeply engrained biases that shape our perspective on the world, events, others, and even ourselves.

Of the many mysteries housed within our brains, none has been more elusive than conscious awareness. Cognitive neuroscience cannot explain what conscious awareness is, how it happens, or what function it serves. However, to the extent that conscious awareness can be parameterized and measured, cognitive neuroscience can speak to the coincidental brain processes and shed light on how to more or less effectively consciously engage humans in various activities.

Conscious versus Nonconscious Engagement

We frequently have experiences that reveal the presence of our unconscious brains operating alongside and in parallel with our conscious experience of the world. In an exercise that I routinely do during classes, I ask students to raise their hands and instruct them to consciously not think about anything and when the first thought pops into their heads, to lower their hands. Most lower their hands in the first few seconds. Very few are able to make it past 20 s and these are generally individuals who practice meditation and have some familiarity with trying to clear their minds of the ongoing stream of thoughts. This exercise demonstrates that despite a conscious attempt to quiet the internal voice emanating from our brains, we can only do so for a brief period of time. I like to say that, "the mind influences the brain, but it cannot control the brain."

There are many other situations familiar to all of us that illustrate the limits of our conscious mind's ability to control the unconscious brain (see Table 3.1). For instance, we may attempt to focus our thoughts and attend to our surroundings or the tasks in which we are engaged, yet without warning, often without even realizing it, our mind wanders and we begin to think about something else. This is particularly true when something is bothering us or we are worried about something and despite our efforts to ignore

TABLE 3.1

The Mind May Influence Many Facets of Our Psychological Experience, But Does Not Exercise Control over the Brain and Its Operations, Which Frequently Intrude on Our Psychological Experience

Mind Influences	But Does Not Control Brain
Focus thoughts	But cannot suppress intrusive, obsessive thoughts
Focus senses	But can be distracted
Force ourselves to stay awake	But still doze off under the right circumstances
Try and remember	But become preoccupied and forget
Know what to do/say	But do not do it/say something else
Tell ourselves to ignore and forget	But are still bothered

it or let it go, we cannot suppress the intrusive thoughts, which repeatedly emerge. Here, we know what we want to do, or actually, what we want our brain to do, but our brain seems oblivious to these intents and does exactly what we do not want it to do. Not only that, some time may pass before we realize that we have slipped and have become consumed with the thoughts we had sought to suppress.

When engaged in a task that requires some degree of concentration (e.g., reading) or sustained attention (e.g., driving), we may tell ourselves to ignore the surrounding distractions. However, certain sensory events capture our attention. For instance, while sitting on a train trying to focus on the book or paper that we are reading, it can be effortful, if not impossible, to ignore an intriguing conversation nearby. When drowsy, we may try to stay awake, but under the right conditions, despite our best intentions, we still fall asleep. Maybe it is a sign of an aging brain or just absentmindedness, but it is a personal struggle for me to leave the house without forgetting something. I tell myself to not forget and may even place items by the door so that I will see them as I am walking out, but to my undoing, I become distracted and forget. Similarly, when I need to do something that is outside my ordinary routine, such as making a stop on the way to work, I am as likely to become distracted and forget as I am to remember. The conscious mind has goals and intentions, and we like to think of ourselves and others as purposeful, goal-directed beings. But not only are our brains prone to distraction, the conscious mind may not realize that the brain has gotten off track until it is too late to recover and we are left to undo what the unconscious brain has done.

Slips of the tongue are particularly interesting. In our conscious mind, we know what we want to say. But, the words that we hear coming out are not the words we had intended to say. Usually, it is explainable in that the slip corresponds to something that we had recently been thinking. Prior to any action, whether speech or otherwise, the brain makes preparations to carry out the act. These preparations have been likened to a software program that contains the instructions necessary to elicit the appropriate muscle activity (Adams, 1971). With slips of the tongue, it is believed that the brain simultaneously prepares multiple programs, yet executes the wrong program (Moller et al., 2007). This was illustrated in a study by Moller et al. (2007), in which subjects were induced to commit a certain type of slip of the tongue known as a *spoonerism*. With spoonerisms, one swaps words within a sentence from one position to another. For example, instead of saying, "Go and take a shower," one might say, "Go and shake a tower." In trials in which a subject committed a spoonerism, there was increased activity in the supplementary motor area of the brain. This brain region is believed to serve as a buffer that holds prepared motor programs until it is time for their execution. It was suggested that the increased supplementary motor area activity prior to committing a spoonerism reflected the activation and competition between multiple motor programs.

The anticipatory preparation of motor programs represents a mechanism to increase the efficiency of brain function. This is evidenced by faster reaction times when a subject is able to anticipate and prepare for a forthcoming motor action (Kerr, 1976). The preparation often occurs at an unconscious level and is a product of environmental cues that prime the brain, generally enabling it to be more responsive. Within an engineering context, at an unconscious level, designs that present ambiguous or competing cues prompt the brain to simultaneously prepare multiple programs for carrying out alternative actions. This ambiguity heightens the level of demand imposed on the brain as it must suppress the inappropriate action while carrying out the appropriate action. The competition between actions may occur entirely outside conscious awareness, yet the effects may be felt at a conscious level through the heightened level of effort that is required to complete a task.

With slips of the tongue, a certain helplessness arises when we witness our brain and body operating in a manner that is contrary to our intentions. Nothing makes the division between the conscious mind and the unconscious brain clearer than these experiences. Our brain has the capacity to operate autonomously and often seems to assert this autonomy. At the same time, our conscious mind seeks to curtail that autonomy and direct our brain. However, no matter how much we try, we eventually slip and the brain does what it wants to do.

Vulnerabilities That Arise due to the Limits of Our Conscious Awareness

It is important to understand the distinction between the conscious mind and the unconscious brain because during our everyday experiences, we are constantly receiving messages, whether through our interactions with other people; the materials we read or watch; or our experiences with objects, devices, and even physical spaces. Some messages are directed to our conscious mind and some are directed to our unconscious brain. A certain image may be used in an advertisement because it is likely to elicit an emotional response. A certain policy or procedure may be put in place because it forces people to slow down and think about what they are doing. A device may be constructed so that it creates a certain feel when we hold it in our hands or it produces a certain sound when activated. Whether done knowingly or unwittingly, messages are generally tailored in such a way that they influence and engage either our conscious mind or our unconscious brain.

Likewise, as we interact with others, we are doing the same. We may not always know that we are doing it, or mean to be doing it, but the words we use, the courses of action that we select, and the ways in which we structure and manipulate the world around us influence others. Sometimes we seek to engage the conscious minds of others, and other times we seek to engage their unconscious brains. When suspicious of attempts by others to influence us, it is pertinent to ask, "Are you talking to my mind or my brain?" Similarly, when we seek to influence the thoughts and behaviors of other people, it is pertinent to ask, "Do I want to speak to their conscious mind or their unconscious brain?" The following sections describe several factors that determine whether a message will have a greater effect on the conscious mind or the unconscious brain (see Table 3.2).

Sense of Urgency

The mechanisms that engage the conscious mind are very different from the mechanisms that influence the unconscious brain. For instance, the

TABLE 3.2

Common Mechanisms Used To Engage the Mind and Other Mechanisms That Operate by Engaging the Unconscious Brain

How To Engage the Mind	How To Engage the Brain
Insist on taking time to think (i.e., sleep on it)	Imposed urgency, no time to wait, limited opportunity
Appeal to facts, statistics, data	Appeal to emotions, sentimentality, stereotypes, fear
Minimize distractions, provide solitude, allow isolation	Present distractions, competing demands
Single distinct message	Simultaneous, perhaps nuanced or subliminal messages
Emphasize personal relevance, address individual considerations	Create sense that there is a fad, trend, groundswell, everyone else is doing it, everyone else agrees
Provide structure or logic for making decision	Go with your gut, hunches, rely on instinct

unconscious brain can be impulsive and act without considering the potential consequences. In contrast, the conscious mind can appreciate delayed gratification and after weighing the consequences of alternative actions, keep us on track to achieve our long-term goals. If we want to engage the unconscious brain, we create a sense of urgency and insist that a decision must be made immediately. We regularly experience this when we see advertisements or interact with salespeople who emphasize limited-time offers, where if we do not do it now, we may never have the chance again. In contrast, the conscious mind is able to envision a future where by waiting, we get more, have a better overall experience, or avoid negative consequences.

Placed in a situation where we are encouraged to take some action, particularly when it is an attractive option, the corresponding action is primed within our brains. Whether or not you actually commit the act, at an unconscious level, the brain prepares to do so. Effective salespeople may not only suggest that you buy their product, but they will present a pitch that causes you to imagine yourself going through the actions of making the purchase. At an unconscious level, this process of imagining yourself taking the desired actions primes those actions within the brain. This priming may be observed as increased activation in two brain regions (Forstmann et al., 2008). One is the supplementary motor area discussed previously in relation to the formation of motor programs. The second is the striatum, which functions to map patterns of cues in the environment to specific actions (Wan et al., 2011). Normally, there is some threshold of activation that must be exceeded before an action will be taken. Consequently, as we go through the world constantly being primed to take various actions, we are able to resist these temptations (e.g., passing a row of vendors with various foods on our way to the restaurant where we plan to have lunch). While tempted (i.e., primed at an unconscious level), activation does not exceed the threshold for us to take action. The capacity to resist temptation and withhold a response is a product of inhibitory mechanisms within the brain that serve to suppress competing actions, preventing the corresponding activation from surpassing the threshold that would produce action, allowing us to stay on track as we carry out our intended action.

The effect of time pressure has been demonstrated in experimental settings in which subjects must decide how long to delay a decision. For instance, subjects may be asked to identify an image as details of the image are slowly revealed. A more accurate decision will be made if the subject waits until more details have been provided. Similarly, if subjects are asked to trace a complex figure, their drawing will be more precise if they take longer to do it. In these settings, subjects may be cued to emphasize either speed or accuracy. As shown in Figure 3.1, when subjects are cued to emphasize speed, there is increased activation of the supplementary motor area and striate, indicating a reduction in the inhibitory processes that would normally operate on these regions (Forstmann et al., 2008).

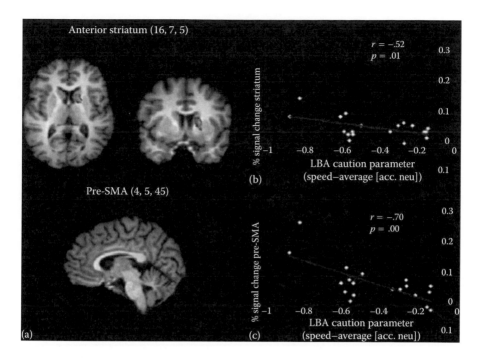

FIGURE 3.1 **(See color insert)**
(a–c) Trials in which subjects were cued to try and produce a speeded response resulted in elevated levels of activity in the striatum and the presupplementary motor areas. LBA, linear ballistic accumulator. (From Forstmann, B.U., Dutilh, G., Brown, S., Neumann, J., von Cramon, D.Y., Ridderinkhof, K.R., and Wagenmakers, E.J., *Proceedings of the National Academy of Science*, 105, 17538–17542, 2008. With permission.)

In contrast, when subjects are cued to emphasize accuracy, there is less activation within these same brain regions suggesting greater involvement of the inhibitory mechanisms associated with increased monitoring and control of ongoing actions.

Whereas the unconscious brain is prone to impulsive action, our conscious mind often supplies an inhibitory influence, keeping the impulses of the unconscious brain in check as we focus on our goals. Time pressure and the resulting sense of urgency can have the effect of not allowing the time necessary for the conscious mind to exert its normal inhibitory influence, causing us to act impulsively. Thus, to engage the conscious mind, you want to insist that there is time to think and that there is no need to make an immediate decision. Although, it should be noted that it is not always certain whether you are better off relying on your conscious mind or unconscious brain. Often, opportunities are limited and in these situations, the deliberations of the conscious mind can be counterproductive and lead to stagnation, missed opportunities, and responses that occur too late to achieve the optimal outcome.

Appeals to Logic

Within Western cultures, where tremendous value has been assigned to logical thought, the conscious mind is predisposed to favor deliberative analytic approaches to interpreting events and making decisions (Nisbett et al., 2001). It is engrained into those of us in the West that when posed with a problem, we resort to a detailed analysis and apply logic to reach a solution. This is what we have been taught that we ought to do. These mental operations are the hallmark of the conscious mind and it has been hypothesized that the capacity for logical thought is one of the factors that promoted the evolution of conscious awareness within humans (Baumeister and Masicampo, 2010). Consequently, when seeking to engage the conscious brain, one should emphasize appeals to logic that are rooted in facts, statistics, and data.

In contrast, the unconscious brain is not predisposed to favor rational thought and is susceptible to appeals based on emotion, sentimentality, stereotypes, and fear. Within Western cultures, these are influences that are looked down on and are treated as weaknesses because they interfere with logical thought. However, emotion allows the brain to almost instantaneously interpret situations and recognize what type of behavior would be appropriate (LeDoux, 1996). When someone knocks on your door in the middle of the night or you walk into a room and are overwhelmed by a disgusting smell, emotions allow you to quickly narrow down your choice of responses and take action with little or no thought.

Stereotypes can be unfair, harmful, and offensive, but there is a reason why the brain is prone to stereotypes. Events can be overwhelming, flooding the brain with more data than it can process. It can become impossible for the brain to individually assess every detail. The brain copes by categorizing so that once something or someone is assigned to a category, everything you know about that category can be attributed to that object or individual (Stevens et al., 2007). Obviously, it becomes problematic when attributes are erroneously associated with a category (e.g., a certain type of person is assumed to always be lazy or dishonest), or categories are applied too broadly allowing people or things to be falsely lumped together (e.g., all vegetables taste bad or all documentaries are boring). However, without this propensity for categorization, the brain would be incapable of coping with the complex world in which we live.

There are many things that brains just do. You may not intend to do it. You do not think about it. Your brain just does it. Categorization is one of them. But there is a reason the brain does these things. Otherwise, it would be incapable of handling the complexities of human existence. Furthermore, the brain is usually right. Yet, the brain sometimes gets it wrong. This makes us vulnerable, whether it is to our tendency to overgeneralize or to the attempts by others to influence us by appealing to false generalities (i.e., stereotypes), particularly those associated with strong emotions (e.g., racial prejudices), whether it is done intentionally or, as sometimes occurs, unknowingly.

Distraction versus Solitude

To deliberate and carefully analyze situations, the conscious mind needs an environment that is free from distractions. The conscious mind is best engaged when offered the opportunity to operate in solitude. When we want to collect our thoughts, we find a quiet room or go for a walk. In contrast, if we want to engage the unconscious brain of another person, we present various distractions. We make it hard to sustain a continuous train of thought. We introduce competing demands so that there is more than one thing to do. We pose some level of threat so that they must contend with the distractions that arise from internal worries and anxieties.

The brain is sensitive to changes in the environment and an involuntary response is generated when it is exposed to either a novel stimulus or an unexpected change in an ongoing stimulus. For example, using the simple task of discriminating even from odd numbers, it was found that reaction times were slower on trials in which an expected background tone (i.e., one that occurred for 80% of trials) was substituted with a natural sound (Alho et al., 1998). Longer reaction times were accompanied by a pronounced neural response in the time frame of 200–300 ms following the unexpected stimulus. Interestingly, in the same study, on some trials (i.e., 10%), the investigators substituted the standard tone with a similar tone, but of a slightly different frequency. This deviant tone did not generate a novelty response and did not slow reaction times, but it did produce a reduction in accuracy for the odd–even number discrimination. The response of the brain to the deviant tone could be seen as a spike in activity at approximately 150 ms following the stimulus. Based on these results, it was concluded that the brain possesses two somewhat distinct mechanisms that involuntarily respond to unexpected stimuli within the environment. One responds to novel stimuli while the other responds to changes to an ongoing stimulus. The involuntary response resulting from either of these mechanisms draws on our limited resources and makes it more difficult for the brain to exert the effort required to consciously focus one's thoughts and attention.

The environment and the associated experiences that we create will influence the extent to which we engage the conscious mind or the unconscious brain of ourselves and others. For instance, there may be situations when for good reason, we do not want to engage the conscious mind. We may want to take a break from whatever weighty matters have dominated our thoughts and allow the brain to take us where it will. I have personally found that nothing accomplishes this goal better than to immerse myself in a busy, noisy, crowded situation. There is a strange but satisfying sensation that comes from walking the streets of a busy city or the multisensory experience of a carnival midway. In these environments, every type of sensory stimulation comes at you from every direction; there are people all around and everywhere you look, there is something different for you to experience. The unconscious brain thrives in this type of environment and it can be a welcome break after a period of prolonged concentration.

Simultaneous Messages

If you want to engage the conscious mind, perhaps you want to convince someone that a certain position, activity, or set of priorities is in their best interest, it is important to present a single, clear, and distinct message. You do not want to confuse them and have them thinking about one thing, then another and not seeing how the different ideas fit together. If their conscious mind cannot latch onto your ideas and, most importantly, begin to operate on them, whether linking to other ideas, appraising the pros and cons, restating your ideas in their own words, and so on, one of two things is likely to happen. Their brains will react to some superficial, unintended facet of what you have said and your message will be misinterpreted, or their brains will drift and they will never hear your message. It is important to never overestimate the capacity of others to consciously attend to what you are trying to communicate to them. They may have the best of intentions and want to give you serious consideration, but if your message is obscure or scattered so that they themselves have to put the pieces together, this may demand more conscious effort than they are willing or able to exert on your behalf.

Our brains are constantly the target of messages. Whereas the conscious mind operates best with a single, distinct message, the unconscious brain can process several simultaneous messages, including the subtle and nuanced implications embedded in these messages. The brain effortlessly processes and reacts to this content, but often, you are not consciously aware of it. For instance, most popular web pages contain advertisements and our general sense is that we effectively ignore them. However, it has been shown that after being exposed to web ads, despite being unable to recall having seen specific ads, subjects reported being more favorably disposed toward the products (Yoo, 2008). Additionally, when asked to generate the names of products, subjects were more likely to list the brands that had appeared in the web ads. Both intentionally and unintentionally, others are influencing us through messages affecting our brains, without our realizing it. This might involve attempts to directly prompt a response (e.g., steer you toward an impulsive purchase), as well as efforts to induce you to bypass the thoughtful considerations of the conscious mind (e.g., appeals to sentimentality or prejudices).

Two common approaches are used to subvert the conscious mind and engage the unconscious brain. The first involves bombarding you with multiple simultaneous messages, which takes advantage of the conscious mind's inability to process more than one message at a time and the brain's capacity to simultaneously process multiple messages. This occurs when a magician diverts our attention in one direction so that we do not notice other activities that are key to the illusion. It occurs where numerous sensory cues are used to create certain experiences, such as at amusement parks, fun houses, and theme-oriented restaurants. It also occurs at a protest, rally, or similar event where signs, slogans, and other messages converge to amplify one another, evoking stronger sentiments in the crowd than exist in all but a few of the more extreme participants.

A second common approach to affect the unconscious brain, while bypassing the conscious mind, embeds triggers within messages that will provoke a response from the unconscious brain, whether through subtle suggestions, hidden associations, or subliminal content. With racial prejudice, it has been shown that following extremely brief exposure (30 ms) to images of faces, within the amygdale, which is a brain region that is sensitive to stimuli that arouse emotions, there is heightened activity when the face is a member of a racial out-group (e.g., White Americans viewing images of African Americans), as compared with faces of individuals from a racial in-group (Cunningham et al., 2004). In crafting a television commercial or a print advertisement, actors and models are selected because their appearance conveys the desired message or because targeted groups will relate to them. Specific words will be used in a slogan or other frequently repeated messages not only because they convey the primary idea, but also because of their association with other ideas, which may include ideas that it would be unacceptable to openly express (e.g., subliminal appeals to racial prejudice). With either approach, the outcome is the same. Your thoughts, ideas, and behavior may be affected without you being consciously aware of the influence others have had on you.

The unconscious brain can be easily influenced; however, many of us might not be alive today if it were not for the capacity of the brain to process simultaneous messages without our conscious awareness. When driving and another vehicle unexpectedly pulls out in front of you, there is no time for the conscious mind to process this situation and decide how to react. Instead, the brain instantly responds, and we slam on the brakes. Afterward, the mind has to catch up, and we become consciously aware of what we have done. While extreme, this example illustrates how beneficial it can be that our brain is constantly taking in sensory input and responding to it, without our being consciously aware of it.

Personal Relevance

To engage the conscious mind, you must first get its attention. Imagine you are in a busy place where there are many people talking at the same time, such as a party or a crowded restaurant. If someone says your name loud enough for you to hear, it immediately captures your attention. It is amazing that one word (i.e., your name) embedded within one of perhaps a dozen conversations will prompt an immediate, involuntary response. As your brain processes the many signals coming from various sources, the brain is particularly sensitive to those that have personal relevance, with there being few signals that have more personal relevance than your name. As illustrated in Figure 3.2, when we hear our name spoken, a combination of brain regions exhibit heightened activation with these being areas associated with speech processing (superior temporal gyrus), one's sense of self or self-consciousness (precuneus), and the monitoring and control of actions

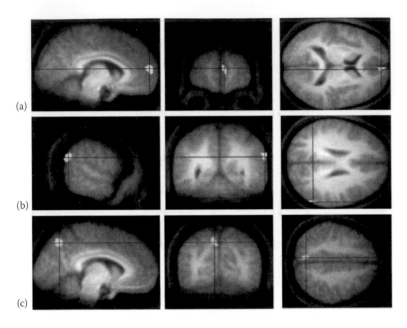

FIGURE 3.2   (See color insert)
When subjects heard their own name, the corresponding electrophysiological response
was correlated with increased activation of the right medial prefrontal cortex (a), right
superior temporal sulcus (b), and left precuneus (c). (From Perrin, F., Maquet, P., Peigneux,
P., Ruby, P., Degueldre, C., Balteau, E., Del Fiore, G., Moonen, G., Luxen, A., and Laureys,
S., *Neuropsychologia*, 43, 12–19, 2005. With permission.)

(medial prefrontal cortex) (Perrin et al., 2005). The broader implication is that
messages that have personal relevance will be more likely to capture your
attention and, consequently, will have preferential access to your conscious
awareness.

To engage the conscious mind, messages should be made personally relevant. While gratuitous acknowledgments can be awkward, there is no more
direct way to get someone's attention than to mention his or her name, ideas,
accomplishments, or similar personal associations. In fact, merely creating an
expectation that there will be a personal reference is often enough to ensure
that you will have the person's attention. The same effect may be achieved by
mentioning places, institutions, people, beliefs, or other references that have
personal relevance. In general, to elicit the thoughtful consideration that is
the hallmark of the conscious mind, an individual needs to sense that a message is personally relevant to him or her, with appeals that are based on personal gains or losses being particularly effective in capturing one's attention.

Two separate cortical networks have been described that mediate the
response of the brain to stimuli based on their personal relevance (Schmitz
and Johnson, 2007). The first network (the ventral-medial prefrontal cortex-
subcortical network) anticipates stimuli that are personally relevant and

orients attention toward these stimuli. Thus, at an unconscious level, the brain senses situations that have the potential to be personally relevant and focuses attention on those situations. The second network (the dorsal-medial prefrontal cortex-subcortical network) engages introspective processes, which may involve self-reflection, evaluation, or recollection. Presented with personally relevant stimuli, this network operates at a conscious level, evoking thoughts that establish and elaborate the personal connection to ourselves. Generally, these networks operate in parallel, with the former capturing our attention and the latter establishing the personal relevance.

Appeal to the Herd

To engage the unconscious brain, you do not want to provoke conscious deliberation, but instead, take advantage of the fact that at an unconscious level, the brain is constantly sensing and being influenced by the world around us. Whether we know it or not, we sense what the people around us are saying and doing, with there being a tendency to mirror what we see in our own actions and what we hear in our own thoughts (Chartrand and Bargh, 1999). This tendency to mirror others has been linked to the brain's "mirror neurons" (Iacoboni, 2009). These neurons and their corresponding circuits are particularly active during situations when an individual is watching another person perform an action and especially when the objective is to imitate that action (Rizzolatti et al., 2002).

At an unconscious level, our brains register the actions of others and exhibit a propensity to imitate those actions. Historically, charismatic leaders have sought to influence the populace through expressions of attitude and beliefs, and calls to action during mass gatherings. Today, the prevalence of various media creates countless mechanisms by which we are similarly being influenced, with the brain willing to transfer the positive affect we associate with celebrities and other popular individuals or groups to various products, activities, and causes (Stallen et al., 2010). The unconscious brain is susceptible to activities that have the effect of creating a sense that there is a trend or a fad, or that everyone is doing, saying, or thinking the same thing. Appeals to the herd can have an inexplicably powerful effect and as chronicled by Charles MacKay (1841) in his classic book *Extraordinary Popular Delusions and the Madness of Crowds*, in retrospect, these attitudes, beliefs, and behaviors may seem irrational, and perhaps even silly. Yet, during most of our endeavors, our propensity for mimicry is highly adaptive, allowing us to effortlessly acquire knowledge that is beneficial in coping with the complexities of everyday life. Actually, the herd is usually right. For example, online recommendations based on the popularity of songs, movies, and so on are usually fairly good. Fortunately, our brains seem to appreciate the wisdom of the crowd. However, it should not be forgotten that sometimes the herd is gullible, and may be steered in directions that are irrational, or perhaps even harmful.

How Do the Pros Do It?

In discussing the distinction between the conscious mind and the unconscious brain, I like to show one or two well-made television advertisements and invite the class to debate whether the intent is to engage the conscious mind or the unconscious brain. One of my favorites is a public service announcement developed for the Canadian Broadcasting Corporation featuring the "house hippo." By searching YouTube for "house hippo," you should be able to easily find it. The commercial begins with the narrator's voice speaking in a deep, serious tone that is typical of a documentary as the camera pans a darkened kitchen with an observant cat sitting on the floor. Then, there is the faint outline of an animal scurrying mouse-like across the floor. However, when the image becomes discernable, it is a miniature hippopotamus. It stands in a grazing posture with a pet's water bowl in the immediate background as the narrator provides a descriptive account wherein the house hippo lives in homes surviving off scraps of food. Subsequent images have the house hippo showing its teeth and backing away from the house cat that towers over it, swimming in a pet's water bowl, and building a nest of threads and lint.

Before the conclusion, which reveals the intended message, I pause the video and ask for opinions as to whether the objective had been to engage the conscious mind or the unconscious brain. There is usually a range of responses. Some will say "mind," and emphasize that the fact that it could not be real makes you rationally contemplate the message. Others cite the cuteness of the miniature hippopotamus as an appeal to the same feelings that are invoked by baby animals and contend that the intent is to engage the unconscious brain.

Either answer is correct. There are facets of this commercial that target the conscious mind and others that target the unconscious brain. In delivering a message, it is not always necessary to select either the conscious mind or the unconscious brain as your target, but a thoughtfully crafted communication may target both. For instance, I believe that the house hippo commercial begins by using surprise (i.e., the animal scurrying across the floor unexpectedly turns out to be a hippopotamus, instead of a mouse) and the cuteness of the miniature hippopotamus to engage the unconscious brain and get the viewer's attention. Afterward, the improbable nature of the subject engages the conscious mind and causes the viewer to think. The commercial ends with a second narrator saying, "That looked really real, but you knew it couldn't be true, didn't you. That's why it's good to think about what you are watching on TV and ask questions, kinda like you just did." Then, we learn that the message is a product of the Concerned Children's Advertisers. This is only one of many strategies that combine mechanisms to engage the conscious mind with other mechanisms to engage the unconscious brain. To be effective in our interactions with others, it is important to consider how to best communicate our message, whether by targeting the conscious mind, the unconscious brain, or both, and craft our messages accordingly.

Reinventing the Television Commercial

In 1984, Apple Computer took an enormous chance in airing an advertisement during the National Football League's Superbowl game that was unlike any of the other commercials that would air that day. Until this time, most television advertisements had been rather direct, with little ambiguity regarding their product or their message. Apple Computer broke with this tradition by hiring a famed science-fiction movie director and airing a commercial that left many wondering exactly what their intent had been.

The commercial began with the mechanism of an oversized clock, followed by uniformed men marching in lockstep. The scenes were entirely in blue-tinted shades of gray. In the background, a speaker bombastically proclaimed idealist slogans. The scene next opened onto a large auditorium where the speaker was projected onto a large screen and rows of men sat transfixed listening to the proclamations. As the commercial switched between perspectives on the assembly, the scene cut to a lone woman running with a sledgehammer in her hands. She had blonde hair and wore red running shorts. As the speaker reached a crescendo and armed security forces marched into the room to intercede, the woman stopped running and, spinning with the sledgehammer in hand, she released the sledgehammer, destroying the screen. An explosion ensued as the speaker fell silent and the faces of the crowd responded in wonderment. An announcer was then heard stating that, "On January 24th, Apple Computer will introduce Macintosh. And you will see why 1984 won't be like 1984."

Whereas most television commercials can be easily ignored, it is difficult to experience this commercial without being affected. The effect occurs at both the level of the conscious mind and the unconscious brain. The images are Stalinesque. They conjure a sense of blind devotion of the masses. For those a generation removed from World War II and the atrocities perpetrated by the Nazi regime, and living through the Cold War and the oppression of Soviet communism, these are powerful images. There is a somber fatalism that harkens to some of the worst fears known to many at the time. The woman connotes a ray of hope symbolized by her interruption of the grayness that subsumes everything else. All these facets of the commercial serve to trigger emotional responses, perhaps felt more strongly at an unconscious level than at a conscious level.

At the same time that the commercial appeals to the unconscious brain, it is engaging the conscious mind. This first occurs with its ambiguity. One is challenged to try and interpret what is being communicated. Then, it introduces the reference to 1984 and makes a connection to Apple Computer. The viewers must first recall what they know and understand concerning the novel *1984* by George Orwell. For most, it has been many years since they read it and they must consciously recall its story and messages. Then, they must link this understanding to the concluding comments, "1984 will not be like 1984" and the reference to Apple Computer. This requires some interpretation, especially given that the personal computer market was in its nascent stages. Most see the message as a call to revolt and to resist the status quo, which was represented by IBM at the time. Apple Computer and their Macintosh brand may be likened to the lone woman confronting overwhelming numbers to strike at tyranny for the sake of personal freedom.

At the time, the Apple Computer commercial was considered to be revolutionary. It did not merely operate at two levels (i.e., conscious mind and unconscious brain), but it did so powerfully. In doing so, it created an image that many in the emerging personal computer market would personally relate to and aspire to. Furthermore, it linked this image to a brand so that those seeking such an image might associate it with the brand. In subsequent years, Apple would continue to embrace this theme, with the "Think Different" campaign being a somewhat more subdued expression. It is perhaps through this ingenious marketing that Apple Computer managed to set the stage within the personal computing market and survive despite overwhelming odds to become one of the most successful companies ever.

Timing of Brain Processes and Conscious Awareness

In 2008, John Dylan Haynes and colleagues at the Max Plank Institute reported a study in which they asked whether the conscious mind can actually keep up with the unconscious brain and, in essence, whether our actions are truly the product of conscious intentions (Soon et al., 2008). We all have the sense that our intentions to do one thing or another arise from our conscious mind, and assume the same for others, holding ourselves and others responsible for the resulting actions. We say that someone was consciously aware of a decision and knowingly acted with the intention to produce a certain outcome.

In the study by Haynes and colleagues, subjects were given two buttons to press and were asked to press one or the other button every so often (see Figure 3.3). Thus, it was the subjects' decision when to press a button and which button they would press. Additionally, during this time, a series of numbers were presented and the subjects were asked to report which number appeared at the time that they made the decision to press the button. During this time, the subjects' brain activity was recorded using functional magnetic resonance imaging (fMRI). Using statistical techniques, the researchers identified distinguishable patterns of brain activity that corresponded to the subjects either pressing one button or the other. Thus, having identified the patterns of brain activity associated with pressing each button, the experimenters could accurately predict which button the subjects had decided to press based entirely on the activity of the subjects' brains.

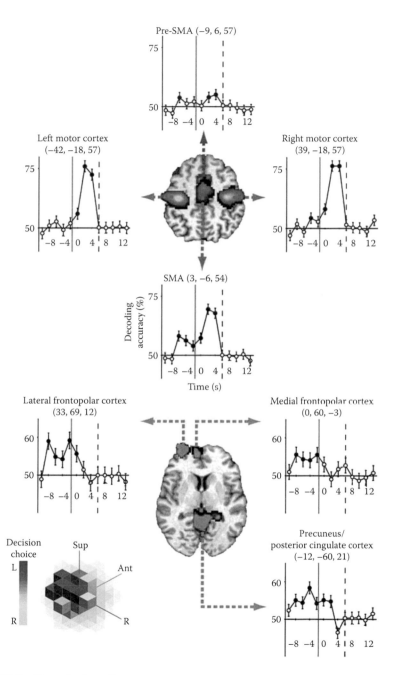

FIGURE 3.3 (See color insert)

Brain regions are highlighted for which patterns of activity predicted forthcoming behavioral responses, with the activity in these areas several seconds prior to conscious awareness of a decision being predictive of the eventual response decision. (From Soon, C.S., Brass, M., Heinze, H.J., and Haynes, J.D., *Nature Neuroscience*, 11, 543–545, 2008. With permission.)

The subjects reported the number that was displayed at the time that they were first aware of having made the decision to act. If the decision to press one of the buttons had been the product of a conscious choice by the mind, then the brain activity associated with choosing the selected button should have appeared at about the same time as the number that the subject reported being present when he or she made the decision to act. Instead, the brain activity preceded the reported number by approximately 7 s. This suggests that the brain had begun preparations to act 7 s before the mind became consciously aware of it. Actually, if you factor in the delay that is inherent in fMRI recordings of brain activity, there was almost a 10 s delay between the point in time when the brain began its preparations and the point that the subject was consciously aware of the brain's intentions.

We have all had experiences equivalent to the one created by the experimental procedure that Haynes and colleagues employed. When slipping on ice, the brain instinctively responds by extending the hands to catch ourselves before we hit the ground. Afterward, there is a moment of confusion and disorientation as the conscious mind catches up, and then we realize what has just happened. Similarly, when we automatically slam on the brakes of our car to avoid an accident, it is only after a moment of thought that we put the pieces together to make sense of what has just happened. Another related example occurs with slips of the tongue where we intend to say one thing, but catch ourselves saying something different. These examples illustrate the momentary delay between when the brain reacts to a situation and the mind becomes consciously aware of it. However, each of these examples also involves a situation that either demands immediate action or is somewhat spontaneous in nature (e.g., the give and take of everyday speech). Most of our actions play out over a longer period of time, allowing ample opportunity for the conscious mind to recognize what the brain is doing and, if necessary, intervene before the action actually takes place. In fact, in the report by Haynes and colleagues, they emphasize that while there may be a delay between the decision to act and conscious awareness of this decision, one is generally quite capable of interrupting before acting on an ill-advised decision.

It is important to realize that this capability of the unconscious brain to get ahead of the conscious mind makes us vulnerable. In this regard, there are at least two ways that we can be tricked into doing things that we know we should not do. Most of us are familiar with the situation where we are driving along a familiar route and, for some reason, we need to deviate from our typical course. Perhaps it is the route that we take to work each morning, but it is the weekend and we are going somewhere else. As we drive along, we become distracted and suddenly realize that we turned at the same place where we would have turned if we were going to work, thereby taking us off our intended route. In this case, there was a well-learned behavior that happened to be inappropriate for the situation. Given that the conscious mind was distracted, the brain ignored the current intentions and went in the familiar direction. In general, whenever people are asked to deviate from well-learned routines, the conscious mind must watch to make sure that the brain does not act out of habit. Unfortunately, our minds can be easily distracted.

Another way to take advantage of the brain getting ahead of the conscious mind involves situations that create a false sense of urgency or prompt a reflexive reaction. Internet scammers frequently employ this mechanism. One popular scam is a pop-up window that appears on the screen saying that a scan of your computer has revealed critical vulnerabilities and offering a link to a report that tells you more. The goal is to trick the computer user into clicking the link, which may take him or her to some type of advertisement or even download malicious software. Some have even elevated the warning to say that the scan has detected that someone else is on your computer. In either case, the scammer seeks to appeal to fear, which causes the computer user to reflexively respond before having actually thought through the situation or the potential consequences of his or her actions. Many find it surprising how often computer users will do things that cause their machines to become infected and spread viruses and other malicious software programs to other computers. However, the scammers and hackers are merely taking advantage of the vulnerabilities that we all share, which emanate from the distinction between our unconscious brain, which sees and reacts, and our conscious mind, which contemplates the consequences of our actions, and the respective time frames in which the unconscious brain and conscious mind operate.

Default Network: Mind Wandering

Whereas one key distinction is that between conscious and unconscious brain processes, a second key distinction exists between whether our conscious awareness is directed internally or externally. Whether daydreaming, fantasizing, or replaying a story or an event, the mind is prone to wander. This is true for all of us, with some exhibiting an even greater propensity for mind wandering, the effects of which are revealed in lower levels of performance in both laboratory studies and everyday life activities (McVay et al., 2009). Neural imaging studies have identified a network of brain regions that tend to be active during periods in which conscious awareness is focused inward (see figure 2 in Mason et al., 2007). This network has been referred to as the "default network" based on a belief that it represents a state of activation that the brain naturally gravitates toward when not attending to external events. Mind wandering occurs effortlessly and often individuals do not realize that their mind has wandered until long after they have ceased attending to surrounding activities. In fact, activity in the default network is most pronounced during episodes of mind wandering in which individuals do not realize that they have allowed their mind to wander (Christoff et al., 2009). Certain conditions and different individuals may be more or less susceptible to mind wandering, and often there is little if any indication that an individual is not paying attention.

More often than not, there is an implicit assumption within systems design that operators, users, and other human components of the system are consciously aware of their surroundings. This is in contrast to an alternative perspective, and perhaps a safer assumption, that at any given point in time, individuals are inattentive and have no conscious awareness of messages presented to them, activities occurring around them, or impending events that may affect them. Within the context of everyday human interactions, there are various mechanisms that allow us to gauge the attentiveness of others and to intervene to ensure that untoward lapses in conscious awareness are avoided. We state that something is important, we ask for verification that we have been heard, and we are attentive to behavior that is unexpected. Few technological systems behave similarly, while often relying on people to be attentive for their successful, and sometimes safe, operation. Furthermore, certain circumstances have the effect of making people more susceptible to mind wandering than they might otherwise be. The following sections summarize some common situations that make mind wandering more likely.

Verbal Rehearsal

Verbal rehearsal, as well as other modes of mental rehearsal, represents a form of mind wandering in that there is little conscious awareness of external events as the mind constructs the right thing to say or imagines an upcoming performance. In general, where situations prompt preparatory activities, one will be prone to mind wandering. A common example occurs during meetings in which everyone is asked to introduce themselves. Anyone who has been in this situation knows that it is often difficult to attend to those who go before you as you imagine what you are going to say.

Threats to Self-Esteem

When one is presented with threats to one's self-esteem, there is a tendency to ruminate. Links have been demonstrated between conditions such as clinical depression and obsessive–compulsive disorder that involve debilitating rumination and heightened activation of the default network (Berman et al., 2011; Gentili et al., 2009). Whereas personal criticism may serve to get someone's attention, it can often have the opposite effect. This is particularly true when the recipient of a critical appraisal does not agree with the appraisal (Heradstveit and Bonham, 1996; Roseman et al., 1990). Any critical appraisal can cause an individual or group to become disengaged. Yet, an erroneous negative appraisal provokes negative emotions that provide a particularly strong catalyst for extended, inwardly focused ruminations.

Physical Discomfort

It is difficult to sustain attention when one is physically uncomfortable. Unpleasant bodily sensations compete for one's conscious awareness. This is evident from studies showing that when experiencing discomfort (e.g., visual discomfort), subjects respond significantly more slowly in measures of sustained attention (Conlon and Humphreys, 2001). It can be quite demanding to try and ignore the sensation of physical discomfort with these demands draining the resources available to attend and respond to external events. Thinking about being hot or cold, how much one hurts, or how bad one feels involves a certain level of conscious disengagement.

Boredom

Perhaps the condition we most commonly think of as being conducive to mind wandering is boredom. Boredom may be thought of as a state of underload during which the brain is inadequately engaged and it becomes exceedingly difficult to sustain attention to external stimuli. I like to say, "the brain wants to be entertained and if not entertained, it will entertain itself." Boredom is most likely to arise when there is a lack of change or novelty, and events, activities, and interactions become repetitious. The brain is unusually sensitive to predictable patterns. Given the complexities of life, this is highly adaptive because limited resources need to be devoted to situations where we know what is going to happen. Consequently, if we know what is going to happen, there is no need to be attentive, and when situations are predictable, there is an opportunity to disengage and turn our conscious awareness inward.

Interestingly, it has been noted that doodling may offer a mechanism to effectively confront boredom and allow the brain to remain engaged in external activities. Andrade (2010) reported a study in which subjects were asked to listen to monotonous telephone conversations for the names of people coming to a party. The subjects were assigned to either a group that was provided with paper and pen and asked to doodle as they performed the task, or a group that was not allowed to doodle. It was found that the subjects who doodled performed significantly better at monitoring the conversations for names and afterward, they remembered more of the names than the group that was not allowed to doodle. This suggests that providing an activity that allows the mind to stay engaged in an externally focused activity may lessen the tendency to become absorbed in internal thoughts, enabling more attention to remain focused on external events.

Often, some degree of mental exertion is required to sustain attention to external events, particularly when events are repetitive and have become boring. The level of default network activity covaries with the level of task engagement. When an individual is engaged in an external task, the transitions between the default network and its counterpart, a network of brain regions that are active when an individual is attending to and responsive to external stimuli, are relatively distinct. In contrast, when an individual is less engaged, the transitions in and out of the default network become somewhat indistinct, with there being greater variability in task performance (Kelly et al., 2008). In a recent study, subjects were shown commercially produced films with it assumed that their appraisal of the films would be correlated with their tendency to mind wander. Thus, subjects who were not interested in the films and grew bored were expected to exhibit more mind wandering. fMRI recordings provided an indication of the level of activity in the default network. The subjects who showed more transitions in and out of the default network, indicating a greater propensity for mind wandering, gave more negative appraisals of the films than the subjects who exhibited fewer transitions. Furthermore, an analysis of the activity within the brain regions making up the default network showed less covariance in the subjects who exhibited more mind wandering and also gave the films poorer ratings. These subjects not only mind wandered more, but their default network was more fully engaged. This suggests deeper levels of disengagement. Furthermore, as their minds wandered, there was greater covariance in the activity of the default network suggesting greater activation of this network (Grubb et al., 2012).

In general, mind wandering corresponds to a state of reduced brain activity. This has been demonstrated by asking subjects to perform a simple, repetitive task for an extended period of time (Smallwood et al., 2008). Specifically, subjects were presented with a series of X's, which served as the nontargets, and their task was to respond when they were presented with a target, which consisted of a number. About 10% of the stimuli were targets. The subjects quickly began to mind wander, which was evident in their frequent failures to respond to targets and their responses to nontargets. Additionally, the subjects were asked to report on their own mind wandering, providing researchers with both performance data and self-reported mind wandering as bases for identifying periods of time in which the subjects had become disengaged from the task. In electroencephalogram (EEG) recordings, there was a pattern of response (i.e., a visual evoked potential) that corresponded to stimulus presentation. During periods in which the subjects exhibited evidence of mind wandering, there was a lower-amplitude EEG response, indicating a relatively reduced baseline level of brain activity.

Inattentional Blindness

Have you ever had the experience where you are looking for something that is right in front of you, but you do not see it until someone points it out to you? Following a collision, motorists often comment that they had looked, but never saw the other vehicle. Designers generally believe that if there is a highly salient signal, it is safe to assume that it will capture people's attention. However, just because the brain is receiving and processing sensory information, with there being activation of brain regions in response to the sensory stimulation, you cannot assume conscious awareness of the sensory information (Logothetis and Schall, 1989; Leopold and Logothetis, 1996).

The phenomenon known as "inattentional blindness" provides a particularly poignant demonstration that salient sensory stimulation may not be perceived at a conscious level, despite being readily available to the sensory system. Demonstrations of inattentional blindness generally involve a complex visual scene with subjects instructed to focus their attention on a specific facet of the visual scene. For instance, one demonstration presents two groups of people in different-colored outfits with each group passing a ball back and forth at the same time (Simons and Chabris, 1999). The observer is instructed to count the number of times that one of the two groups passes the ball. It is a busy scene and one must pay close attention to keep track of the designated group. As the scene unfolds, a highly salient event will occur. For example, a person dressed in a gorilla costume will walk from one to the other side of the scene, stopping in the middle to dance or perform other moves. On first witnessing this demonstration, most observers do not report seeing the gorilla. Then, having had it pointed out to them that a person in a gorilla suit passed through the scene, they are astounded that they had not noticed something so obvious.

Attention seems to be the critical factor in determining the response of the brain to sensory stimuli, with stimuli that are the focus of attention triggering the expected brain response. In contrast, when equally salient stimuli are not the focus of attention, critical higher-level brain processes do not respond, as if the stimuli had never occurred. Rees et al. (1999) demonstrated this effect in a study in which subjects were shown letter strings superimposed onto images. The subjects were instructed to attend to either the letter strings or the images. When attention was focused on the letter strings and they contained meaningful words, as compared with random consonants, there was activation of brain areas that are generally active during language processing. In contrast, the same stimuli produced essentially no activation of these brain areas in conditions in which the subjects were instructed to attend to the visual scene, ignoring the superimposed letters. It should be noted that unattended sensory information triggers activation of initial low-level sensory processes, indicating that the brain senses the stimuli, yet it is in the time period 200 ms or more after the stimulus when higher-level brain processes would normally be active that there is no response (Sergent et al., 2005).

Inattentional blindness occurs when the sensory systems of the brain are presented with competing demands. In these situations, the brain copes by not merely favoring one task over the other, but by actively suppressing activation associated with the competing task (Todd et al., 2005). The effect may be the product of demands to either focus on ongoing sensory events or to hold recent sensory experiences in short-term working memory. For example,

either asking an individual to monitor a complex stream of sensory information or asking them to remember one or more complex sensory experiences
is sufficient to consume the available resources, forcing the brain to cope by
ignoring other ongoing demands. Brain activity elicited by the competing
sensory experiences is transmitted through the lower-level sensory circuits
(e.g., areas within the visual or occipital cortex responsible for distinguishing
shapes, colors, and other physical attributes of a stimulus), but it is suppressed
as it reaches the higher-level brain processes that provide the basis for our
conscious awareness of the sensory events. While the most pronounced demonstrations of inattentional blindness involve a single sensory modality, it
can also occur in situations involving multiple sensory modalities (Sinnett
et al., 2006). For example, by focusing attention on visual information, an individual may fail to perceive auditory information, or vice versa. Yet, it should
be noted that the same brain mechanisms that make us susceptible to inattentional blindness also allow us to listen to a single conversation while standing
in a crowded room where several people are talking at the same time.

These facets of brain function have important ramifications for systems
design. In particular, where there is a reliance on the human to sense and
respond to environmental stimuli, it must be recognized that there is a limited capacity to simultaneously monitor multiple streams of sensory input,
particularly when one of those streams is both demanding and the focus of
attention. Furthermore, in high-demand situations, the brain's mechanisms
for coping operate automatically and at an unconscious level. Consequently,
an individual may have no conscious awareness of actively ignoring potentially significant facets of the overall sensory experience. It cannot be
assumed that the individual has made a conscious decision to ignore some
sensory input in favor of others. Instead, the brain operates outside the individual's conscious awareness to actively suppress competing sensory experiences as a means to enable the individual to cope with the demands of the
task on which his or her attention is focused.

Implicit Operations of the Brain

Previous sections have emphasized that the majority of what the brain does
occurs at an unconscious level. The following sections summarize several
ways in which the unconscious operations of the brain are manifested within
our daily activities.

Implicit Memory

One of the most basic distinctions made regarding human memory concerns that between recall and recognition. Within naturalistic settings, an

individual may be able to recall very little of what he or she has experienced. For example, taken on a tour through an unfamiliar city or building, immediately afterward, and even days or weeks later, people will only recall the most salient and meaningful sights. However, if shown a series of photographs and asked if they had or had not seen various objects or features, people will respond with accuracy far above chance, despite being unable to recall the same objects or features. During the tour, an individual may have paid little attention to many of the sights, yet the visual images were processed at an unconscious level and memories were formed that, while they could not later be consciously recalled, were sufficient to produce a sense of familiarity. It should be noted that this effect does not contradict the previous discussion of inattentional blindness where there is no subsequent awareness of certain sensory experiences. Inattentional blindness occurs when attention is focused on one stream of sensory experience and the associated demands cause the brain to suppress input from competing streams of sensory experience. The phenomena being addressed here occurs when attention is focused on a given stream of sensory experience, yet some information is processed at a conscious level, while the rest may be momentarily processed at a conscious level, but is primarily processed at an unconscious level.

The mechanism whereby we are capable of recognizing items from our past experience that we are unable to intentionally recall has been referred to as implicit memory and serves as the underpinnings for otherwise unaccountable feelings of familiarity with certain objects, people, and places, as well as sensory experiences such as sounds, smells, and so on. Within the brain, parallel processes are activated by sensory experiences, with one providing the basis for explicit memory and the other providing the basis for implicit memory. The distinction is apparent in cases where brain damage has left explicit memory intact with there being little or no accompanying implicit memory, or has left implicit memory intact with there being little or no accompanying explicit memory (Gabrieli et al., 1995). Three patterns of brain activity occur when test subjects are shown a series of stimuli, and are later shown a second series of stimuli and are asked to indicate which items from the second series appeared in the first series (i.e., old) and which did not (i.e., new) (Rugg et al., 1998). One pattern appears with words correctly classified as having not appeared in the first list (i.e., new), a second for words that appeared in the first list and are correctly recognized, and a third for words that appeared in the first list, but are not correctly recognized (i.e., false negatives). This latter pattern of neural activity where the brain seems to recognize the word at an unconscious level, yet the subject does not consciously recognize the word, has been linked to the common experience of "familiarity." This is the experience where we see something that seems personally relevant, yet we do not immediately realize what connection may exist.

In the design of information displays, it is worth asking whether the objective is for information to be later recalled or merely recognized. A comparison of the brain regions that are most active during recall and recognition reveals a greater engagement of executive functions during recall (Cabeza et al., 1997). In contrast, there is a greater engagement of the brain regions associated with perceptual processes during recognition. Consequently, where the objective is for information to later be recalled (e.g., a code that must be read and later entered, or an instruction that is given at one time and must be executed at a later time), there is the need to present information in a way that will engage executive functions and facilitate those executive functions when the time comes to recall the information. For instance, this occurs when we prepare a hint or use some form of pneumonic device to help us later recall a password, procedure, or other information. In other cases, the objective may be for information to later be recognized (e.g., recognizing the path through a building or a menu system) or the objective may be for there to merely be a sense of familiarity (e.g., designers may want a new product design to evoke the positive sensations associated with a popular predecessor). In these situations, one might want to use perceptual features that will help bolster a sense of familiarity. This could occur through a variety of mechanisms such as the formatting of information, the background against which the information is presented, the context in which the information is presented, or the shape and feel of a product.

Behaviorally, implicit memory is often manifested through priming. Priming occurs when incidental exposure to a stimulus (e.g., a word) activates associated memories within the brain, yet this activation is slight and there may be no conscious awareness that the brain is responding to the stimuli (Schacter and Buckner, 1998). Experimentally, the effect of priming may be demonstrated through studies in which subjects who are exposed to words for durations that are so brief there is no opportunity to consciously process the word and its related meaning, react faster when later presented with semantically similar probes (Schacter, 1992). For example, if primed for an extremely brief exposure to the word "fire," and later presented with a series of words and asked to indicate which words describe a common injury, subjects will respond faster to "burn" than words not related to fire (e.g., sprain, burp). With implicit memory, there may be no conscious awareness of the stimuli that are the source of the memory. Yet, there is activation of the brain processes associated with the stimuli and this activation prepares the individual to respond more readily or more robustly to the stimuli, or associated stimuli, at a later time.

In the design of systems, priming offers a mechanism to better prepare individuals to respond to upcoming events (Crundall and Underwood, 2001; Navarro et al., 2007). This may occur through overt mechanisms such as instructions or videos that prepare an individual for an upcoming activity. For example, in many airports, prior to entering the security screening area, passengers are shown videos that depict the screening procedures. These videos serve as an overt prime reminding passengers of the rules and procedures and readying them to carry out these procedures more efficiently once they have reached the screening area. Priming may also be used in ways that are much more subtle. For example, with assembly operations, the parts and tools that will be needed may be laid out in the order that they will be used. Seeing the parts and tools associated with the upcoming steps serves to prime memories for those steps, allowing the operator to be better prepared on reaching those steps in the operation. Whether done overtly or through more subtle mechanisms, priming may be effectively used to elicit activation in neural circuits associated with knowledge or activities that will be required at a later point in time, allowing the individual to respond more quickly and effectively when the time arrives.

Implicit Learning

I like to say that "learning is one of the things that brains just do." Learning is a by-product of brain function and occurs whether or not there is a conscious intent to learn. As designers, we are constantly engineering experiences and when people encounter these experiences, learning will occur. This can be beneficial in many circumstances. However, one must be attentive to what might be learned and, specifically, what unintentional learning might occur.

Often, training involves the use of simulators that emulate the experiences of actual operational systems. Yet, for the sake of expediency, trainees may be allowed to skip procedural steps that are essential with the operational system, but are unnecessary with the simulation-based trainer. Similarly, trainees may be required to perform a modified procedure to accommodate the peculiarities of the simulation-based trainer or the training protocol. In either case, trainees are acquiring patterns of behavior, as well as developing expectations regarding the behavior of the system and how the system will respond as the trainees take various actions. This illustration highlights a rather obvious example. Incidental, unintended, or implicit, learning certainly may occur with salient tasks or facets of the environment. However, implicit learning may also occur for more subtle experiences, with much of what shapes implicit learning occurring outside conscious awareness. Consequently, one is often unaware of what the brain is learning. As designers, we must attend to the subtle patterns, sequences, and associations that are embedded within the experiences created by our products and, specifically, opportunities for potentially counterproductive implicit learning.

In engineering systems, there is an imposition of order where order might not have otherwise existed. Thus, within any engineered system, there is an inherent orderliness from which certain rules of operation may be extrapolated. Many years ago, I was part of a research team that undertook the job of developing a capability to use the data generated while operating an automobile (e.g., steering wheel rotation and lateral acceleration) to make real-time inferences concerning the ongoing driving context (e.g., approaching an intersection and executing a lane change). Initially, I had some concern that driving was such an open-ended task that we would have little success applying the machine learning techniques that had worked well within laboratory settings for relatively constrained activities. However, I was pleasantly surprised when our algorithms did quite well in predicting a wide range of driving contexts (Dixon et al., 2005). In retrospect, I later realized that I had underestimated the extent to which driving is a highly constrained activity. The structure of the roadways imposes many constraints that limit the realm of possibilities. Furthermore, the rules of the road and the behavior of other drivers impose further constraints. Finally, the automobile itself offers even more constraints. There is an implicit orderliness and corresponding rules associated with driving that through our experiences we have all learned. Yet, like me, unless we are given a reason to consciously think about these rules, they rarely enter our awareness, although they are constantly shaping our behavior and experiences. Implicit learning refers to the process whereby our brains unconsciously recognize patterns and infer the relevant rules that emanate from those patterns during our day-to-day experiences.

Experimentally, implicit learning has been examined in studies that present subjects with a series of meaningless stimuli that may or may not follow a consistent pattern. For example, subjects may be presented with the letters "A," "B," "C," and "D," with a different finger assigned to each letter and the instructions to press a key with the corresponding finger whenever a letter is presented (Eimer et al., 1996). When the letters are presented randomly, the reaction time associated with each letter is approximately the same. However, when the letters are presented in a sequence (e.g., A,C,D,B,A,C,D,B,…), reaction times decrease over a series of trials, although often subjects cannot accurately report the sequence. The fact that the reaction times decrease implies that the subjects have learned the sequence, although implicitly, at an unconscious level. When an individual prepares to execute a motor response, there is increased activation of the brain regions on the side of the brain opposite the limb that will execute the response (i.e., lateralized motor potential). With implicit learning of sequences, this increased activation occurs prior to the presentation of the stimulus, implying that the individual anticipates the response that will be triggered by the next stimulus. Furthermore, once an individual has learned a sequence, if an unexpected stimulus (i.e., deviant) is inserted (e.g., instead of the A,C,D,B pattern, the series, A,B,D,B is presented), a wave of activity spreads across the brain in response to the out-of-sequence stimulus. This occurs whether the subject can or cannot consciously report the sequence, although there is a larger-magnitude response to a deviant stimulus if the subject is consciously aware of the sequence than if the subject is not consciously aware of the sequence.

With experimental paradigms such as the one described in the previous paragraph, if subjects are provided with enough exposure to a recurrent sequence of stimuli, they will generally recognize the sequence and will be able to accurately report it. Thus, learning progresses from an initial stage in which there is implicit knowledge of the sequence as evidenced by reduced reaction times, to a later stage in which there is explicit knowledge as evidenced by the ability to correctly report the sequence. This transition is marked by an accompanying transition in the activation of neural circuits (Honda et al., 1998). During the implicit learning stage, decreases in reaction time are correlated with activation in the primary sensorimotor cortex. This activation may be interpreted as priming where expectations regarding the next stimulus–response pairing in the sequence lead to anticipatory activation of the corresponding neural circuits. In contrast, during the explicit learning stage, there is a correlation between the accuracy with which subjects report sequences and activation across a broad area that encompasses the parietal cortex, precuneus, and premotor cortex. This latter pattern of activation may be interpreted to indicate greater awareness of the stimulus–response sequence with increased conscious control of task performance.

Implicit Perception

Much has been said about the potential influences of subliminal messages and their use within various contexts. Subliminal stimuli are perceptual cues that are either of too low a magnitude or too short a duration to be perceived at a conscious level (i.e., subthreshold), yet they may have a psychological or behavioral influence (Dehaene et al., 2006). It has been shown that presenting words with either a positive or a negative connotation for as little as 1 ms is enough to produce a measurable response in the brain (Bernat et al., 2001). Furthermore, unpleasant words produced a larger-amplitude response and a somewhat different pattern of response than pleasant words. This illustrates that at an unconscious level, verbal stimuli that one has only been exposed to for an instant can evoke patterns of brain activity associated with either pleasant or unpleasant sensations. Whereas we generally think of subliminal stimuli as messages that are engineered to affect recipients in a certain way, we are constantly being bombarded by stimuli that our brains process at an unconscious level. Some of these may be subthreshold or subliminal, but most are of a magnitude and duration that would be readily perceived if they were the object of our attention.

As designers, there is a tendency to only consider the facets of a design that are related to the functions of a product, environment, or system. However, other incidental factors will create perceptual sensations that may not be consciously perceived, but will influence how our design is experienced. It has been said that, "99% of design is invisible" (99% Invisible, 2012). This expression conveys the idea that when people interact with a design, they may only be consciously aware of 1% of the overall design. However, their experience is shaped by the entirety of the design and the resulting sensations created by the design. This serves as a caution that otherwise good designs can go awry without sufficient attention to detail. For example, a restaurant may place trash at a location such that the patterns of airflow result in the dining area being permeated by imperceptible odors of food waste. Customers may not consciously recognize the odor, but find their dining experience inexplicably unpleasant. Likewise, subtle details of design may be used to create a positive impression. Automobile makers appreciate the effect of the sound that a car door makes when it is closed and electronics makers understand that devices need to produce a solid snap when they are closed. Many years ago, when commercial airlines regularly served meals on lengthy flights, a persistent meme revolved around the poor quality of the meals served on flights. When passengers were asked to rate various facets of their travel experience, it was found that a correlation existed between how well passengers rated the quality of the meals that an airline served and the associated service, and how well they rated the safety of the airline (Rhoades and Waguespack, 1999). This is a particularly telling example because safety is an aspect of the airline that passengers have very little evidence to judge how well an airline is doing. Yet, passengers seemed to have made the assumption that if the airline got the meals and meal service right, they were probably doing a good job with safety.

The phenomenon whereby a stimulus that is processed at an unconscious level has a measurable effect on behavior and psychological experience is known as *implicit perception*. It is often difficult to distinguish implicit perception from implicit memory given the mutual dependence of perceptual and memory processes within everyday activities. Perhaps the clearest illustration of perception without conscious awareness occurs with motor behavior, where perceptual processes construct an internal representation of the environment as a basis for guiding actions with respect to specific goals (Rossetti, 1998). While perception is essential to most motor actions, there is little conscious awareness of the corresponding perceptual experience. We carry out motor acts that are continuously mediated by perceptual knowledge and ongoing perceptual input; however, we are rarely aware of the corresponding perceptual experiences.

An extreme example of implicit perception occurs with the phenomenon of *blindsight* (Milner and Goodale, 1995). Blindsight is observed in patients suffering damage to the primary visual processing regions of the brain. These patients have no conscious awareness of some portion of their visual field. For example, they may have no conscious awareness of the right side of their overall visual field, with their awareness of the left side remaining intact. However, if shown a target in the portion of the visual field for which they have no conscious awareness and are asked about its presence or absence or approximate location, or are asked to reach for the target, these patients perform far better than chance. This performance indicates that the brain remains capable of processing the sensory information, yet there is no conscious awareness. Blindsight has been attributed to the distinction between two separate visual pathways. The dorsal or *how* pathway processes information concerning how to act toward objects and the ventral or *what* pathway processes information about the identity and characteristics of the object (Milner and Goodale, 1995). In blindsight, the dorsal pathway remains intact, allowing the individual to execute appropriate motor responses, while damage to the ventral pathway impairs the individual's ability to consciously recognize the target.

In everyday activities, a wide array of brain processes are engaged in a seamless, somewhat symphonic, accord. The degree of conscious awareness devoted to an activity may vary, as well as the facets of the activity that are the object of our conscious awareness. Yet, generally, for familiar activities, there is little conscious awareness of the countless brain processes that combine to enable us to perform the activity. The proficiency with which we perform these activities testifies to the depth and breadth of the brain's capacity to process perceptual information at an unconscious level. It is important to remember that this unconscious processing involves some level of appraisal of attributes such as pleasantness, goodness, and so on. Consequently, as designers, we must assume that every detail matters. Every detail will be sensed and appraised. No matter how removed a facet of our design may be from the direct operation of a device or system, if users have any exposure, whether conscious or unconscious, it will shape their experience of the product.

Automaticity

Within the course of everyday life, we engage in countless activities that involve a repetitive routine that does not change from one occurrence to the next. For instance, my morning routine on workdays generally involves taking a shower, shaving, getting dressed, eating breakfast, brushing my teeth, and finally, collecting the things I will need for the day, telling my wife goodbye, and leaving the house. This routine has not only been learned, but the learning is so deeply engrained that much of the time, my mind is consumed with other thoughts, and I devote little attention to these activities. The level of automaticity becomes apparent when something causes me to deviate from the routine. In these cases, I am likely to forget a step in the sequence. For instance, on more than one occasion, I have gotten in the shower and found that there was no soap. The mere variance of turning off the water to get a new bar of soap and starting over again has been sufficient to cause me to forget to shampoo my shaved scalp. Similarly, my wife asking me to do something during breakfast has been enough to cause me to forget to finish my breakfast and leave the dirty dishes on the table, instead of my usual routine of taking them into the kitchen and rinsing them. Without any effort, our brains learn these repetitive sequences of behavior and are capable of carrying them out with little or no conscious thought.

When learning a new skill, there is a progression from the initial stages where there is the need for conscious attention to later stages in which the activity can be performed effortlessly with little or no conscious attention. With tasks that are primarily sensory-motor (e.g., manual tracking), the initial stages involve increased activation of the cortical regions (frontal cortex, somatosensory cortex, and parietal cortex) associated with executive functions, processing somatosensory feedback, and motor planning (Floyer-Lea and

Mathews, 2004). Once the task has been well learned, activation shifts to the subcortical regions (cerebellum and basal ganglia) associated with the coordination and execution of motor actions. Similarly, where learning involves a series of actions performed in a specific order, a shift in activation from regions associated with conscious control of actions to regions involved in the execution of learned sequences of actions (supplementary motor area, and putamen and globus pallidus of the basal ganglia) occurs (Poldrack et al., 2005). Within the subcortical regions of the brain (i.e., basal ganglia and associated areas), there are specialized circuits that enable well-learned actions to be carried out with little or no conscious awareness. This automaticity allows conscious attention to be focused on other facets of the environment or, as often occurs, to be turned inward. Automaticity also serves as an essential interim step in constructing sequences of complex actions. In this case, initially, each action may require significant attention during learning, but once learned, may be treated as a chunk and combined in a sequence with other similarly complex actions. This occurs with combinations of chords in music; in sports activities such as the combinations of step sequences, postures, attacks, and defenses in martial arts; and with professional activities that involve sequential series of actions (e.g., detailed assembly operations).

While the brain processes underlying automaticity have been extensively studied for sensorimotor activities, the potential for automaticity extends to a broad range of cognitive activities. For instance, proficiency in reading (Wolf et al., 1986), speech comprehension (Friederici et al., 2000), and mathematics (Dehaene and Akhavien, 1995) have each been linked to the automaticity of basic operations within the brain. Furthermore, these processes underlie the formation of many habits and ritualistic behaviors (Graybiel, 2008). From a systems design perspective, one might consider the overall array of behaviors that might occur in achieving various objectives and ask, "what is the potential impact of automaticity?" In many cases, automaticity may allow increased efficiency and allow individuals to focus their attention on other more important events. In this case, a designer may look for opportunities to create repetitive activities, as well as opportunities to combine repetitive sequences into longer series of actions. However, automaticity can also prompt conscious disengagement. Thus, where the potential for disengagement poses risks, designers should be sensitive to this potential and introduce design features that intentionally engage conscious processes (e.g., system probes that require nonstandard responses). When implemented effectively, operators may continue to experience the benefits of automaticity, but are occasionally reminded to think about what they are doing so that they do not become completely disengaged from ongoing activities.

Unconscious Cognition

When presented with a challenging problem, there may be a period in which we are consciously focused on solving the problem. Yet, when our attention is directed elsewhere and we are no longer consciously focused on the problem, does our brain continue to work on it? It has been asserted that the ah-ha phenomenon, where the solution to a problem occurs to us spontaneously at a time when we may not actually be thinking about the problem, suggests that the brain has continued to work on the problem, but at an unconscious level (Metcalfe and Wiebe, 1987).

Jung-Beeman et al. (2003) used a common paradigm for studying creativity—defined as the solution of problems through insight, as opposed to analytic strategies—known as the remote associates test. In this test, subjects were presented with three problem words (e.g., pine, crab, and sauce). Their task was to identify a word or a phrase that connected the three problem words. In this example, the correct answer would be "apple." In this study, the subjects were asked to respond by pressing a button when they had attained a solution and then report their solution. After each trial, the subjects were asked to indicate whether or not the solution involved insight (i.e., came to them suddenly). fMRI recordings found that the feature that most clearly distinguished trials in which subjects reported an ah-ha experience was an increased level of activity in the right hemisphere of the brain (i.e., right anterior superior temporal gyrus). Using the same procedure, a second experiment showed that in the time period immediately prior to their response on trials involving insight, subjects exhibited a burst of high-frequency brain activity in approximately the same area of the right hemisphere.

Interestingly, it was also noted in the study by Jung-Beeman that prior to the burst of high-frequency activity that corresponded with the ah-ha experience, there was a period marked by slower frequency, or alpha activity. In this context, alpha activity was interpreted to reflect the suppression of neural processes. It was suggested that the suppression of interference from competing attentional processes may be essential for the right hemisphere to make distant semantic connections. Thus, it was suggested that the mechanisms underlying the ah-ha experience involve a period during which there is activation of diverse semantic connections, which occurs at an unconscious level. This may occur in parallel with more analytic processes involving the left hemisphere of the brain, which is normally associated with language-related processes, with these analytic processes dominating one's conscious awareness. It may be essential that the broad activation of semantic connections within the right hemisphere that gives rise to a problem solution be accompanied by a momentary suppression of competing activation. The suppression of competing activation may serve to amplify the potential solution. This is then followed by a burst of high-frequency activity, which accompanies the emergence into conscious awareness of the solution and the corresponding ah-ha experience.

It appears that in problem solving, the brain is capable of carrying out somewhat separate processes at both a conscious and an unconscious level, and often the solution arises as a product of unconscious problem solving. However, to realize the benefits of unconscious problem solving, individuals must be capable of relinquishing their focused attention on the problem long enough for a solution that is attained through unconscious processes to emerge into their conscious awareness. This suggests that certain environments may be more conducive to creative problem solving than others. In particular, an environment rich in engaging external stimulation will make it difficult to turn one's conscious awareness inward long enough to allow a solution to arise from unconscious processes. Likewise, an environment that serves to keep an individual engaged in analytic problem-solving strategies will similarly dampen the individual's awareness of ongoing unconscious problem-solving processes. In contrast, an environment that makes it easy to momentarily disengage from the immediate problem should have the effect of interrupting ongoing, conscious problem-solving strategies long enough for solutions to pop into one's conscious awareness. One can only wonder how many ingenious ideas have been lost due to single-minded dedication to an analytic problem-solving strategy or the constraints imposed by organizational or other contexts to rely solely on or to operate within an environment that favors analytic problem-solving strategies.

What Is the Downside of Unconscious Brain Processes?

On the surface, it seems great that the brain is continually working and that we do not need to be consciously engaged, yet benefit from the products of our ongoing unconscious brain processes. However, while we can usually report our conscious thought processes with some accuracy, what we have learned or experienced implicitly is often inaccessible. Consequently, where there is a reliance on implicit learning, one often has a poor sense of what one has learned and how well one has learned it. Likewise, you do not know when you have forgotten something that you may have once learned. When asked to explain how you do something, your report will orient around those facets for which you have conscious awareness. Knowledge and skills that are the product of implicit knowledge will be reported unreliably and if pressed for an answer, as often occurs with expert accounts, individuals can only make their best guess as to exactly what they are doing and why they do it that way. In general, while unconscious brain processes may significantly impact the things that we do and how well we do them, we have very little conscious access to those brain processes, or the associated knowledge.

Unconscious Impact of Cognitive State on Decisions

Recently, Jonathan Levav and colleagues reported a research study that illustrates the extent to which unconscious brain processes shape conscious decisions and, particularly, may bias our decisions in ways that we do not appreciate (Danziger et al., 2011). In this study, they looked at the parole decisions of judges in Israeli courts. These decisions involved a prisoner going before a judge and an argument being made for the judge to reduce the prisoner's sentence due to good behavior or other mitigating circumstances. Data were analyzed for a 10 month period and consisted of 1112 hearings, with prisoners from four different prisons and decisions made by eight different judges.

The researchers considered whether parole was granted (i.e., the prisoner received a reduced sentence) relative to where a hearing occurred within the overall order of hearings on a given day. It was striking how the probability of being awarded parole varied over the course of a day. On any given day, there were three sessions. At the beginning of any one of these three sessions, the likelihood of a prisoner receiving parole was approximately 65%. However, by the end of a session, that likelihood had dropped to nearly zero. It did not matter how severe the crime was, the amount of time that the prisoner had already served, whether the prisoner had previously been incarcerated, whether rehabilitation services were available, or the nationality or gender of the prisoner. The likelihood of being awarded parole was driven primarily by placement within the order of hearings within a given session.

The researchers attributed these results to the unconscious effects of fatigue on the cognitive processes of the judges. Specifically, it was asserted that as one becomes increasingly fatigued, one tends to choose the easier option and in this case, awarding parole was the more difficult decision because it involved incurring the risk that the prisoner would again commit a criminal offense. In contrast, it was an easy decision to deny parole because the prisoner returned to prison and there was no risk to society of his or her continuing to commit crimes. The key point is that the judges' decisions were systematically biased and they had no conscious awareness of this bias. At a conscious level, one may believe that one is operating in a consistent, unbiased manner. However, various biases operating at an unconscious level to shape our conscious deliberations may be in effect, and we may never know how strongly we have been influenced by these unconscious brain processes.

Acknowledgments

Sandia National Laboratories is a multiprogram laboratory managed and operated by Sandia Corporation, a wholly owned subsidiary of Lockheed Martin Corporation, for the US Department of Energy's National Nuclear Security Administration under contract DE-AC04-94AL85000.

References

99% Invisible. (2012). A tiny radio show about design with Roman Mars, December 12, 2012, http://99percentinvisible.org/.

Adams, J.A. (1971). A closed-loop theory of motor learning. *Journal of Motor Behavior*, 3, 111–150.

Alho, K., Winkler, I. and Naatanen, R. (1998). Neural mechanisms of involuntary attention to acoustic novelty and change. *Journal of Cognitive Neuroscience*, 10(5), 590–604.

Andrade, J. (2010). What does doodling do? *Applied Cognitive Psychology*, 24(1), 100–106.

Baumeister, R.F. and Masicampo, E.J. (2010). Conscious thought is for facilitating social and cultural interactions: How mental simulations serve the animal-cultural interface. *Psychological Review*, 117(3), 945–971.

Berman, M.G., Peltier, S., Nee, D.E., Kross, E., Deldin, P.J. and Jonides, J. (2011). Depression, rumination and the default network. *Social, Cognitive and Affective Neuroscience*, 6(5), 548–555.

Bernat, E., Bunce, S. and Shevrin, H. (2001). Event-related brain potentials differentiate positive and negative mood adjectives during both supraliminal and subliminal visual processing. *International Journal of Psychophysiology*, 42(1), 11–34.

Cabeza, R., Kapur, S., Craik, F.I.M., McIntosh, A.R., Houle, S. and Tulving, E. (1997). Functional neuroanatomy of recall and recognition. A PET study of episodic memory. *Journal of Cognitive Neuroscience*, 9(2), 254–265.

Chartrand, T.L. and Bargh, J.A. (1999). The chameleon effect: The perception-behavior link and social interaction. *Journal of Social and Personality Psychology*, 76, 93–110.

Christoff, K., Gordon, A.M., Smallwood, J., Smith, R. and Schooler, J.W. (2009). Experience sampling during fMRI reveals default network and executive system contributions to mind wandering. *Proceedings of the National Academy of Sciences*, 106(21), 8719–8724.

Conlon, E. and Humphreys, L. (2001). Visual search in migraine and visual discomfort groups. *Vision Research*, 41(23), 3063–3068.

Crundall, D. and Underwood, G. (2001). The priming function of road signs. *Transportation Research Part F: Traffic Psychology and Behavior*, 4(3), 187–200.

Cunningham, W.A., Johnson, M.K., Raye, C.L., Gatenby, J.C., Gore, J.C. and Banaji, M.R. (2004). Separable neural components in the processing of Black and White faces. *Psychological Science*, 15, 806–813.

Custers, R. and Aarts, H. (2010). The unconscious will: How the pursuit of goals operates outside of conscious awareness. *Science*, 329(5987), 47–50.

Danziger, S., Levav, J. and Avnaim-Pesso, L. (2011). Extraneous factors in judicial decisions. *Proceedings of the National Academies of Science*, 108(17), 6889–6892.

Dehaene, S. and Akhavien, R. (1995). Attention, automaticity and levels of representation in number processing. *Journal of Experimental Psychology: Learning, Memory and Cognition*, 21(2), 314–326.

Dehaene, S., Changeux, J.P., Naccache, L., Sackur, J. and Sergent, C. (2006). Conscious, preconscious, and subliminal processing: A testable taxonomy. *Trends in Cognitive Sciences*, 10(5), 204–211.

Dixon, K., Lippitt, C.E. and Forsythe, C. (2005). Supervised machine learning for modeling human recognition of vehicle-driver situations. In *Proceedings of the IEEE/RSJ International Conference on Intelligent Robots and Systems*, pp. 604–609, August 2–6, Edmonton, AB.

Eimer, M., Goschke, T., Schlaghecken, F. and Sturmer, B. (1996). Explicit and implicit learning of event sequences: Evidence from event-related brain potentials. *Journal of Experimental Psychology: Learning, Memory and Cognition*, 22(4), 970–987.

Floyer-Lea, A. and Mathews, P.M. (2004). Changing brain networks for visuomotor control with increased movement automaticity. *Journal of Neurophysiology*, 92(4), 2405–2412.

Forstmann, B.U., Dutilh, G., Brown, S., Neumann, J., von Cramon, D.Y., Ridderinkhof, K.R. and Wagenmakers, E.J. (2008). Striatum and pre-SMA facilitate decision-making under time pressure. *Proceedings of the National Academy of Science*, 105(45), 17538–17542.

Friederici, A.D., Meyer, M. and von Cramon, Y. (2000). Auditory language comprehension: An event-related fMRI study on the processing of syntactic and lexical information. *Brain and Language*, 74(2), 289–300.

Gabrieli, J.D.E., Fleischman, D.A., Keane, M.M., Reminger, S.L. and Morrell, F. (1995). Double dissociation between memory systems underlying explicit and implicit memory in the human brain. *Psychological Science*, 6(2), 76–82.

Gentili, C., Ricciardi, E., Gobbini, M.I., Santarelli, M.F., Haxby, J.V., Pietrini, P. and Guazzelli, M. (2009). Beyond amygdale: Default node network activity differs between patients with social phobia and healthy controls. *Brain Research*, 79, 409–413.

Graybiel, A.M. (2008). Habits, rituals, and the evaluative brain. *Annual Review of Neuroscience*, 31, 359–387.

Grubb, M., Wallisch, P., Hasson, U. and Heeger, D.J. (2012). A neural signature of covert disengagement during movie viewing. In *Proceedings of Annual Meetings of the Cognitive Neuroscience Society*, March 31, Chicago, IL.

Heradstveit, D. and Bonham, G.M. (1996). Attribution theory and Arab images of the Gulf War. *Political Psychology*, 17, 271–292.

Honda, M., Dieber, M.P., Ibanez, V., Pascual-Leone, A., Zhuang, P. and Hallett, M. (1998). Dynamical cortical involvement in implicit and explicit motor sequence learning: A PET study. *Brain*, 121, 2159–2173.

Iacoboni, M. (2009). Imitation, empathy and mirror neurons. *Annual Review of Psychology*, 60, 653–670.

Jung-Beeman, M., Bowden, E.M., Haberman, J., Frymaire, J.L., Arambel-Liu, S., Greenblatt, R., Reber, P.J. and Kounios, J. (2003). Neural activity when people solve verbal problems with insight. *PLOS Biology*, 2(4), e97.

Kelly, A.M.C., Uddin, L.C., Biswal, B.B., Castellanos, X. and Milham, M.P. (2008). Competition between functional brain networks mediates behavioral variability. *NeuroImage*, 39(1), 527–537.

Kerr, B. (1976). Decisions about movement direction and extent. *Journal of Human Movement Studies*, 3, 199–213.

LeDoux, J. (1996). *The Emotional Brain*. New York: Touchstone.

Logothetis, N.K. and Schall, J.D. (1989). Neuronal correlates of subjective visual perception. *Science*, 245, 761–763.

Leopold, D.A. and Logothetis, N.K. (1996). Activity changes in early visual cortex reflect monkey's percepts during binocular rivalry. *Nature*, *379*, 549–553.

MacKay, C. (1841). *Extraordinary Popular Delusions and the Madness of Crowds*. New York: Harmony Books.

Mason, M.F., Norton, M.I., Van Horn, J.D., Wegner, D.M., Grafton, S.T. and Macre, C.N. (2007). Wandering minds: The default network and stimulus-independent thought. *Science*, *315*(5810), 393–395.

McVay, J.C., Kane, M.J. and Kwapil, T.R. (2009). Tracking the train of thought from the laboratory into everyday life: An experience-sampling study of mind-wandering across controlled and ecological contexts. *Psychonomic Bulletin and Review*, *16*(5), 857–863.

Metcalfe, J. and Wiebe, D. (1987). Intuition in insight and noninsight problem solving. *Memory and Cognition*, *15*, 238–246.

Milner, D.A. and Goodale, M.A. (1995). *The Visual Brain in Action*. Oxford: Oxford University Press.

Moller, J., Jansma, B.A., Rodriguez-Fornells, A. and Munte, T.F. (2007). What the brain does before the tongue slips. *Cerebral Cortex*, *17*(5), 1173–1178.

Navarro, J., Mars, F. and Hoc, J.M. (2007). Lateral control assistance for car drivers: A comparison of motor priming and warning systems. *Human Factors*, *49*(5), 950–960.

Nisbett, R.E., Peng, K., Choi, I. and Norenzayan, A. (2001). Culture and systems of thought: Holistic versus analytic cognition. *Psychological Review*, *108*(2), 291–301.

Perrin, F., Maquet, P., Peigneux, P., Ruby, P., Degueldre, C., Balteau, E., Del Fiore, G., Moonen, G., Luxen, A. and Laureys, S. (2005). Neural mechanisms involved in the detection of our first name: A combined ERPs and PET study. *Neuropsychologia*, *43*(1), 12–19.

Poldrack, R.A., Sabb, F.W., Foerde, K., Tom, S.M., Asarnow, R.F., Bookheimer, S.Y. and Knowlton, B.J. (2005). The neural correlates of motor skill automaticity. *Journal of Neuroscience*, *25*(22), 5356–5364.

Rees, G., Russell, C., Frith, C. and Driver, J. (1999). Inattentional blindness versus inattentional amnesia for fixated but ignored words. *Science*, *286*, 2504–2507.

Rhoades, D.L. and Waguespack, B. (1999). Better safe than service? The relationship between service and safety quality in the US airline industry. *Managing Service Quality*, *9*(6), 396–401.

Rizzolatti, G., Fogassi, L. and Gallese, V. (2002). Motor and cognitive functions of the ventral premotor cortex. *Current Opinion in Neurobiology*, *12*(2), 149–154.

Roseman, I.J., Spindel, M.S. and Jose, P.E. (1990). Appraisals of emotion-eliciting events: Testing a theory of discrete emotions. *Journal of Personality and Social Psychology*, *59*(5), 899–915.

Rossetti, Y. (1998). Implicit short-lived motor representations of space in brain-damaged and healthy subjects. *Consciousness and Cognition*, *7*, 520–558.

Rugg, M.D., Mark, R.E., Walla, P., Schloerscheidt, A.M., Birch, C.S. and Allan, K. (1998). Dissociation of the neural correlates of implicit and explicit memory. *Nature*, *392*, 595–598.

Schacter, D.L. (1992). Priming and multiple memory systems: Perceptual mechanisms of implicit memory. *Journal of Cognitive Neuroscience*, *4*(3), 244–256.

Schacter, D.L. and Buckner, R.L. (1998). Priming and the brain. *Neuron*, *20*, 185–195.

Schmitz, T.W. and Johnson, S.C. (2007). Relevance to self: A brief review and framework of neural systems underlying appraisal. *Neuroscience and Biobehavioral Reviews*, *31*(4), 585–596.

Sergent, C., Baillet, S. and Dehaene, S. (2005). Timing of the brain events underlying access to consciousness during the attentional blink. *Nature Neuroscience, 8,* 1391–1400.

Simons, D.J. and Chabris, C.F. (1999). Gorillas in our midst: Sustained inattentional blindness for dynamic events. *Perception, 28,* 1059–1074.

Sinnett, S., Costa, A. and Soto-Faraco, S. (2006). Manipulating inattentional blindness within and across sensory modalities. *Quarterly Journal of Experimental Psychology, 59*(8), 1425–1442.

Smallwood, J., Beach, E, Schooler, J.W. and Handy, T.C. (2008). Going AWOL in the brain: Mind wandering reduces cortical analysis of external events. *Journal of Cognitive Neuroscience, 20*(3), 458–469.

Soon, C.S., Brass, M., Heinze, H.J. and Haynes, J.D. (2008). Unconscious determinants of free decisions in the human brain. *Nature Neuroscience, 11,* 543–545.

Stallen, M., Smidts, A., Rijpkema, M., Smit, G., Klucharev, V. and Fernandez, G. (2010). Celebrities and shoes on the female brain: The neural correlates of product evaluation in the context of fame. *Journal of Economic Psychology, 31*(5), 802–811.

Stevens, S.T., Guise, K., Christiana, W., Kumar, M. and Keenan, J.P. (2007). Deception, evolution and the brain. In S.M. Platek, J.P. Keenan and T.K. Shackelford (eds), *Evolutionary Cognitive Neuroscience*, pp. 517–540. Cambridge, MA: MIT Press.

Todd, J.J., Fougnie, D. and Marois, R. (2005). Visual short-term memory load suppresses temporo-parietal junction activity and induces inattentional blindness. *Psychological Science, 16*(12), 965–972.

Vedantam, S. (2010). *The Hidden Brain: How Our Unconscious Minds Elect Presidents, Control Markets, Wage Wars and Save Our Lives.* New York: Spiegel & Grau.

Wan, X., Nakatani, H., Ueno, K., Asamizuya, T., Cheng, K. and Tanaka, K. (2011). The neural basis of intuitive best-move generation in board game experts. *Science, 331*(6015), 341–346.

Wolf, M., Bally, H. and Morris, R. (1986). Automaticity, retrieval processes and reading: A longitudinal study in average and impaired readers. *Child Development, 57*(4), 988–1000.

Yoo, C.Y. (2008). Unconscious processing of web advertising: Effects on implicit memory, attitude toward the brand, and consideration set. *Journal of Interactive Marketing, 22*(2), 2–18.

4

Perceptual Experience

Engineering design is generally focused on the objectives of a system and the mechanisms for accomplishing those objectives. However, engineering design also involves the experience that is created by a system. Whether an operator or user or those otherwise affected by a system and its operations, the experiences that are created will determine whether objectives are met, and how well they are met. Technically, a system may provide the mechanisms to achieve its objectives, yet due to confusion, frustration, annoyance, fatigue, or other effects, the system may fail. While key facets of a system may operate as designed, there may also be unintended effects. For example, artifacts associated with simulation-based trainers may result in learning that proves counterproductive when students must function within real-world settings. To successfully engineer systems that accomplish their stated objectives, it is important that designers attend to the experiences that are created by these systems. Furthermore, there are opportunities to engineer experiences that will produce more positive outcomes than would be expected, given only the mechanics of the system. Within many contexts, a functional system that meets the basic operational objectives may be readily achievable. However, by also attending to the experience created by a system, there is a differentiating opportunity to create a level of satisfaction and a subsequent desire that will translate into high regard and loyalty toward one's products.

Our brains recreate the world around us within our heads. Everything that we experience is an abstraction that arises through transduction as energy flows from sensory receptors through intermediate neural circuits, eventually resulting in an integrated internal representation of the external world. This is perception, at least from our brains' perspective. Perception concerns the processes whereby we experience the world around us based on our creating an abstract representation of the external world within our heads. It is worth noting that the majority of this experience may never enter into our conscious awareness. However, whether experienced at a conscious or an unconscious level, one's experience of a system and its design will arise through perceptual processes.

Traditionally, from an engineering perspective, perception has mainly been discussed with respect to the capacity for a human to effectively sense, process, and use various information to achieve task objectives. Certainly, effective task performance is essential to achieving system objectives, and there are many excellent accounts of the principles underlying effective information presentation and display (Boff and Lincoln, 1988; McBride and Schmorrow, 2005; Salvendy, 1997). However, in the following sections of this chapter, there will be little emphasis on engineering information displays for task performance, with the primary focus placed on engineering design that engages perceptual processes to create certain experiences within operators, users, and others affected by a system. Each of the following sections discusses general principles concerning the mechanisms and organization of perceptual processes within the brain that determine how systems will be experienced and the resulting efficacy with which people will operate within those systems.

Our Minds Attend to a Small Slice of What Our Brains Sense

At some time, we all learned about the five senses: sight, hearing, taste, smell, and touch. This idea of five primary senses is a simple, practical means of teaching children about how our bodies use specialized organs to sense the world around us. These are also the senses that dominate our conscious awareness. This is particularly true for vision and audition, as our conscious experiences tend to be dominated by these two senses.

I recall the day that my daughter came home from school and told me that they had learned about the five senses. I could not help myself and pointed out to her that there were at least three other important senses that she should know about. First, there is proprioception, which concerns the movement of our joints. Second, there is kinesthesis, which concerns the movements of our muscles. And third, there is equilibrium, or our sense of balance. Then, I pointed out that there are probably at least 40 other distinct senses.

The exact number of senses we have is unknown. This is partly due to disagreement about the definition of a sense. However, in addition to the eight senses mentioned so far, we can add temperature, with heat and cold being separate senses; nociception or pain due to either nerve damage or tissue damage; and chronoception or the sense of time. There are also a number of senses that respond to the internal state of the body. For example, pulmonary stretch receptors in the lungs help to control the rate of breathing and sensory receptors in the urinary bladder and rectum give us the sense of being full with the need to go to the bathroom. There are still other senses that respond to the molecular concentration of specific chemicals. For example, there are sensory receptors that respond to the relative concentrations of carbon dioxide and oxygen within the brain and are responsible for the sense of suffocation when carbon dioxide levels become too high.

While our conscious awareness is focused on the sights and sounds around us, our brains have a substantially richer sensory experience, although this primarily occurs at an unconscious level. Consequently, it is common that when we experience some sensation such as the wind blowing in our face or the aroma of a certain spice, it triggers a memory from long ago. We may or may not make a conscious connection between the immediate sensory experience and the memory that has been triggered. Nonetheless, it is important that we understand that our experiences involve sensory sensations that go well beyond our conscious experience, and include much more than sights and sounds. This can be important when attempting to create a high-fidelity representation of an actual system for simulation-based training. For instance, subtle sensory sensations such as the smell of a straining engine or the saltiness of the ocean air may be important cues that the student must learn to correctly interpret key events. Likewise, in entertainment, there is the opportunity to enhance experiences by reproducing subtle sensory sensations, or to confuse and disorient the audience by introducing unexpected sensory sensations. There has been relatively little research exploring the use of alternative sensory channels to affect experiences at an unconscious level; however, based on fundamental biology, there should be numerous opportunities to produce richer sensory experiences, while leveraging unique channels of communication to create more engaging experiences.

Our Judgment Is Shaped by Unconscious Sensory Experiences

In the previous chapter concerning conscious awareness and the preceding section of this chapter, I have made the point that a tremendous amount of sensory information is relayed to the brain and is processed at an unconscious level, yet very little enters our conscious awareness. This raises the question, "Does sensory information processed at an unconscious level affect our judgments?"

A series of studies reported by Josh Ackerman and colleagues indicate that our judgments are not only affected by unconscious sensory processes, but they are also affected in ways that we are not consciously aware of (Ackerman et al., 2010). In one study, subjects were asked to watch videos of individuals participating in a job interview and subsequently to rate each job candidate on a number of attributes. The subjects were provided with a clipboard that held the sheets that they were to use for their ratings. One group of subjects was given a relatively heavy clipboard, whereas a second group was given a relatively light clipboard. The subjects who received the heavier clipboard on average rated the job candidates as being more serious and more interested in the job. Similarly, in a second study, subjects were asked to read a story involving a social interaction. They were then asked to assemble the pieces of a puzzle. For one group, the puzzle pieces that they had been given had a rough texture, whereas the second group was given puzzle pieces with a smooth finish. Afterward, the subjects were asked to rate the social interaction with regard to various attributes. On average, the subjects who had been given the puzzle pieces with a rough texture rated the social interaction as being harsher and less pleasant than did the subjects who had been given the smooth puzzle pieces. Ackerman and colleagues noted that their findings mirror expressions that occur in everyday language. For instance, weight is associated with seriousness in expressions such as, "thinking about weighty matters" or "the gravity of the situation." Similarly, roughness is associated with difficulty or harshness in expressions such as, "having a rough day" or "coarse language." These expressions reflect implicit associations that under certain circumstances may affect our judgments without our having any conscious awareness that largely irrelevant sensory experiences have had an effect on our thinking.

In a somewhat different study, researchers considered how sensory experiences associated with environmental surroundings affect our judgments (Woods et al., 2010). Part of the sensation associated with eating potato chips derives from their crunchiness. Subjects wore headphones and ate potato chips in one of three conditions. In one, there was silence; in the second, there was soft white noise; and in the third, there was loud white noise. On average, when asked to rate the tastiness of the potato chips, the subjects in the loud condition gave lower ratings than did the subjects in the quieter conditions. This suggests that there is a sensory experience that is associated with eating potato chips and that if other sensory experiences interfere with this experience, the overall experience is diminished. In this case, there was no direct association between the level of background noise and the flavor of the potato chips. However, when the background noise overshadowed the expected auditory sensations (i.e., the crunchiness of the chips), the overall experience, including the flavor of the chips, was less satisfying.

Within design, unconscious sensory experiences can be used to affect judgment. These unconscious sensations offer an alternative channel of communication. For instance, the information display of a device may serve as a primary mode of communication that is task oriented. At the same time, the shape and feel of the device may be used to convey an overall sense of seriousness, or a sense of whimsicalness. Similar effects may be accomplished through the design of the environment. This is not a new idea. However, a consideration of unconscious brain processes suggests mechanisms for more systematically achieving such effects. The studies discussed above address two mechanisms. The first takes advantage of semantic associations. The language used to describe sensory sensations carries with it associations to other attributes. Heaviness is associated with seriousness. Its opposite, lightness, is associated with airiness and freshness. Second, there may be unconscious sensory experiences that we have learned to associate with unrelated positive experiences. For instance, there may be no direct link between a product's packaging and its quality. However, a well-packaged product may be assumed to be of higher quality than a product that is not as well packaged. If some event interferes with our unconscious sensory experience (e.g., someone else removes the packaging of the otherwise well-packaged product for us), without that association, the overall experience may be critically diminished.

Perception Is Multisensory

As is true with other animal species, our perceptual systems are specialized to sense stimuli that are biologically significant for given modes of survival within the context of certain environments. There is considerable debate surrounding the environment(s) and the mode(s) of survival that most shaped the development of humans as a species (Potts, 1998). Furthermore, some senses are more primitive than others (e.g., internal senses associated with basic life functions such as respiration), as evidenced by their being largely the same in many diverse species (Hodos and Butler, 1997). Yet, for any given sensory system, there is a range of stimuli for which the human sense organs and the associated neural circuitry are most responsive.

One perspective that explains the differential emphasis that is placed on the different senses points to the energy demands associated with sustaining the sensory organs and the associated neural processing (Niven and Laughlin, 2008). Sensory systems with broader ranges or higher levels of acuity or both, exact a greater cost than those that are sensitive to a smaller range of stimuli or provide lower levels of acuity or both. It is asserted that the specialization of sensory systems within any given species reflects a balance between the costs of sustaining a sensory capability and the benefits derived from that sensory capability. These pressures may be combined with trade-offs that are imposed by basic anatomical and physiological characteristics. For example, the frequency range of sounds to which humans, as well as other mammalian species, are most sensitive corresponds to the range of sound affording the optimal localization of sounds given the size and shape of our head (Masterton et al., 1969). It has been said that "the brain is not a well-designed machine, but a magnificent compromise" (Krubizer, 2007). This principle is reflected in the relative emphasis that is placed on different sensory systems and for any given sensory system, the relative sensitivity to the stimuli to which it responds.

From the perspective of engineering design, human sensory processes have been fairly well characterized (Boff and Lincoln, 1988). This is particularly true for vision, audition, and touch, with somewhat less data existing for the chemical senses (i.e., taste and smell) and secondary senses such as proprioception and equilibrium. Given the available resources (e.g., Department of Defense, 2012), there is little excuse for the design of products that do not accommodate the basic strengths and weaknesses of the human sensory systems.

Design may go beyond merely matching the sensory signals that are used to communicate information to the relative acuity of different sensory systems. An alternative perspective sees design as the creation of a sensory ecology. Analogous to ecologies in nature where different animal and plant species coexist by occupying and exploiting different niches, one may similarly think about sensory signals as different species and the various sensory systems as different niches. Applying this analogy, different sensory signals may exist side by side, each exploiting a different channel of sensory communication. For instance, as we visually navigate our surroundings, auditory signals may be used to both entertain and communicate important information. This presents the opportunity to create rich, multifaceted sensory experiences that communicate and engage individuals through a variety of mechanisms, some operating at a conscious level and others at an unconscious level.

In practice, the design of a sensory ecology should begin by considering the impressions that a designer hopes to make on users, operators, and others affected by a system. The clearest examples occur with environmental design. In the design of a grocery store, the intent may be to create the sense of freshness, which may be addressed through air exchange and ventilation. To create a sense of quality, items may be neatly stacked and well organized. Clean floors, shiny surfaces, and bright lights may be used to create the sense that meats and produce are fresh and free from contaminants. Well-constructed carts that roll easily across the floor suggest efficiency. Happy, perky music evokes a sense of impulsiveness. Shoppers may only be consciously aware of the immediate tasks of remembering and locating what they need to purchase, making selections, deliberating over costs, and so on. However, the sights, sounds, and smells of their surroundings and the physical sensations associated with their actions impinge on their senses and create an overall sensory experience. A shopper may be totally unaware of the various aspects of the environment that are shaping their experience. Yet, if something changed or they went to another grocery store, they would likely sense that something was different, although they might not be able to say exactly what it was.

As stated above, environmental design offers tremendous opportunities to structure a sensory ecology to achieve certain experiential effects. However, most designers are only tasked with the development of specific elements or components of the overall environment. For example, a designer may only have responsibility for a single electronic device that is to be combined with several other electronic devices within a vehicle's electronics console. In this case, the designer likely has no control over the totality of the sensory ecology. The designer's device is analogous to a single species that must find a niche where it may flourish alongside other species that are filling adjacent niches. In such a situation, the potential exists for conflicts where multiple devices are competing for the same limited resources. Recently, I was talking on my cell phone in a busy airport where there were many different sounds occurring all around me. My phone beeped to warn me that the battery was running low. I heard the sound, but failed to recognize that it came from my phone. Consequently, I continued my phone conversation, ignoring two additional warnings, until the battery could no longer power the phone and I was disconnected. In this case, there was a clearly discernible signal, yet because there were other simultaneous signals in the same range of frequency and intensity, I failed to correctly localize the source of the signal, and therefore failed to recognize the relevance of the signal. In this example, several signals are in competition for a limited resource (i.e., the range of audio frequencies for which my hearing is sensitive). While the low power warning on my phone was detectable, I failed to distinguish it from other similar auditory signals. It is unlikely that this would have been the case had the auditory signal been combined with a brief vibration creating a compound stimulus for which there were no comparable competing stimuli.

Within the brain, the processing of sensory input for a given sensory modality follows a progression from lower to higher levels of detail. For example, at the lowest levels of visual processing, an analysis of visual signals involves the detection of features such as the color and orientation of visual stimuli. Similarly, the lowest levels of auditory processing distinguish features such as sound frequency and pitch. As processing progresses from lower to higher levels, there is both an integration of low-level features (e.g., for the detection of objects, features are combined and distinguished from the surroundings) and an increasing influence from top-down processes or expectations (e.g., a round object in the context of a child's room takes the form of a ball). Accompanying this progression from lower to higher levels of processing, there also occurs an integration of the input from different sensory modalities, as well as the modulation of the input from one sensory channel based on the input from other sensory channels. This serves to disambiguate the input from a given sensory channel, enhancing the clarity of the signal.

The capacity for effective sensory integration has been linked to attaining superior levels of performance within certain domains. For example, using a task that required subjects to stand immobile, Vuillerme et al. (2001) compared expert gymnasts with individuals who had attained notable levels of performance in other sports. As the subjects attempted to maintain a stationary posture, proprioceptive input from the ankle was disrupted by applying vibration to the tendon. Gymnastics requires an ability to effectively integrate proprioceptive with visual, kinesthetic, and vestibular input to establish and sustain balance. Enhanced skills were evidenced in the gymnasts' ability to recover faster and they were less affected by the disruption in proprioceptive input. Further research has demonstrated that in expert gymnasts, the multisensory processes associated with sustaining balance demand less attention, as evidenced by their faster reaction times while simultaneously balancing on one leg (Vuillerme and Nougier, 2004). Similarly, it has been shown that with dancers, there is an enhanced capacity for the integration of visual and proprioceptive input, as evidenced by the performance of manual tasks with and without disruption of sensory input (Jolla et al., 2011). This research points to a differential capacity for sensory integration, with individual differences manifested in measurably higher levels of performance for tasks placing similar demands on the capacity for sensory integration exercised during gymnastics or dancing.

Our conscious awareness is generally focused on the dominant sensory modality for a given type of signal. For example, during conversation, our awareness is primarily focused on the sounds being produced. However, at an unconscious level, we are also processing visual signals, whether it is the movement of the speaker's mouth or his or her gestures and facial expressions. All the while, the brain is combining all of these signals to produce an integrated perceptual experience. This is illustrated by the *McGurk Effect* (Massaro and Stork, 1998; McGurk and MacDonald, 1976). If watching a person speak the syllable "ga" while hearing an audio recording of the syllable "ba," the listener will likely report having heard the syllable, "da." Similarly, if watching a speaker say the expression, "My gag kok me koo grive" combined with an audio recording of the expression, "My bab pop me poo brive," the listener will likely report having heard the expression, "My Dad taught me to drive." In both cases, the listener consciously attends to the audio recording. Yet, at an unconscious level, the listener is processing the visual signals from the speaker's mouth movements and combining the auditory and visual inputs to produce a conscious experience that is the integrated product of inputs from the two sensory channels.

Traditionally, it was believed that in higher cortical areas of the brain, input from the brain regions that are responsible for processing specific sensory channels converge, with higher cortical processes integrating signals from multiple sensory modalities. These regions of the cortex have been referred to as sensory association areas. Numerous regions of the brain's cerebral cortex have been attributed with this function (Baylis et al., 1987; Desimone and Ungerleider, 1986; Lewis and Van Essen, 2000). Additionally, there are subcortical areas with functional connections to higher cortical areas, such as the thalamus and amygdala, where sensory integration also occurs (Mesulam and Mufson, 1982; Turner et al., 1980).

Yet, the integration of input from specific sensory channels is not limited to higher-level cortical processes, but also occurs early during the initial low-level processing of sensory input. It has been shown that there are projections from areas that are responsible for the low-level processing of auditory signals to areas that are responsible for the low-level processing of visual signals (Ettlinger, 1990; Falchier et al., 2000). Through these connections, the brain is able to use auditory input to signal the visual processing areas regarding the likely presence of important visual cues. Likewise, low-level projections from the visual cortex, as well as the somatosensory cortex (i.e., regions responsible for processing signals from tactile, or touch, sensors), to the auditory cortex have also been demonstrated (Schroeder and Foxe, 2002).

With our visceral senses (i.e., those associated with the internal organs of the body), integration occurs at an even lower level within the spinal cord, with the sensory signals reaching the brain having already undergone some degree of integration (Cervero and Tattersall, 1987). These observations of integration at nearly every level of sensory processing suggest a conceptualization of the brain wherein input from different sensory modalities may enter the brain through separate pathways, yet almost immediately, the brain begins to construct a multisensory representation of the world. The limitations on the amount of processing that can occur at a conscious level may bias our awareness to emphasize one or more dominant sensory modalities. However, at an unconscious level, the brain is experiencing the world as an integrated fabric combining input from all of our sensory systems to create a multisensory representation.

The Brain Responds More Strongly to Some Stimuli than Others

While at a low level, the brain may exhaustively process the stimuli impinging on sensory receptors, relatively few stimuli provoke a pronounced response. While registered, most stimuli merely serve to fill in the background. To elicit a strong enough response to distinguish a given stimulus from the background of accompanying stimuli, it is not sufficient to merely be detectable. A conspicuous signal must be distinct from its surrounding environment (Enquist and Arak, 1998).

As previously discussed, a given signal exists within a sensory ecology and competes against other signals, with some provoking a more pronounced response than others, and some provoking a sufficient response to capture one's attention and enter into one's conscious awareness. Within nature, various approaches are employed by different species to enhance the conspicuousness of the signals that they produce. For instance, stimuli that sharply contrast with their environment tend to be more conspicuous. This is evidenced in the evoked response of the brain to visual stimuli of varying levels of contrast measured using an electroencephalogram (EEG). In particular, the overall amplitude of the brain's response tends to be greater for higher-contrast stimuli (Campbell and Kulikowski, 1972).

Viewed at a finer level, the response of the brain to stimuli of varying levels of contrast reveals an interesting property of the brain. It is a misnomer to think of the brain as either active or inactive because there is constant activity throughout its entirety. In the absence of a prominent stimulus, this activity takes the form of spikes that occur at varying locations, with waves of activity emanating from these spikes that diminish as they travel further from their origin (Nauhaus et al., 2008). As shown in Figure 4.1, this

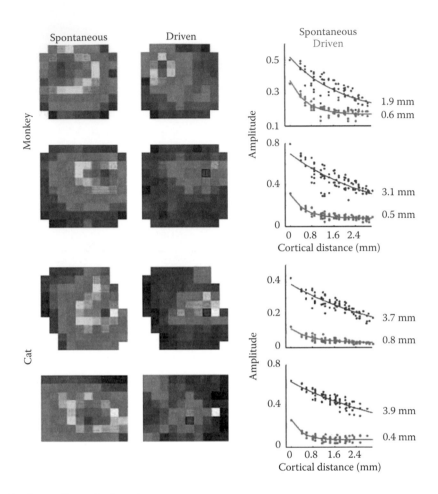

FIGURE 4.1   (See color insert)
The differential trajectory of the spread of cortical neural activation in response to visual
stimulation is depicted with regard to spike-driven versus spontaneous activity. (From
Nauhaus, I., Busse, L., Carandini, M., and Ringach, D.L., *Nature Neuroscience*, 12, 70–76, 2008.
With permission.)

produces relatively constant, yet somewhat diffuse levels of activity. When
presented with a stimulus, diffuse activation patterns are transformed, with
pronounced activity localized to areas involved in processing the stimulus
(Nauhaus et al., 2008). This transformation and the subsequent localization
of activity varies in response to the stimulus contrast with there being a
greater disruption of diffuse activation patterns and heightened localized
responses with increasing stimulus contrast. Thus, the brain's response to a
conspicuous stimulus does not involve a generalized increase in activation,
but instead an increased coordination of activation.

While the contrast between a stimulus and its background may be the key
to its conspicuousness, there are many mechanisms for achieving contrast.

For instance, visual stimuli may vary in size, shape, intensity, and color, as well as other more complex dimensions such as flicker and frequency gratings. In nature, it has been observed that signals that elicit pronounced responses tend to be very different from one another, and are often much more distinct than necessary for them to merely be discriminated from one another (Brown, 1975). Darwin referred to this observation as the *principle of antithesis* (Darwin, 1872). This principle is consistent with the fact that when processing a given stimulus, generally the brain simultaneously analyzes the stimulus with regard to different dimensions. For instance, with visual stimuli, their orientation, color, and location are simultaneously processed somewhat separately and are later integrated to form a coherent visual representation (Hubel and Wiesel, 1959, 1962). This opens a range of opportunities for designers to take advantage of different stimulus qualities as a basis for creating contrast between the stimulus and its background, thereby enhancing the conspicuousness of the stimulus. This may be realized through signals that vary along multiple dimensions. For example, auditory signals may vary with respect to their pitch, tone, volume, rhythm, and cadence, as well as the sound source. Variation along each of these dimensions should serve to heighten the contrast between the stimulus and its surroundings.

Another method that may be used to enhance the conspicuousness of a signal involves the simultaneous activation of multiple sensory modalities. For instance, alarms often combine a flashing light with a loud sound. Certain combinations of stimuli will elicit a more pronounced response from the brain than any one stimulus by itself. Furthermore, this response may be parlayed into enhanced behavioral performance. For example, it has long been known that faster reaction times occur for a visual stimulus if the stimulus is combined with an auditory stimulus (Todd, 1912), with similar facilitating effects having been reported for the combination of auditory and tactile stimuli (Loveless et al., 1970). Furthermore, sensitivity to stimuli that are slightly below the normal threshold for detection may be enhanced if there is simultaneous stimulation of another sensory modality (Frassinetti et al., 2002). To achieve these effects, the stimuli must be synchronized in a manner that allows them to merge into a compound stimulus. Where visual and auditory stimuli are combined, a brief offset in the time that the two stimuli are presented or the location of the two stimuli will lead to a diminished effect, with the effect no longer occurring once there is sufficient separation of the stimuli (Stein et al., 1989). Thus, stimulus facilitation effects are contingent on stimuli being merged such that they are perceived as a single compound stimulus.

The response to multisensory signals is modulated by attention with a more robust response to attended stimuli than unattended stimuli. Using auditory and visual stimuli, EEG measures indicated a larger amplitude response to multisensory stimuli that were the focus of attention, as compared with stimuli that were not the focus of attention (Talsma and Woldorff, 2005). This effect occurred from the very earliest stages of the response, beginning within 100 ms of the stimulus presentation. Furthermore, the facilitating effect may not occur with noncongruent stimuli (i.e., stimuli that one would not expect to occur together), with the overall response often being of a reduced magnitude. For example, in a functional magnetic resonance imaging (fMRI) investigation of sensory integration with taste and smell, Small et al. (2004) found that unexpected combinations (e.g., vanilla and salty) produced less activation, with the incongruity producing an apparent suppression of the brain's response.

Within the midbrain, the superior colliculus is a structure that possesses receptive fields for multiple sensory modalities including audition, vision, and touch, with it significantly involved in directing attention to focus on significant stimuli. It has been observed that within the superior colliculus, cells responsive to each sensory modality overlap and that when there is simultaneous stimulation of multiple senses, there is a pronounced amplification of the overall electrophysiological response (Stein and Meredith, 1993). This amplification may be as much as twelvefold, as compared with the activation observed when the same sensory modalities are activated one at a time. The response is often greatest when the intensity of the sensory stimulation is relatively low, suggesting that the response amplification may serve to facilitate our reaction to somewhat weak, yet potentially significant, sensory signals. Furthermore, the response amplification diminishes with the separation of the stimuli in space or time or both, with response suppression once there is a sufficient degree of separation between stimuli (Kadunce et al., 1997). Consequently, under certain conditions, one stimulus may actually suppress the response to a second stimulus. While other brain regions involved in sensory integration do not show as distinct a response as the superior colliculus, in general there is an enhanced sensitivity to multisensory stimuli, particularly with respect to capturing and orienting our attention toward certain sensory events. From a design perspective, if a multisensory stimulus is designed correctly, it can trigger a marked response that increases its conspicuity. However, any disparity in the timing or other facets of the multisensory presentation can diminish the response and, under certain circumstances, can actually produce the opposite effect (i.e., signal suppression).

Finally, there is a class of stimuli that have been referred to as *supernormal* stimuli. A supernormal stimulus is one that compared with other comparable stimuli, produces a disproportionate response. With a supernormal stimulus, there are physical properties of the stimulus (e.g., combination of size and shape) for which there is an unusual sensitivity with the propensity to evoke an amplified electrophysiological and behavioral response. Supernormal stimuli were first observed in animals (Enquist and Arak, 1998). Researchers noted that sometimes animals would respond more strongly to the dummies used in their experiments than to the natural objects being mimicked by the dummies. For example, in a study of egg recognition in a species of bird known as the ringed plover, it was observed that the birds preferred higher-contrast dummies that were white with black spots than their actual eggs, which were brown with dark spots. Similarly, with another bird, the herring gull, it was observed that chicks pecked more enthusiastically at a rod with three white bars at the tip than at a realistic replica of the parent's bill and head.

In contrast to animal studies, there has been little research to identify supernormal stimuli to which people respond. Human infants seem to find low-frequency murmuring sounds calming. In a study by Hutt et al. (1968), infants were presented with artificially produced murmuring sounds that had a specified structure (i.e., square wave) and low-frequency components. The skin conductance of infants was measured, which provided an indication of the infants' emotional response to the tones. It was observed that the infants were more responsive to the artificially produced tones than to an actual voice.

Another example of supernormal stimuli in humans involves facial features. Humans are uniquely sensitive to faces and within the human brain there is a region known as the fusiform gyrus that is particularly responsive to images of faces and face-like stimuli (McCarthy et al., 1997). This sensitivity to certain facial features was illustrated in a study that presented subjects with facial caricatures (i.e., cartoonlike drawings). To produce the caricatures, an average or prototypical face was obtained based on a statistical analysis of numerous faces and the development of a model containing 20 physical dimensions along which human faces differ from one another (Brennan, 1985). A caricature was created using a drawing that faithfully depicted the facial features of former US President Ronald Reagan, exaggerating specific features that corresponded to dimensions identified in the model. When subjects were shown either a drawing with a relatively accurate representation of the facial features or the caricature, they were faster and more accurate in recognizing the caricature than the drawing of the actual face (Dewdney, 1986). This study suggests that the face processing area within the brain is unusually sensitive to exaggerated facial features. Similarly, related studies have demonstrated a heightened sensitivity to other human physical features. For instance, men have been shown to prefer women whose physical characteristics vary more from the average male form, with women preferring men whose physical features vary more from the average female form (Ridley, 1993).

In general, supernormal stimuli involve naturally occurring, biologically significant stimuli (e.g., the sound of a mother's voice, facial expressions, or the physical form of a potential mate). For designers, there is an opportunity to emulate these physical forms so that certain features of design stand out from the surroundings. The key lies in identifying which physical features of the stimuli are essential to the brain's perceptual representation and the associated dimensions along which these features may be exaggerated to produce an amplified response. Then, the stimuli must be placed within surroundings where the exaggerated features contrast with the physical features of other stimuli. It should be noted that contrast is important because the exaggeration of physical features is relative, and if the environment is filled with similarly exaggerated stimuli, the response to any one of these stimuli will be diminished.

Vulnerabilities Arising from Our Perceptual Processes

The previous sections have described how designers may use the physical properties of stimuli to enhance our sensitivity to those stimuli. These same properties may also be applied from an adversarial perspective. It is often the intent to be inconspicuous and avoid being noticed. The same mechanisms that may be used to enhance the contrast between a signal and its surroundings may be applied in reverse to minimize the contrast so that a stimulus blends into its surroundings. This can be seen with camouflage where there is an attempt to match the colors, patterns, and other physical properties of the surroundings. Likewise, if attempting to conceal a signal, one should avoid properties discussed in the preceding sections that enhance sensitivity to a stimulus (e.g., stimulation of multiple sensory modalities or physical features for which there is a heightened sensitivity).

The exception occurs with mimicry. With mimicry, there is a known, or mimicked, signal that is either assumed to be harmless or is associated with danger and is generally avoided. The known, or mimicked, signal may be quite conspicuous, as often occurs when it is associated with danger or some other hazard. The objective is not to avoid detection, but to deceive. Mimicry may be found in nature where to avoid being attacked by predators, a species assumes a form that resembles another species that is either poisonous, known to taste bad, or is dangerous. For example, with certain butterflies, black spots on their wings make them visually distinct. However, this coloration serves to repulse predators due to the black spots resembling eyes, creating the appearance of an owl or other large predator.

Internet phishing attacks can take mimicry to extraordinary lengths in an effort to confuse intended victims and cause them to inadvertently download nefarious software. In this case, the objective is to recreate the properties of a signal that would generally be considered harmless and potentially even helpful or to disguise the phishing attack as a signal that would otherwise be trusted. Likewise, the same occurs with cyber social engineering where individuals convince their victim that they can be trusted or that they are harmless, and they use this trust to gain access to computer systems and facilities that they would not otherwise be allowed to access. In each of these cases, the secret lies in recognizing the critical properties of the signal being mimicked. These properties may be physical (e.g., the presence of corporate logos or the layout of an official email) or social (e.g., the language used in legitimate emails or the demeanor of a genuine computer support technician), with the corresponding features faithfully recreated and perhaps exaggerated.

One means of mimicry is to assume the identity of someone who would otherwise be trusted. In a study of email phishing, college students' social networks were combed to construct phishing emails disguised to be from people within each student's social network (Jagatic et al., 2005). The students responded to 72% of the emails that had been sent from the spoofed address of a friend, as compared with only 16% who received equivalent emails from an anonymous individual. This finding illustrates the level of trust that is placed in personal relationships and how susceptible one can be when an adversary has the capacity to mimic an individual or group that would otherwise be trusted.

An analysis of phishing attacks revealed a variety of approaches that take advantage of perceptual processes to deceive email recipients (Dhamija et al., 2006). These approaches include the following: (1) "typejacking," where the letters of a web address are substituted with letters that appear similar (e.g., with www.paypa1.com, the letter "l" may be replaced with the number "1"); (2) images masked as text, where what appears to be text linking to a website is actually an image of that text with the image linked to a different website; (3) images that look like legitimate windows or dialog boxes, with buttons, menus, or links, but are actually surreptitious links; (4) illegitimate windows that appear adjacent to or overlay legitimate windows; and (5) replicas of legitimate websites that contain links to nefarious software or data entry fields where users may voluntarily enter personal information.

The Cyber Watering Hole

It is a familiar scene. On the arid plains, everyone needs water. Sooner or later, everyone must visit the watering hole. Predators know this, and they know that if they wait long enough, their prey will come. We have seen images of lions lurking in the shadows as their prey come to get water and then, suddenly, they quickly and violently attack. The hackers had expropriated this idea. They had established a valuable resource on the Internet that was openly available to anyone. Their prey had discovered the resource and regularly visited the website. In this case, the website offered content that was of value to those working in the tech industry and visitors came from companies around the world. Yet, much like the lion quietly sitting in the shadows, the site contained seemingly legitimate links that if clicked, executed an attack. In this case, this involved the surreptitious uploading of nefarious software onto the visitor's computer.

This is how the incident began. Employees of Google, as well as US defense contractors and other companies, unknowingly downloaded the nefarious software onto their computers. The standard virus detection software was in place, but due to the hackers having used multiple levels of encryption, it was not detected. Actually, some of the exploits that were employed had been known for some time. Once the software had infected the machines, it then established a portal back to the hackers who then began to scour the networks looking for other vulnerable machines. The primary attack and data exfiltration were timed to occur in mid- to late December, coinciding with the Christmas holidays, so the hackers could take advantage of lightly staffed information technology departments.

The hackers had taken precautions to not just avoid detection, but to also conceal their identity. Prior to commencing operations, they had stolen accounts from a service known has Rackspace that provides companies with remote servers. Using these accounts, the hackers were able to command and control software on the infected machines through these remote servers. When analysts began to look for the trail leading back to the hackers, it took them to these stolen accounts, which resided on servers in Illinois, Texas, and Taiwan.

As the hackers scanned the company networks, they searched for machines with vulnerabilities that they could exploit. This could be a machine that had not been regularly patched and could be accessed through vulnerabilities in common desktop software applications. They searched for databases of source code and other intellectual property from the companies, as well as credentials that could be used to gain access to other computers and resources on the network.

Perhaps most significantly, Google is the proprietor of Gmail, which is used by individuals and groups of all stripes. When the US Federal Bureau of Investigation (FBI) and other law enforcement agencies suspect someone of committing criminal activity, they often obtain a court order that allows them to access the person's Gmail accounts. For these cases, Google had established a backdoor to Gmail for use by law enforcement. The hackers managed to gain access to this backdoor. Consequently, they gained knowledge of who the FBI was investigating, including individuals suspected of espionage. From an intelligence perspective, this was an incredible achievement in that with one cyberattack, information had been gained for which traditionally the intelligence agencies would have invested tremendous amounts of time and resources to secure. Additionally, the hackers gained access to the Gmail accounts of individuals in whom they had an interest, with these being primarily individuals considered to be dissidents and activists opposed to their government.

This incident illustrates how perceptual features can be used in an adversarial manner. The watering hole was designed to resemble a legitimate website. It served as a lure to attract prey, concealing the underlying danger. Furthermore, the link that surreptitiously uploaded the nefarious software was actually a legitimate link. The prey never realized that they had become victims. Encryption served as a basis for concealment, preventing detection by mechanisms that would have ordinarily recognized the threat, blocked it, and warned computer security personnel. Using the stolen computers as an intermediary allowed the hackers to cover their tracks, making it difficult for authorities to link the crime to its perpetrators. While there are suspicions, there has been no definitive attribution. This was a well-orchestrated, sophisticated attack that has come to be known as the Google Aurora incident and provides an illustration of the manner in which hackers take advantage of perceptual processes as an intrinsic element in their strategies.

Dhamija et al. (2006) conducted a study in which they presented subjects with either spoofed versions of actual websites or authentic websites, and asked the subjects whether they believed the websites were real or fraudulent. They found that, on average, the subjects were fooled about half the time, with there being no relationship between the likelihood of being fooled and the reported number of hours using a computer or experience using Internet browsers. It is particularly striking that the best-spoofed websites fooled 90% of the participants, with one of these spoofed websites being that for a bank. This research illustrates the extent to which people are vulnerable to relatively simple mimicry within the context of their everyday lives. It should also be noted that this occurs despite mechanisms that are meant to lessen users' vulnerability to deceptive activities. For example, Dhamija et al. (2006) reported that 68% of their subjects ignored pop-up windows warning them that a website appeared to be fraudulent.

Decoys are a variant on mimicry. Often, a decoy may serve as a source of distraction. In martial arts, an important skill is the ability to perform an effective feint. A feint involves pretending to attack (e.g., pretending to throw a punch) and once the opponent moves to defend against the feigned attack, the attacker takes advantage of the resulting opening with his or her actual attack. For a feint to be effective, it should not only have the same perceptual properties as a real attack, but it should also exaggerate those properties to help ensure that it gets the attention of the opponent and, ideally, elicit a reflexive reaction. In Shaolin-style kung fu, which is a sport in which I have participated for many years, one of my favorite techniques involves feigning a sweeping ridge hand to the side of the head. I execute the ridge hand with my lead hand as a big circular movement so that it not only can be readily detected, but it also draws my opponent's attention to the side. Then, my real attack comes from the rear hand and involves a reverse punch (i.e., palm of fist facing upward) to the abdomen, which my opponent usually never senses, since my decoy (i.e., the ridge hand) has drawn my opponent's attention away from his or her midsection. I have always believed that the key to the effectiveness of this technique lies in the exaggerated movement associated with the ridge hand. As this example illustrates, a decoy may be made more effective by exaggerating or amplifying the perceptual cues that trigger a response in a way that may begin to resemble a supernormal stimulus.

What does the brain see when presented with a decoy? Essentially, it sees the same thing it would see if presented with the object being mimicked by the decoy. In a study of the early stages of visual processing, Ress and Heeger (2003) presented subjects with images of gratings composed of contrasting dark and light tiles that either did or did not contain an embedded figure (see Figure 4.2). As the subjects viewed the images and indicated whether they believed a figure was or was not present, fMRI measurements of their brain activity were recorded. As shown in Figure 4.3, an analysis of the fMRI data allowed the researchers to distinguish the patterns of activation in the visual cortex that corresponded to trials in which a figure was present (i.e., hits) from trials in which a figure was not present (i.e., correct rejections). The researchers then considered trials in which the subjects made a false positive response, meaning that they said a figure was present when the image did not actually contain a figure. In these trials, the level of brain activation was similar to that observed in the trials in which the subjects correctly responded that a figure was present. Thus, from the perspective of brain activation, there appeared to be little distinction between images in which an actual object was present and images in which an object appeared to be present, yet was absent. It may be conjectured that in the trials in which the subjects exhibited a false positive, there were some elements of a figure present (e.g., a few tiles arrayed in a configuration

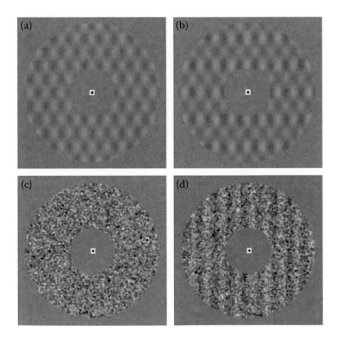

FIGURE 4.2
(a–d) The stimulus conditions used in Ress and Heeger (2003) involved gradients in which a pattern was either present or absent. (From Ress, D. and Heeger, D.J., *Nature Neuroscience*, 6, 414–421, 2003. With permission.)

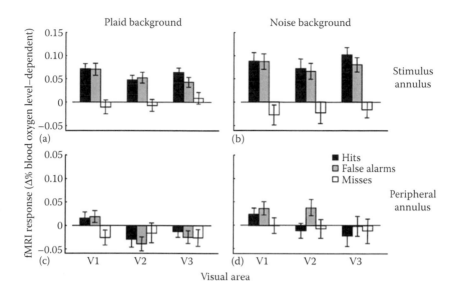

FIGURE 4.3

(a–d) The fMRI response from brain regions associated with processing perceptual stimuli was similar for trials in which the target was present and there was a false positive in which subjects falsely reported the presence of the target when the target was actually absent. (From Ress, D. and Heeger, D.J., *Nature Neuroscience*, 6, 414–421, 2003. With permission.)

that resembled a figure), but not the entire figure. In these trials, once the brain had detected a few cues that a figure might be present, it may have filled in the remaining details, creating the perceptual experience that the figure was actually present. This principle applies to decoys. If the brain is presented with a few essential cues, it has the propensity to fill in the missing details, creating the sense that the actual object is present, when in fact it is merely a decoy.

Perceptual Activities the Brain Does Well

The preceding sections have addressed facets of perception that can cause an individual to misinterpret situations. Yet, with respect to perception, there are some activities for which the brain is surprisingly adept. In the following sections, I describe several of these innate aptitudes.

Associations between Perceptual Form and the Actions Afforded by an Object

The brain has a natural capacity for recognizing how an object might be used based on its perceptual form. The association between an object's perceptual form and the actions made possible by the object is referred to as an *affordance* (Gibson, 1979). After standing for a long time, one may look around and recognize that any one of a number of surfaces offers a place to sit down. It might be a rock, a tree stump, or a concrete block. Each of these objects has physical characteristics that afford sitting. In particular, they are solid, have a relatively flat horizontal surface, and are sufficiently elevated from the ground to accommodate a seated posture. None of them is designed to be a chair, yet given the impetus to sit down, any surface with the right characteristics will be recognized to afford sitting, whether or not it was designed for this purpose. In fact, architects often incorporate these features into buildings or landscaping (e.g., slabs of concrete may be placed near ground level outside a building where people are expected to spend time milling about). Likewise, by observing the unintended uses of certain architectural features, it is often evident what unanticipated needs are being addressed by people in an *ad hoc* manner. For example, impromptu footpaths in otherwise grassy lawns suggest points at which designers did not appreciate the most efficient flow of foot traffic and provide suitable walking surfaces. As a result, seeing a surface that afforded walking, people created shortcuts.

Within the brain, the motor cortex issues commands to the musculature of the body to enable us to carry out various actions. For common actions, memories are established within the motor cortex (i.e., motor programs) that consist of the corresponding neuromuscular commands. As shown in Figure 4.4, it has been observed that when presented with an image of an object that affords certain actions (e.g., a hammer), there is activation of the motor cortex comparable with the activation that would occur if the person was actually using the object (Buccino et al., 2009). Furthermore, merely looking at a picture of an object is sufficient to trigger activation of the motor cortex. Through this activation, perceptual processes have the ability to prime the motor cortex, readying an individual for the potential actions that an object might afford.

Affordance-based priming may extend beyond physical actions to similarly prime memory representations of language. Costantini et al. (2011) showed subjects three-dimensional (3-D) pictures of various objects. Afterward, the subjects were presented with a verb and were asked to indicate if the verb was appropriate for the object. The verbs either conveyed a function, a manipulation, or an observation. For example, shown a drinking glass, the function verb might be "to drink," the manipulation verb might be "to grasp," and the observation verb might be "to look at." They found that the subjects responded fastest to the manipulation verbs, suggesting that the images had primed the corresponding motor actions, enabling the subjects to respond slightly faster to these verbs. Interestingly, this effect was strongest when the 3-D objects were presented at a reachable distance, as compared with their being presented at a distance that was slightly out of reach.

Fischer and Dahl (2007) demonstrated that affordances can affect performance for tasks that bear no relevance to the actual affordance. Their subjects

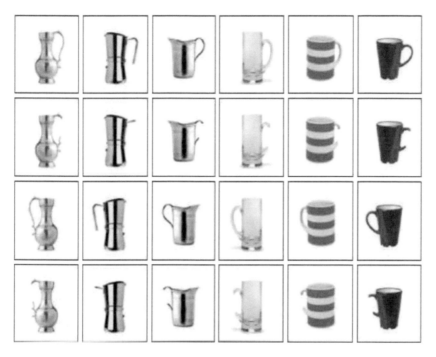

FIGURE 4.4
The stimuli used in the study by Buccino et al. (2009) consisted of objects oriented to accommodate either a left or a right hand grasp and presenting a normal handle that could be easily grasped or a broken handle. (From Buccino, G., Sato, M., Cattaneo, L., Roda, F., and Riggio, L., *Neuropsychologia*, 47, 3074–3078, 2009. With permission.)

viewed a coffee cup that rotated so that the handle came in and out of view. The subjects were asked to indicate when a dot changed color. The dot was always at the center of the image and was always visible, despite the orientation of the cup's handle. The subjects responded faster when the cup's handle was in view than when the handle of the cup was obstructed. These findings suggest a top-down influence in which the recognition of an affordance produced more efficient processing of perceptual features that had no relevance to the affordance.

The propensity for the brain to recognize and respond to affordances provides an opportunity for designers to use perceptual features as a means to both ready individuals for forthcoming actions, as well as to attain higher levels of task engagement. Affordances are a wonderful tool that, used judiciously, can enhance design by engaging users through triggering unconscious perceptual-motor processes. Affordances may also provide a basis for influencing the behavior of an adversary. For instance, by providing a forum that facilitates and encourages communication, accompanied by an admiring audience, one might be lured into divulging sensitive or incriminating information. This can be seen in situations where criminals are identified as a result of their having boasted of their deeds within the context of an online community. In other cases, an affordance may serve as a distraction. For example, with medieval fortifications, passageways were often structured in a maze-like configuration where paths doubled back on one another as a means to delay an adversary's assault and lure them into traps or ambushes. While an affordance may not always elicit the desired response from an adversary, often the mere presence of the affordance is sufficient to cause indecision, and in the right circumstances, achieve an effective misdirection.

The Brain Orients toward Moving Stimuli

The capacity to recognize moving objects is one of the most basic mechanisms by which perceptual processes contribute to the survival of many animal species. We are uniquely sensitive to movement. With vision, our eyes are automatically drawn to moving objects. Similarly, a moving sound source or tactile stimulus can readily elicit an orienting response. Moving stimuli are not merely detected, but a special significance is assigned to them that often results in their entering conscious awareness, even if for a fleeting moment (e.g., the fleeting awareness of an insect flying past our face), while equivalent stationary stimuli go unnoticed.

Our heightened sensitivity to movement allows us to quickly recognize those facets of our environment that are dynamic and changing and, consequently, may signal the need for an imminent response. Furthermore, movement is interesting and stimulating. Adults and infants will preferentially turn their attention to a moving object, with multiple independently moving objects being more interesting than a single moving object or multiple moving objects that move in unison (Rochat et al., 1997). There is a specific region within the visual cortex that may be distinguished from the surrounding regions due to it sensitivity to moving stimuli (Watson et al., 1993). However, the brain does not merely respond to movement, but it also has areas that differentially respond to objects moving at different velocities (Orban et al., 1981). The visual perception of movement is quite complex due to the timescale at which the neural circuitry of the brain must operate. Specifically, in the 30–100 ms required for cells in the retina to convert light energy into neural signals and the subsequent relay of those signals from the eye to the brain, an object may move a considerable distance. This problem is resolved through mechanisms that allow the cells of the retina, as well as the visual cortex, to anticipate the direction of an object's movement, enabling minimal delay in their response (Berry et al., 1999). Yet, the perception of movement goes beyond the immediate psychophysics of the stimulus. Moving stimuli can evoke activation of brain regions associated with inferring the intent and mental state of other individuals (Castelli et al., 2000). Thus, embedded within our perception of movement, there is an appraisal of the relevance of the movement to one's self based on attributions concerning associated intentions and causation.

Movement can be used to make design more engaging. For example, with computer screen savers that cycle through a series of pictures, the software feature that simulates a camera panning across the images can be compelling. In this case, the object of the picture does not move, but instead the perspective changes. Likewise, I have seen the animation features within PowerPoint used with tremendous effectiveness to illustrate the dynamic aspects of a topic (e.g., the flow of information through a system or an organization). However, movement for the sake of movement can often backfire. I cringe when I see presenters use animation to make the content of their PowerPoint slides enter and exit like performers coming on and off stage. Movement not only captures an audience's attention, but it can also be quite compelling when it emulates something that actually does move through space. However, when movement is attributed to objects for which movement is not an inherent characteristic (e.g., bullet points on a PowerPoint slide), the movement is distracting and an annoying source of unnecessary sensory stimulation.

Movement suggests that something is changing. From an adversarial point of view, it forces the opponent to pay attention. Movement can serve as a source of distraction, drawing attention away from more critical activities. Following an extended period of inaction, it may be assumed that sensitivity to movement will be at its greatest. This is particularly true if the movement occurs within a context of uncertainty. Perhaps, more importantly, movement may or may not be of significance. As discussed previously, a good decoy captures the attention of an opponent. However, an even better decoy sustains an opponent's interest. Movement may cause an opponent to attend to a decoy, but if the opponent must then devote additional resources to ascertain whether the movement is of significance to them, the decoy has occupied the time and resources of the opponent, and distracted him or her from other activities. However, the ultimate decoy not only sustains attention, but it also misleads its opponent, causing him or her to infer false patterns or intents based on a sequence of movements. The key is to tap into the brain's unique sensitivity to movement to create the impression that something of importance has changed.

Certain Stimuli Have a Biological Significance

A previous section discussed supernormal stimuli, which are a class of biologically significant stimuli that are marked by their capacity to evoke a disproportionate response relative to other comparable stimuli. Biologically significant stimuli involve objects or actions that have been ascribed special significance due to their being critical to the survival of an animal species (e.g., a gosling's capacity to imprint on its mother). There are various stimuli that seem to have a biological significance to humans and thus we exhibit an innate capacity for recognizing corresponding patterns of sensory stimulation.

Many of the stimuli that might be classified as biologically significant involve objects that evoke fear or a general unease. For example, the
experience of a physical drop-off or a cliff presents a somewhat universal
approach–avoidance dilemma. There is a curiosity and allure to experiencing an expansive view of one's surroundings, but an accompanying uneasiness that may cause mild dizziness, weakness in the knees, and even heart
palpitations, as well as mental images of going over the edge and falling to
one's death. In a recent paper, Bracha (2006) described four types of fear-
related brain circuits. Each circuit is rooted in different stages of human
evolution and highlights separate classes of biologically significant stimuli.
The first type is the Mesozoic or mammalian-wide fear circuits. These are
the most deeply rooted and are presumed to be shared by all mammalian
species. The fear of heights falls into this category, with extensive evidence
accumulated since the original visual cliff experiments (Gibson and Walk,
1960) to establish that this fear is manifested in the absence of prior learning
(Poulton et al., 1998). It has been noted that some individuals exhibit a capacity to operate effectively in high places (e.g., skyscraper construction workers). The apparent absence of a fear of heights seems to run in families and it
is difficult for nonblood relatives to acquire this. Throughout the centuries,
there have been examples where people have taken advantage of the human
proclivity to fear long drop-offs by constructing fortifications on high moun-
taintops where an aggressor would be forced to mount an assault on precari-
ous terrain, confronting his or her fear of heights at every step.

While we generally think of separation anxiety within the context
of young children, it has been argued that it reflects a deeply rooted
emotion–motivation system that influences behavior throughout a lifetime.
Specifically, Fisher et al. (2002) described three such emotion–motivation
systems, each mediated by a different corpus of neurotransmitters within
the brain: (1) lust, which evokes courtship behaviors; (2) attraction, which
steers one to appropriate mates; and (3) attachment, which leads to greater
parental involvement in caring for children. Bracha identified separation
anxiety as a Mesozoic mammalian-wide fear circuit, pointing to evidence of
separation anxiety in the young of mammalian, and even marsupial, species. However, as discussed by Fisher et al. (2002), separation anxiety can be
seen as the avoidance end of an approach–avoidance continuum that may
serve to promote enduring bonds. Conceived of as an approach–avoidance
continuum, each of the three emotion–motivation systems described by
Fisher et al. may be leveraged as a means to promote certain behaviors and,
at the same time, diminish the likelihood of other behaviors. For example,
in relation to attachment, online social media sites such as Facebook promote the development of communities and through "friending" and "lik-
ing," allow users to cultivate and sustain enduring relationships and, at
some level, satisfy their needs for affiliation. In contrast, a popular mechanism used by spammers is to insert a message onto a webpage alerting the
user that he or she has been "unfriended" by several individuals. Rejection,

and its extension to banishment and exile, evokes profound emotions in people. The spammers use these emotions to capture their victims' attention and lure them, offering the promise that they can find out exactly who has rejected them. The ability of these mechanisms to elicit a reaction in individuals, many of whom may not even participate in online communities, illustrates the capacity to provoke a behavioral response through signals that trigger brain circuits underlying the emotional and motivational foundations of attachment.

The second type of fear circuit is the Cenozoic or simian-wide fear circuits. These fears are shared by all the great ape species (i.e., gorillas, orangutans, chimpanzees), as well as lesser apes (i.e., gibbons and siamangs) and many species of monkey. Included in this type is the fear of snakes and reptiles. The innate propensity to fear these animals was demonstrated in studies by Cook and Mineka (1989, 1990), which used laboratory-bred rhesus monkeys that had never had any experiences outside the laboratory. One group of monkeys observed a video in which other monkeys exhibited a fear response to either a toy snake or a toy crocodile. Later, when presented with either the toy snake or the toy crocodile, these monkeys reacted fearfully. In contrast, a second group of monkeys were shown a video in which other monkeys exhibited similar fearful responses to either a toy rabbit or an artificial flower. After observing this video, the monkeys did not behave fearfully when they were later exposed to the same toy rabbit or artificial flower. These studies reveal a biological preparedness to recognize and fear certain animals. Related to this fear, Bracha (2006) also includes the preparedness to respond fearfully to teeth and being bitten. With most primates, the primary means of attack involves biting, which is also true for many of the animal species that might prey on primates. Consequently, an image of sharpened teeth and fangs has the capacity to evoke an emotional response and, similarly, showing one's teeth serves as a universally recognized expression of aggression (Ekman, 1993).

Cenozoic or simian-wide fears also include fear of the dark and fear of confined spaces. While the human visual system is not well suited for nighttime activities, our avoidance of the dark goes beyond practicality. This is evidenced in connotations associated with darkness. Darkness is associated with evil, as in "the Dark Lord," and misfortune as in "these were dark times." The color black carries the same connotations. It might be said that someone has "a black heart." Likewise, black attire has traditionally been used to convey a sinister quality. For instance, adversarial hackers are referred to as "Black Hats." The discomfort that is often experienced in response to confined spaces has been linked to the sensation of being trapped and having nowhere to escape (Kendler et al., 2001). Within a confined space, flight is not an option. Similarly, this fear also manifests itself within our common language. We talk about "the world closing in on" someone who has run out of options or a person being "trapped" and having "nowhere to go." These expressions tap into a universal recognition that darkness and confined spaces, which often occur together, as in caves, basements, and prison cells, present danger and should be avoided.

Bracha (2006) mentioned two additional Cenozoic or simian-wide fears, both of which harken back to an earlier section of this chapter concerning the breadth of our senses, including the capacity to sense the internal states of our body. One of these fears is triggered by elevated carbon dioxide (CO_2) levels in the body and is associated with the sensation of suffocation. This fear is related to another simian-wide fear discussed by Bracha, the fear of being immersed in water. Again, there is an approach–avoidance spectrum where at one end, there is a strong attraction to water with respect to playing and bathing, yet many rituals involve having one's head dunked in water, in some cases symbolizing the act of cleansing (e.g., Christian baptism) and in others symbolizing the act of drowning (e.g., hazing-related activities). Furthermore, much symbolism surrounds waterfalls, which simultaneously portend the experience of being swept away in a rapid rush of moving water and falling over the edge of a steep cliff. Still, despite having all the ingredients to evoke a fearful reaction, large dramatic waterfalls are an enormous attraction for tourists around the world.

The second of these internally based simian-wide fears is induced by lactate accumulation resulting from extended physical exertion. In certain individuals, high lactate levels can trigger a panic attack with profuse levels of anxiety and associated physiological reactions (e.g., sweating, accelerated heart rate). While lactate-induced panic attacks are uncommon, most people are familiar with the sense of helplessness that accompanies conditions when the body reaches a level of physical exhaustion such that it is impossible to continue activities.

The next class of fears identified by Bracha (2006) is believed to have arisen late in the evolutionary history of the human species and is referred to as *Homo sapiens* specific. These fears would have arisen following the split of humans from the other great apes and reflect conditions that uniquely affected early humans. Bracha discusses the fear of bloodletting as one illustration. People are unusually sensitive to bloody images and often exhibit anxiety when receiving a shot or having blood withdrawn that exceeds what would be proportionate to the actual pain. Modern horror movies highlight graphic depictions of bloody violence and it is generally this quality of visual imagery that distinguishes relatively tasteful depictions of violence from depictions of violence that many find senseless and unnecessarily horrific.

Also included in the *H. sapiens*–wide fears are fears implied by compulsive behaviors that occur with unusually high frequency in individuals seeking clinical care for obsessive–compulsive disorders and phobias. It should be noted that in most of these cases, the compulsive behavior involves an exaggeration of a behavior that is otherwise highly adaptive. Bracha (2006) identified the following examples of unusually common compulsions and phobias:

- *Compulsive lock checking*: Barriers and security have a special significance for people and there is a profound sense of violation associated with the experience of someone or some creature (i.e., wild animal) intruding on one's domain. Stove checking is another common compulsive behavior that similarly emanates from anxiety associated with the security of one's dwelling.

- *Compulsive washing/cleaning and obsessive fear of contamination*: Human excrement has been a common mechanism for the spread of disease within human populations, historically as well as in modern times. Consequently, a deeply rooted concern for cleanliness and disgust in response to the smell and sight of human excrement would seem natural.

- *Compulsive hoarding*: Human archeological sites reveal that hoarding appears to be a long-standing pattern of behavior in humans. For example, human Paleolithic sites often contain large hoards of stone tools and axes that exceed what would actually be needed based on the estimated size of the group inhabiting the site (LeBlanc and Register, 2003). This pattern of behavior has been linked to the prevalence of warfare in ancient times. With regard to the hoarding of food and other objects that are essential to daily survival, hoarding may represent an otherwise adaptive pattern of behavior in response to past and anticipated shortages. Whether the hoarding of weapons, as is more common in men, or the hoarding of food and clothing, as is more common in women (Samuels et al., 2002), hoarding is an intrinsic behavioral response that is prone to arise in response to certain conditions (i.e., suspected threats or potential shortages).

- *Irrational fears of insects and mice*: As noted above, the hoarding of food is adaptive as a means of preparing for anticipated shortages. However, food caches generally attract insects, mice, and other small rodents. Animals that are drawn to human food caches are also prime mechanisms for the transmission of disease. Thus, a distaste for insects and small rodents reflects a response to conditions that might undermine one's own health and that of one's family.

- *Irrational fears associated with social situations*: The fear of being in the presence of strangers or the fear of meeting new people lies at the root of commonly reported social phobias. Within human history, the experience of being in the midst of a large group of non-blood-related individuals, especially individuals who differ from one's self, while being observed and scrutinized by them, would generally warrant some degree of anxiety. However, in modern civilized societies, this same anxiety may be amplified to the point that it becomes a source of dysfunction.

Other research has addressed biologically significant stimuli that are not linked to fear circuits and an approach–avoidance continuum, or at least not to the extent of those identified by Bracha (2006). For instance, it has long been established that humans are uniquely sensitive to the visual patterns associated with a human gait and can easily distinguish a pattern corresponding to someone walking from other seemingly similar patterns (Johansson, 1973). Similarly, there is pronounced sensitivity to looming stimuli consistent with a rapidly approaching object that has been demonstrated at early stages of child development (Schiff, 1965).

From the perspective of design, there is the opportunity to incorporate biologically significant stimuli into design as a means to shape behavior associated with a product. This is particularly true for the biologically significant stimuli discussed by Bracha (2006) in that these stimuli imply an approach–avoidance continuum. The fears that are somewhat universal across human populations emanate from stimuli that have a shared significance, accompanied by privileged access to the neural circuitry underlying our experiences of fear, anxiety, and uneasiness. At the same time, many of these fears present an inverse that lies on the approach end of the continuum, which may be employed to enhance the attractiveness of a product. Likewise, within social settings, whereas one may be easily put off by situations that involve forced interactions with strangers, this can be alleviated through mechanisms that highlight the similarities and common interests of individuals (e.g., common uniforms, mechanisms that indicate shared interests, acquaintances, or backgrounds).

We Adjust to the Habitual and Become Sensitized to the Provocative

In my office, I have a speaker and a docking station that allow me to continuously play music from my iPod. I always have the speaker set to a relatively low volume so that my music does not disturb the people in the adjacent offices. On a daily basis, I have an experience that never fails to amaze me. I will step out of my office for a few minutes and when I return, I will be unable to hear the music coming from the speaker. Then, after waiting a minute or so, I will start to hear the music again. There are continuous background noises in my office from the fluorescent lights and ventilation system. This background noise is sufficient to drown out the music coming from the speaker. However, it takes only a minute or so for me to habituate to the continuous background noise and once my auditory system has habituated, I can again hear the sounds coming from the speaker. This example illustrates a basic principle of the human sensory systems. There is a propensity to habituate to continuous stimuli, particularly when those stimuli convey little or no meaning.

When a stimulus occurs repeatedly (e.g., auditory tone, visual pattern), it begins to trigger less and less activation of the cortical regions that are involved in processing the stimulus. For instance, when subjects are shown a visual pattern repeatedly, there is a reduction in the activation observed within the occipital, or visual, cortex (Hakan et al., 2000). This reduction in cortical activation is accompanied by an increase in the activation of the thalamus, a region of the brain associated with early processing and subsequent relaying of sensory information. Hakan et al. (2000) suggested that the thalamus might operate to modulate the activation of upstream cortical circuits in response to redundant stimuli. Yet, despite there being a muffled response to redundant stimuli, the brain continues to process the stimuli and is sensitive to unexpected changes (Naatanen et al., 1989). When the brain is presented with a redundant stimulus (e.g., a recurrent tone of a specific volume and frequency) and, unexpectedly, there is some change to the stimulus (e.g., the tone becomes louder or switches to a higher or lower pitch), a pronounced wave of activity extends across much of the brain. This phenomenon has been referred to as mismatch negativity and it has been reported for many different types of stimuli. The brain appears to habituate to redundant stimuli, but at the same time, it is unusually sensitive to any change in a stimulus. Furthermore, it has been shown that habituation not only occurs with perceptual processes, but there is also habituation in brain regions that underlie the formation and retrieval of memory, specifically the hippocampus (Grunwald et al., 2003). This habituation is manifested in a similarly diminished response following repeated exposure to cues triggering memory retrieval. However, habituation within the neural circuits that give rise to memory manifests on a much slower timescale than habituation associated with perceptual processes. Consequently, stimuli that one may exhibit a diminished response to at a perceptual level may continue to trigger activation of the neural circuits associated with memory and become incorporated into the memories of the corresponding experiences.

With design, it can be assumed that there will be habituation in response to features of a product that are relatively insignificant. However, this will only occur if the features remain constant. Any change in these same features will not only evoke a response, but will also trigger an orienting response that calls attention to the feature. For example, this often occurs as features of a product begin to wear down due to age or excessive use. Thus, straps, mountings, and supports that go unnoticed throughout the early lifespan of a product may break, loosen, or become discolored and, as a result, become a focal point and a potential source of discontent with the product.

The inverse of habituation is sensitization. With sensitization, there is an amplified response following repeated exposure to a stimulus. The distinction between habituation and sensitization primarily lies with the significance of the stimulus. Habituation occurs when a stimulus is relatively insignificant (e.g., the background noise in my office). In contrast, sensitization occurs with stimuli that are somewhat meaningful. For instance, sensitization occurs in response to stimuli that produce pain or discomfort. A piece of clothing that does not fit well or chafes will become increasingly uncomfortable over time. A person who has irritating habits will find that others are less and less tolerant of him or her as they become increasingly sensitized to the annoying behavior. In general, following repeated exposure to a stimulus, the brain becomes increasingly less responsive to stimuli of little significance, while it becomes more responsive to stimuli that are significant.

Much of the research concerning sensitization has concerned stress and addiction. With stress, as has often been described in the context of post-traumatic stress disorder, one becomes sensitized to stimuli associated with a traumatic experience and as a result, those same stimuli, or similar stimuli, elicit a disproportionate response within the brain (Stam, 2007). In addiction, various cues are associated with the addictive behavior, with addicts becoming sensitized to these cues. As a result of this sensitization, the cues that addicts have associated with their addictive behavior are amplified to the point that they become difficult to ignore, leaving them unable to resist the urge to satisfy their addiction (Robinson and Berridge, 1993). For example, individuals attempting to recover from a gambling addiction might find that merely being in the vicinity of a casino, with the surrounding context, is enough to squash their willpower and overcome their intentions to restrain from further wagering.

With sensitization, there is an amplified brain response to stimuli that extends over broad regions of the brain. In a study conducted by Hugdahl et al. (1995), subjects participated in a classical conditioning paradigm in which a tone was presented in combination with an electric shock. Once the subjects had learned the association between the otherwise neutral tone and the aversive stimulus, the electric shock, mere presentation of the tone was sufficient to elicit broad activation of the right cerebral hemisphere of the brain. As a result of the electric shock, the subjects had become sensitized to the tone and exhibited a pronounced response that engaged many different regions of the brain. Sensitization appears to be largely rooted in the arousal mechanisms of the brain. A stimulus for which one has become sensitized activates neural circuits associated with perceptual processes, but additionally, it activates arousal mechanisms within the brain. This has been demonstrated through research showing differential activation of regions of the brain stem associated with arousal in situations involving sensitization to pain (Lee et al., 2008). Thus, with sensitization, due to the influence of arousal, brain activation associated with perceptual and other related neural processes is amplified.

Generally, sensitization is associated with negative consequences and is something that a designer would seek to avoid. Consequently, where one might anticipate there being discomfort, displeasure, or pain, a designer might seek to isolate aspects of the design so as to minimize the formation of associations with the unpleasant experience, and the resulting sensitization. However, sensitization may also be used to achieve design objectives. For instance, where there are experiences that are known to be enjoyable, one might expect to see some degree of sensitization for stimuli associated with those experiences. Thus, certain peripheral experiences become part of the pattern of behavior that leads to the desired experience. For example, going to an amusement park or a sports arena is generally associated with positive, enjoyable experiences. By placing advertisements in the path of those visiting these venues so that they become a peripheral part of their routine, there is an opportunity to capitalize on the positive experiences.

A second means by which a designer may apply sensitization to achieve design objectives relies on the arousing properties of stimuli for which there has been sensitization. Stimuli for which one has become sensitized evoke a generalized arousal. This can be effectively put to use in situations where one wants to capture someone's attention or ensure that people are alert. For instance, standup comedians, or any other presenters, might begin their presentation with a provocative assertion. The comedian may care nothing about the assertion and it may be irrelevant to his or her subsequent material; however, it serves to get the audience's attention. While such techniques can quickly become ineffective, if used sparingly and with care, one can take advantage of topics for which there is considerable sensitivity as a means to get people's attention and ensure that they are alert.

We Fill in the Pieces to See the Whole

The term *gestalt* has become incorporated into common vernacular to convey the idea of seeing the whole of any object or situation, rather than a mere collection of its parts. Formally, this idea has been expressed as a collection of principles that describe various perceptual phenomena (e.g., the *law of proximity*, which states that similar objects that are close to one another will be perceived to constitute a group). Yet, in general, it is a basic property of the brain that when presented with various pieces of a recognizable figure, the brain fills in the missing pieces and perceives a whole figure.

One of the most common illustrations of the gestalt principles of perception involves what is referred to as a *bistable* figure. A classic example is Rubin's vase, in which, depending on one's perspective, the figure appears as either a vase or two faces looking toward one another. Within the brain, fast frequency, gamma-band activity is associated with active perceptual or cognitive processing. When Rubin's vase, or other bistable figures, is rotated, there is an orientation at which the vase or faces are seen most clearly (see figure 1 in Keil et al., 1999). Within the visual areas of the brain, gamma-band activity increases when the figure is in the vertical orientation that most clearly affords seeing either the vase or the two faces (see figure 6 in Keil et al., 1999). This indicates an increased coordination of fast frequency neural activation when the figure appears at an orientation at which specific objects are perceived, in contrast to other orientations of the figure in which no discernible object is perceived. Furthermore, as demonstrated using the Kanizsa square (i.e., a figure with four darkened circles arranged in a grid with slices removed from each circle to suggest the image of a square), the increased coordination of activity is combined with an amplification of activity in response to seeing the illusionary square (Hermann and Bosch, 2001). This research demonstrates that given perceptual ambiguity, the brain tends to separately process the various elements of a scene, but once the brain is able to put the pieces together to form a recognizable object or shape, there is an amplification and coordination of the corresponding neural activation.

Where the common experience of an object involves multiple sensory modalities (e.g., the sight and sound of an object), the propensity to fill in the missing pieces spans the relevant sensory modalities. In a study reported by Meyer et al. (2010), subjects were presented with muted video clips that depicted familiar objects without the accompanying sounds. It has been demonstrated that within the auditory regions of the brain that process sound, memories for the sound of objects from certain categories of objects are localized to specific areas. For example, memories for the sounds made by different animals will be grouped together within a distinct area of the auditory cortex. Likewise, the sounds associated with different musical instruments will be grouped together. For this study, the researchers used three categories: animals (e.g., howling dog, mooing cow, crowing rooster), musical instruments (e.g., violin, bass, piano), and general objects (e.g., chainsaw cutting wood, glass vase shattering, coin being dropped). Each of these categories of objects could be distinguished on the basis of their activating a specific area of the auditory cortex. When the subjects viewed the video without sound, it was observed that there was activation in the region of the auditory cortex that would ordinarily have been activated in the presence of the corresponding sound. For example, when watching the muted video of the dog howling, there was activation in the area that would have been active had the subject been presented with the sound of a dog howling, without the video. Here, the brain had expectations that spanned multiple sensory modalities, and when sensory information from only one modality was presented, the brain filled in the missing pieces.

For designers, there is a risk that patterns may be observed inadvertently, giving rise to the perception of objects or symbols that are not relevant to the actual design, and may serve as a basis for distraction or misinterpretation, or even offense. For instance, there is almost no limit to the objects that have been attributed phallic symbolism and there are frequent occurrences in which architectural features are found to contain patterns that resemble the Nazi swastika. On the other hand, there is an artistic allure to designs that imply yet do not actually depict familiar symbols or patterns.

More practically, the capacity of the brain to fill in the missing pieces offers an opportunity for economies in design. This is well illustrated with simulation-based training where, to reduce costs, the key features of a system are replicated, but many details are omitted. In many occupations, there is a desire to train individuals using conditions that closely resemble actual operations. However, while actual operations may be simulated with tremendous fidelity, this comes at a great cost. By using low- and medium-fidelity trainers that only replicate the critical details of an actual system or operations, training may be provided at a much lower cost. I have often been asked to comment on the importance of fidelity in simulation-based training. Fidelity refers to the extent to which a simulated system matches the real system or actual operations. Speaking solely from the perspective of knowledge of the brain, I can say that there is a propensity for the brain to fill in the elements that are missing in low- and medium-fidelity simulators. However, the trainee must have sufficient experience with the actual system to expect those elements that have been omitted in the simulator and fill in the missing pieces. This suggests that for experts, low- and medium-fidelity simulators may be adequate because these individuals know what to expect and their brains fill in the missing pieces. In contrast, novices have little or no experience with the actual system and are unable to fill in these missing elements. As a result, novices are more likely to be surprised when their experiences with the actual system do not correspond to the experiences they have had during training or they fail to generalize what they have learned during training to actual operations.

Brains Naturally Categorize

If every object was distinct and it was necessary to appraise every object individually, this would make our everyday lives intractable. The brain has greatly simplified the problem through categorization. If an object can be recognized as a member of a known category, then all the knowledge that has been accumulated concerning this category can be attributed to the object. On seeing an object for the first time, individuals may immediately draw on knowledge that they have acquired over their lifetime. For example, birds are common objects for which almost everyone has some familiarity. When we go to the zoo and see a species of bird that we have never seen before, we know what to expect. We know that they have wings and can fly, and that they lay eggs and raise their young in a nest. It is the exceptions to the category that usually generate interest (e.g., birds that do not fly) and we take notice of evolutionary vestiges, such as the wings possessed by chickens and other birds that have lost the capacity for flight.

When presented with a familiar object, activation occurs within neural circuits of the brain that underlie our knowledge of that object. Generally, this activation is quite diffuse, spanning broad regions of the brain. However, using brain imaging techniques, it may be observed that brain activity tends to be most intense within specific areas. Numerous reports have illustrated that areas that are activated by specific categories of objects may be isolated (see Thompson-Schill, 2003 for review). For instance, in one of the earlier studies (Spitzer et al., 1995), subjects were shown pictures of different items from one of four categories (i.e., furniture, fruit, animals, or tools) and were asked to name each object. When comparing the brain regions that were most active, it was found that there was a somewhat different pattern of activation for each of the four categories. The regions that were activated varied for each subject, with this attributable to life experiences having differentially shaped the brains of each individual. However, during tests that were administered on different days, the areas that were activated by a given category were essentially the same for a given subject. Other studies have reported similar findings when comparing activation with living versus nonliving objects (Mummery et al., 1996); animals versus tools (Martin et al., 1996); and animals, tools, faces, and houses (Chao et al., 1999). These findings indicate that the brain not only distinguishes between objects, but it also makes distinctions based on the similarity of objects with regard to known categories, with these distinctions evidenced through there being localized activation of brain regions associated with different categories.

More recent research has suggested that the dimensions along which categories of objects differ are reflected in the organization of the brain areas that are activated by these objects (see figures 2 and 7 in Connolly et al., 2012). In one study, fMRI was recorded as subjects viewed images of six different species of animals, with two each from the categories of primates, bugs, and birds. In a second study, there were 12 species with 4 each from the categories of mammals, reptiles, and bugs. When the regions that were activated by each category were compared, there were two primary dimensions. One spanned from primates to bugs and the second spanned from mammals to bugs. Interestingly, the areas associated with primates and mammals were close to one another and closer to the areas found to be associated with animate or living objects. In contrast, bugs were more distant and closer to the areas found to be associated with inanimate objects. Thus, a primary dimension along which categories of objects differ involves the degree to which we think of an object as a living being similar to ourselves, as opposed to it being more similar to inanimate objects.

Within the brain, the organization of different categories of objects is somewhat dynamic and reflects learning that occurs over the course of a lifetime. These categories embody both the perceptual properties of objects and their semantic relationships to similar objects. The propensity to form categories and then differentially respond to the world in relation to these categories is an intrinsic property of the brain. Furthermore, it is an ongoing work in progress with new categories being formed and existing categories being revised, with a continuous reorganization of the corresponding neural circuitry (Linden et al., 2011; Carlson et al., 2012).

Placed in a given environment, individuals will invariably cope by calling on their categorical knowledge of the world. They will look at objects, people, and situations, and relate them to categories that are already known, reacting to them accordingly. Yet, at the same time, they will update and revise their knowledge of the world based on these experiences. This may entail the formation of new categories, or the refinement and elaboration of existing categories. From the perspective of design, our understanding of systems, products, and experiences has an underlying categorical organization. However, in the earliest stages of design when a product has not yet been realized, it is necessary for the designer to imagine ways in which people will interact with his or her design. Ideally, the design would embody the mental model of the designer and that mental model would correspond to the mental models of the people who will interact with the product. In reality, the categories that people use to organize the world may not comply with those of the designer. Furthermore, the ways in which people engage with a product may vary from that imagined by the designer, resulting in their developing a mental model of the product that is contrary to that of the designer. Through their interactions with a product, people will infer relationships and sense patterns, and based on these relationships and patterns, they will form an understanding of the product that will guide their beliefs, expectations, and interactions with the product. Furthermore, over time, this knowledge will increasingly crystallize to the point that it may become difficult to see the product in any other way.

What can the designer do? First, one might leverage existing, commonly shared categorical relationships. For example, stores are generally organized so that there are separate sections for men's, women's, and children's clothing, which leverages the fact that in our homes, families usually keep their clothes separate. Second, one might structure design to facilitate the formation of certain categorical knowledge, while discouraging the formation of irrelevant categorical relationships. Within a graphical user interface, related functions may be grouped together and nonrelated functions may be separated, thus requiring the user to open a new window or menu to access those nonrelated functions. This serves to tell the user that some items belong to the same category and that other items are different. Third, where practical, people may be allowed the opportunity to customize the design in a way that makes sense to them with respect to how they use the product. For example, the desktop environment of most computing systems allows users to place the objects that they want on the desktop and organize them in a way that makes sense to them and corresponds to how they use the system. Finally, there is much to be said for keeping the design simple so that one minimizes both the need and the potential for the development of complex, diverse, and perhaps inappropriate categorical understandings of a system.

How to Trick, Confuse, and Otherwise Baffle the Brain

The objective with system design is generally to recognize and orient human–systems interactions to take advantage of the intrinsic strengths of the human perceptual systems and avoid interactions that rely on activities for which human perception is ill-suited. It is worthwhile considering the inverse. One might ask, "How might I present a signal that is well within the bounds of what the human perceptual systems can sense and recognize, yet will likely go unnoticed?" In other words, setting aside the earlier discussion of decoys and mimicry, how can one take advantage of the weaknesses inherent in human perception?

Imagine that the intent is to conceal an auditory signal. For example, one may want to signal one's presence and intent to an ally without an adversary knowing about it. First, if the same sound is being emitted from different locations, it becomes difficult to distinguish one instance of the sound from another. Likewise, if different sounds are being emitted from the same location, it may be difficult to separate the sounds and recognize the one that is serving as a signal. Both these mechanisms take advantage of limitations in the ability to segregate sensory stimulation. It can be confusing when the same sound comes from different locations or when the sound for which one is listening must be distinguished from other sounds that are all originating from the same location.

Second, one can assume that an adversary is sensing patterns, whether this is occurring at a conscious or an unconscious level. Thus, as the predictability of a signal increases, it will become more easily recognized. To successfully conceal a signal, one must strike a balance. The presence of a discernible pattern within a stimulus will draw attention to the stimulus. However, an unpredictable signal, within the context of an otherwise predictable background, will also draw attention to the signal. Consequently, the regularity of a signal should mimic the regularity that is naturally present within the background so that the regularity of the signal does not provide a cue for recognizing the signal.

Third, people are sensitive to boundaries. Boundaries demarcate the beginning and end of meaningful units. Distinct stops and starts within a signal serve as boundaries and alert a listener to the beginning and end of something that may be potentially meaningful. To conceal a signal, continuity, with there being no distinguishable starts and stops, will deny the listener the boundaries that would otherwise facilitate his or her ability to recognize the presence of a signal.

Similarly, the presence of dead spaces where there is little or no stimulation creates a contrast against which any signal that intrudes will be particularly noticeable. Thus, the broadcasting of a signal should be timed and placed so that it does not coincide with a dead space. In this regard, one might broadcast continuous background noise that has the effect of eliminating the presence of any dead spaces.

As previously noted, it can be difficult to isolate a specific signal when similar sounds are being emitted from multiple sources. Likewise, a moving source can be difficult to discern. Distinguishing the "what" of the signal and the "where" of the signal involves somewhat different perceptual mechanisms. In challenging situations, while it may be possible to discern one, it can be difficult to simultaneously discern both. Consequently, when the signal is emitted from a moving source, conditions may arise where distinguishing the location of the source prevents recognition of the content of the signal, and vice versa.

Finally, when an individual is distracted and faced with other perceptual and cognitive demands, it becomes more difficult to recognize a signal.

Many years ago, I had the opportunity to work with one of the major automobile makers. We were experimenting with technology that would use data that were available on the car to recognize when the driver was in a challenging driving situation (e.g., changing lanes to overtake another car or merging onto a busy highway). One of the ideas considered was to lower the volume of the radio when the driver was in a difficult situation so that the radio did not serve as a source of distraction. There was an unusually profound effect that when driving, one did not notice that the volume had been reduced and subsequently returned to its original setting. However, as a passenger, the automatic volume adjustment was quite apparent. This example illustrates how task demands can affect our sensitivity to perceptual input. Consequently, if a signal can be timed to coincide with periods in which an adversary is distracted by other task demands, then the adversary should be less likely to recognize the signal.

These are a few means by which an auditory signal may be concealed. This does not speak to what may be accomplished given the technology to augment human perceptual processes, but assumes that the adversary must recognize the signal using only his or her perceptual systems. This example has focused on the concealment of an auditory signal. With other sensory modalities, these mechanisms may be more or less effective, and there may be other mechanisms that can be used. It is important to recognize that the human perceptual systems have certain strengths that can be leveraged in design. Likewise, the human perceptual systems have certain weaknesses that can be leveraged in adversarial situations.

Perception Is Not a Continuous Process

Historically, there has been a tendency to conceive of human perception as a continuous, ongoing process in which bottom-up processing of stimulus information gives rise to perceptual experiences, which then feed into cognitive processes. This assumed continuity is understandable given that our conscious experience is continuous and free of periodic disruptions. Likewise, we have extensive experience with machines and electronic devices that function on a continuous basis, whether it be a gear that rotates at a speed that is proportionate to the energy supplied from a drivetrain or an electronic device that produces transmissions that are proportionate to the input signal. However, these experiences can be misleading when trying to understand the functioning of the human brain. For example, consider vision, where our experience is of a continuous stream of visual input corresponding to the world around us. The reality is that the visual signals from the eyes are intermittent, coming and going with the saccadic twitches of the eyes, yet the brain fills in the holes to produce a continuous experience. Perception is best described as a multiphase process, with the operations at each phase being subject to ongoing modulations of the corresponding neural circuitry, and the results manifested through variability in our moment-to-moment performance of tasks reliant on perceptual processes.

Using EEG-based electrical recordings of the activity of the brain, the coordinated activity of neural circuits can be observed in the frequency characteristic of the EEG signal. If variations in the amplitude of the signal over time are charted, these variations will form waves with recognizable peaks and troughs. Frequency describes the number of waves that occur within a given time frame. For example, if the time between the peak of one wave and the peak of the next wave is 100 ms, then in the period of 1 s, 10 of these waves will occur. This signal would be said to have a frequency of 10 Hz. When looking at the signal emanating from a given recording site, there are generally many different frequencies simultaneously present within the signal. However, often there will be a dominant frequency with the signal strongest for this frequency. This is indicative of a large population of neurons that are pulsing in a coordinated manner. Research has shown that the timing of a stimulus relative to the dominant waveform impacts the likelihood that the signal will be detected and the subsequent salience of the signal (Wyart and Sergent, 2009).

When at rest, the rear region of the brain, which is largely involved in visual processing, is dominated by activity with frequencies of approximately 10 Hz. In research by van Dijk et al. (2008), it was shown that the amplitude of this activity correlated with the likelihood that subjects would detect a visual stimulus for which the intensity of the stimulus was near the threshold for detection. Faint stimuli were more likely to be detected if the populations of neurons within the visual cortex were pulsing, or oscillating, in coordination with one another, with the likelihood that a faint stimulus would be detected correlated with the degree to which there were coordinated oscillations.

Subsequent research has considered the timing of the stimulus relative to the phase of the dominant frequency (Busch et al., 2009; Mathewson et al., 2009). In other words, at the time that the stimulus was sensed, was the waveform rising toward its peak or falling toward its trough? These researchers have reported that when the amplitude of the waveform is lowest, or the wave is on its downswing, subjects are less likely to report having seen a faint stimulus. Comparing the phase of the waveform with the greatest likelihood of detection (i.e., the upswing) to that with the lowest (i.e., the downswing), there was a 12%–16% difference in the likelihood of detecting the stimulus. This same effect has been shown for auditory stimuli in studies that have used transcranial direct current stimulation (tDCS) of the brain to manipulate frequency characteristics. By manipulating the waveform through direct electrical stimulation of the brain, the likelihood of detecting an auditory stimulus could either be increased or decreased (Neuling et al., 2012).

In the design of systems, one must constantly contend with the variability in performance that is intrinsic to human operators. The research described here points to one source of variability. Specifically, the human brain undergoes continuous fluctuations and these fluctuations may translate into moment-to-moment variations in performance. Perhaps more importantly, this research highlights how the variability that is intrinsic to the human brain can affect recognition of stimuli that are near the threshold for detection. The human brain is unlike a machine that operates in a continuous manner. Instead, the human brain is in continuous flux. Consequently, there will be a certain range of variability in the performance of operators that cannot be eliminated through training or other related mechanisms. This suggests the need for systems to be designed so that they are tolerant of a range of variability in the performance of human operators, with this being particularly true when systems require that operators function near the limits of their capacities.

Perceptual Processes May Be Flexibly Adapted to Circumstances

Chapter 2 discussed the inherent plasticity of the human brain and made the point that through experience, we continuously shape our brains over the course of a lifetime. With perceptual processes, plasticity is evidenced in the expansion of brain regions following extensive practice of an activity that relies on a particular sensory modality. For instance, in individuals who are blind, there is activation of brain regions normally associated with vision during the performance of a task that requires the sense of touch (Sadato et al., 2002). This activation of visual areas during a tactile task was not observed in individuals with normal vision. Furthermore, the extent to which the visual areas were engaged by the tactile task was much greater in individuals who lost their sight prior to the age of 16 years, as opposed to those who lost their sight later in life. Similarly, in deaf people, it has been shown that visual stimuli activate areas of the auditory cortex that would ordinarily be responsive to sound stimulation (Finney et al., 2001). Thus, in extreme cases, the processing of one sensory modality can encroach on brain regions associated with the processing of other sensory modalities, taking over the associated neural circuits.

Less pronounced illustrations of brain plasticity associated with perceptual processes have been described in musicians. When one plays a musical instrument, one engages sensory processes linked to fine motor control. Research has demonstrated anatomical differences in the brains of musicians as compared with nonmusicians. In musicians, areas involved in listening and producing music are more extensive and show denser connectivity (Gaser and

Schlaug, 2001). Yet, in addition to the anatomical differences, it has similarly been shown that musicians' brains function somewhat differently, exhibiting extreme sensitivity to minor variations in stimuli associated with musical performance (Russeler et al., 2001). With trained musicians, when notes were off by a mere 20 ms, a response was triggered within their brains that would normally occur with an unexpected, surprising, or deviant perceptual stimuli. At 50 ms, nonmusicians responded to the mistimed performance. However, at 50 ms, the brain response of the musicians was still much more pronounced than that of the nonmusicians. These studies illustrate that the experience that one attains within the course of extensive practice produces measurable differences in both the structure and functional capabilities of the brain.

Many activities for which individuals may gain expertise involve brain functions that are unlike those of activities that would have naturally occurred prior to the advent of modern technology. For these activities, the intrinsic functional capabilities of the brain may be harnessed and adapted to fulfill the new roles. This often involves co-opting brain circuits that were originally specialized for other functions. This was recently demonstrated in a study of 8- to 10-year-old children who had expressed intense levels of interest in Pokemon cards (James et al., 2012). When these children were compared with other children who did not share this interest, fMRI recordings revealed pronounced activation of the fusiform gyrus, an area linked to human face recognition. These children had co-opted the areas of the brain that would normally be employed in the recognition of human faces for the processing and recognition of the images found on the Pokemon cards. When adult experts in Pokemon were studied, they showed the same pattern of activation of the fusiform gyrus face recognition region of the brain as the child experts. In fact, the level of activation associated with the Pokemon cards in both the child and adult Pokemon experts was greater than the activation of the face recognition region when viewing actual faces. These findings suggest that with expertise, the brain applies neural circuitry relevant to the activity (i.e., in the case of the Pokemon experts, this was the neural circuitry associated with recognizing faces) and these neural circuits may become finely tuned to the trained activity, even to the extent that brain regions respond more robustly to the trained activity than the activity for which the brain regions are presumed to be specialized.

The brain is remarkably flexible and can adapt to a broad range of activities, many of which would not exist if it were not for the demands of modern technology. The brain does not develop new functional capabilities, but instead applies existing capabilities, perhaps in new ways, and then hones and elaborates those capabilities to attain increasing levels of skill. The designer might ask "what perceptual, cognitive, and motor skills are essential to successful performance within the context of a system and what existing skills might be leveraged in developing these skills?" Understanding that face recognition might be leveraged in recognizing abstract symbols or that language skills might be leveraged in learning and remembering otherwise meaningless codes (e.g., computer passwords), the design can then accommodate the ability to leverage these functions. Assuming that the designer has found a good match, the brain can then be relied on to facilitate this process through adaptation and specialization of the corresponding neural circuits, enabling skills to emerge that have little precedent within individuals' previous activities.

The External World Is Replicated within the Brain

That our brains are so adept at capturing memories of events that we can later recall is a wonderful gift, allowing us to reexperience the sensations of our most pleasant experiences. Granted, these recollections are not exact replicas and, over time, they diminish in clarity and detail. But still, whether consciously recalled during a quiet moment or brought to life within a dream, perceptual experiences can be strong enough to trigger many of the same emotions that we experienced during the original event.

When our brain imagines a sensory experience, it reengages the neural circuitry that would normally be engaged if we were directly experiencing the same event. For instance, if one is asked to visualize a face, activation occurs in the brain regions that would normally be active if attending to someone's facial features (O'Craven and Kanwisher, 2000). Similarly, imagining being in a specific place generates activation of the brain regions associated with the recognition of places. Thus, the same neural circuitry that is associated with the original experience is reengaged when later imagining that same experience. However, the activation that occurs during imagination is not as pronounced as that which occurs during an actual experience. Yet, this is consistent with the sensation that the imagined experience is never quite as vivid as the actual experience.

The capability for mental imagery has utility that goes beyond our occasional daydreams. Often, in performing tasks, we need to create an image in our mind as a means to recall specific information about an object or an event. For instance, if I am giving someone directions, I might recall my perceptual experience from the last time I made the same journey. Similarly, if I am asked a factual question (e.g., does a turtle have pads on its feet?), I may rely on perceptual recollections to produce an answer. In these situations, performance depends on the ability to accurately re-create perceptual experiences (Kan et al., 2003). It has been shown that the cognitive mechanisms that are used to actually perform a task are comparable to those that are used to visualize performing the task. For example, subjects were shown faint images and were later asked to make perceptual judgments (e.g., is the object taller or wider) after having been again shown the image or only allowed to imagine the image. Comparing these two conditions, there was greater overlap in the activation of the brain regions associated with making a comparative judgment than there was for visual areas of the brain (Ganis et al., 2004). Thus, in both conditions, the same cognitive mechanisms were employed, whether the judgment was based on actually seeing the object or merely visualizing the object.

Given that the brain responds to imagined events in the same way that it responds to actual events, imagery offers a mechanism to create richer experiences and perhaps bolster learning. However, it is worth noting that during imagery, the brain mechanisms involved in performing various cognitive operations may be more engaged than the brain regions associated with sensory processes. This suggests that when asked to imagine a given situation, the brain regions associated with cognitive operations, whether solving a problem or performing some physical activity, will exhibit a more pronounced level of engagement. Consequently, it is important that when creating experiences involving some degree of imagination, these experiences ask individuals to actively engage in the situation, as opposed to being mere bystanders.

Activity in the Brain Does Not Mean There Was a Conscious Perceptual Experience

If a group of people are placed in a given situation, perhaps a train station, and all are exposed to the same sensory experiences without any distractions or other interferences, one might assume that there would be a common perceptual experience. Everyone should be exposed to the same sensory stimulation with activation of the associated regions of their brains responsible for processing signals from the corresponding sensory pathways. Within the brain, there may be activation that is consistent with the recognition of specific objects or the recognition of events. However, this does not mean that each individual has had an equivalent perceptual experience. Just because there is activation in the brain consistent with the perception of a given sensory experience, this does not mean that a person has consciously had that experience. For a group of people standing in a train station, exposed to exactly the same sensory stimulation, each having a fully functioning set of sensory systems, the perceptual experiences for which they are conscious will vary from one individual to another. Each individual will have his or her own unique perceptual experience, despite having been exposed to exactly the same sensory stimulation.

In research conducted by Moutoussis and Zeki (2002), subjects were presented with images of a face and a house in rapid succession, with the duration of each exposure being extremely brief. For a given trial, the researchers could tell that the subjects had perceptually processed both stimuli because of the activation in the brain regions that would normally be activated if presented with an image of either a face or a house. However, because the stimuli were present for such a brief duration, it was not possible for the subjects to consciously recognize both the face and the house. The subjects routinely reported seeing one of the two stimuli, but not the other. Another group of researchers (Pasley et al., 2004) conducted a similar study, except that some of the faces exhibited a distinct expression of emotion (e.g., fear, anger, happiness). Their subjects routinely failed to report having seen the face. However, not only was there activation of the region of their brains responsible for recognizing faces, but there was also activation of a region associated with processing emotional stimuli (i.e., amygdala). In this case, the subjects had no conscious awareness of having seen a face, but the neural circuits of their brains that are responsible for recognizing and responding to facial expressions of emotion were triggered (Figure 4.5).

The fact that one cannot rely on different individuals presented with the same sensory experience to have similar perceptual experiences presents a dilemma for the designer, particularly where it is important to the operation of a system that individuals sense and behave in a predictable manner. The situation is different in art and entertainment where the propensity for

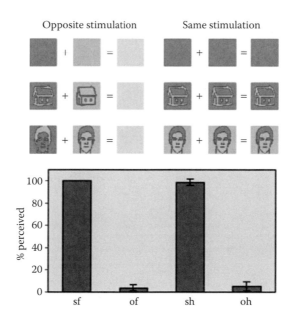

FIGURE 4.5   (See color insert)
Simultaneous stimuli used by Moutoussis and Zeki (2002) in their study illustrating brain activation in response to stimuli that are not perceived at a conscious level. sf, same faces; of, opposite faces; sh, same houses; oh, opposite houses. (From Moutoussis, K. and Zeki, S., *Proceedings of the National Academy of Science*, 99, 9527–9532, 2002.)

different individuals to have the same sensory experience, yet perceive it differently, can be used to create a more interesting and engaging product. In situations where there is a need for people to respond predictably, there are many things that can be done to lessen the extent to which individuals experience a situation differently. For instance, certain stimuli may be made more salient or individuals may be primed to expect and respond to certain stimuli. Similarly, individuals may be engaged in ways that elevate certain stimuli to conscious awareness. Actions may be required that cannot be completed without having consciously processed essential stimuli or mechanisms may be employed that serve to verify conscious awareness of certain stimuli (e.g., it may be necessary to enter a code that cannot be attained without having consciously attended to essential stimuli).

On the other hand, one might also ask what can be done to encourage people to experience situations differently. In art, this may be done through ambiguity and abstraction. The procedure used by Moutoussis and Zeki (2002) illustrates another approach in which stimuli are presented in rapid succession such that there is only time to consciously process a subset of the available stimuli. Another approach involves engaging individuals on a personal level so that the experience of each individual is uniquely shaped by his or her own personal history. The key point is that in designing the sensory ecology that emerges as the product of a given design, there is a need to manage the perceptual experience. This may involve a management strategy that emphasizes the need for consistency and predictability, with the design structured accordingly, or it may involve a management strategy that encourages diversity and distinct individual experiences.

Our Brains Are Specially Tuned to the Actions of Others

Previous sections have discussed the brain's special sensitivity to certain stimuli, particularly those that have biological significance. The actions of people around us have special significance. Another person's actions may have a direct bearing on our own goals and actions (e.g., as we are walking across a room to sit on a bench, someone else may take the seat that we had intended to sit on); gestures and facial expressions may be used to communicate (e.g., someone may motion for us to stay away); and certain actions may be specifically directed toward us (e.g., we are handed a plate of food). But, perhaps most importantly, it is through watching the actions of others that we learn many essential behaviors. While there has been debate regarding whether there is a particular neural circuit within the brain that is specialized for recognizing and responding to the actions of others (Hickok, 2009), it is clear that the brain is sensitive to the actions of others (Iacoboni et al., 1999). Furthermore, certain brain regions that would ordinarily exhibit activity when performing a given action, display comparable activity when watching another person perform the same action.

The neural circuits that selectively respond to the actions of another person have been referred to as *mirror neurons*. Mirror neurons were first identified in monkeys when researchers realized that the neural circuits associated with reaching and grasping for objects, which were the subject of their studies, exhibited comparable activity when the monkeys observed the human experimenters perform similar actions (Di Pellegrino et al., 1992). Subsequently, these findings were extended with demonstrations that the human brain exhibits a similar response (Iacoboni et al., 1999). The activity in the mirror neurons seems to involve a simulation of actually performing the same activity. This is evidenced by findings showing that the progression and time course of the neural activity are comparable with those that would occur if the observer was performing the action (Gangitano et al., 2001). This helps to explain the finding that when a person observes another person perform an activity, the individual is primed to perform the same activity, as evidenced by faster reaction times when prompted to perform an observed activity, as compared with an equivalent activity that has not been observed (Brass et al., 2000). With respect to learning through imitation, when experimental subjects observed chords formed on a guitar and were instructed to either merely watch or to watch with the intent to imitate the hand positions, there were similar patterns of activation in the brain (Rizzolatti and Craighero, 2004). This suggests that the activity within mirror neurons that results from observing an act, with or without the intent to imitate the act, may serve as a precursor for reproducing the same act.

In the presence of others, as we observe their actions, our brains respond to these observations, producing patterns of activation comparable with our performing the same activity. This primes us to behave in the same way as the people around us. In the design of systems, certain behaviors may be promoted by creating a situation where people observe others performing the desired behavior. In contrast, where there is a risk of unruly behavior (e.g., during sporting and other live events involving tremendous levels of excitement and emotion), a demonstration of riotous or other undesirable behavior may serve as a trigger to prime and elicit similar behavior from others. A wonderfully benign example can be seen in a YouTube video from Derek Sivers entitled "First Follower: Leadership Lessons from Dancing Guy." This video involves an outdoor concert where a member of the audience who stands out because he is shirtless begins dancing wildly. Shortly, the dancing guy is joined by a couple of others, and then, more and more, until there is a large crowd all dancing together. Sivers uses this video to illustrate the importance of the *first follower*, or the individual who recognizes that someone else has a good idea and joins him or her in advancing the idea. However, this example also illustrates how watching someone can prime the same behavior in others. This is a property of the brain that can be applied to achieve productive ends when attempting to steer the behavior of a crowd, teaching various skills, or within the context of entertainment, creating experiences where the audience becomes immersed in events. Yet, the same propensity within the brain to mirror the behavior of others is also present in situations where behavior is potentially dangerous or offensive, or merely counterproductive.

Our Sense of the World Is a Product of Our Social Environment

Our brains intrinsically sense the actions of others. Yet, does this sensitivity to others manifest in how we perceive the world, and is it evident in our own actions? The answer is "yes," and the effect may largely occur at an unconscious level. When we see someone yawn, it is often difficult to suppress a yawn ourselves. Likewise, when watching another person laugh, we may find ourselves laughing with them, or at the least, we may find it hard not to smile. We similarly mimic the posture and gestures of others. In a group of people, see what happens if you assume a posture that is rather typical (e.g., hands behind the head while slightly leaning backward), yet is not being exhibited by anyone in the room. It is quite likely that shortly, one or more others will assume the same posture. With babies, it is quite common that after one begins to cry, others will soon also start to cry. Having lived for many years in the southern United States, at times during my life, I have had a distinct southern accent, although this accent has now largely faded. However, I have often noted that after talking to my parents, who retain a strong southern accent, hints of my former accent return. All these examples illustrate the concept of a *contagion*. A contagion refers to behaviors, mannerisms, gestures, emotions, or attitudes that, after observing their expression in others, people tend to mimic.

Research by Fowler and Christakis (2008) illustrates the practical impact of contagions on our everyday perspectives of the world. Their research utilized data that were collected through the Framingham Heart Study, which involved extensive data collection from three generations of participants linked to one another as family, friends, and coworkers. Data were regularly collected from over 4000 subjects over several decades. Included in the surveys were several questions that asked individuals to rate various responses concerning their individual well-being, such as "I felt hopeful about the future," "I was happy," "I enjoyed life," and "I felt that I was just as good as other people."

The analysis by Fowler and Christakis found that happiness tended to cluster such that individuals who were happy tended to associate with other individuals who were happy. With a given individual, for every happy friend, his or her likelihood of being happy increased by 9%, whereas every unhappy friend decreased his or her likelihood of being happy by 7%. Furthermore, the contagion extended beyond one's immediate relationships. On average, an individual was 15% more likely to be happy if he or she were closely related to another happy person. Yet, an individual was 10% more likely to be happy if he or she was the friend of someone who was happy and 6% if one of his or her friends was friends with someone who was happy. It appeared that happiness operated as a contagion, much like a virus, spreading throughout networks of individuals linked through their social relationships.

These findings point to the influence that our awareness of the people around us can have on our perspective of the world. When the people around us perceive the world in a certain way and act accordingly, there is a certain propensity for us to take a similar perspective. This suggests that close social networks will have a tendency to produce homogeneity in the perceptual experiences of their constituents. In contrast, looser networks in which individuals freely come and go, bringing with them diverse perspectives, should result in less homogeneity. Accordingly, to the extent that we structure the world in which we live, choosing to affiliate with certain individuals and avoiding others, we set the stage for our own perceptual experiences. Likewise, in the design and management of systems, we create an environment that may lead to an organization assuming a certain personality, with the persistence of that personality being a function of the extent to which the organization is insular, with few outside interactions, or open to numerous diverse interactions with people from outside the organization.

Acknowledgments

Sandia National Laboratories is a multiprogram laboratory managed and operated by Sandia Corporation, a wholly owned subsidiary of Lockheed Martin Corporation, for the US Department of Energy's National Nuclear Security Administration under contract DE-AC04-94AL85000.

References

Ackerman, J., Nocera, C.C. and Bargh, J.A. (2010). Incidental haptic sensations influence social judgements and decisions. *Science, 328*(5986), 1712–1715.

Baylis, G.C., Rolls, E.T. and Leonard, C.M. (1987). Functional subdivisions of the temporal lobe neocortex. *Journal of Neuroscience, 7*, 330–342.

Berry, M.J., Brivanlou, I.H., Jordan, T.A. and Meister, M. (1999). Anticipation of moving stimuli by the retina. *Nature, 398*, 334–338.

Boff, K.R. and Lincoln, J.E. (1988). *Engineering Data Compendium: Human Perception and Performance*. Wright-Patterson Air Force Base, OH: Harry G. Armstrong Medical Research Laboratory.

Bracha, H.S. (2006). Human brain evolution and the "Neuroevolutionary Time-depth Principle:" Implications for the reclassification of fear-circuitry related traits in DSM-V and for studying resilience to warzone related post-traumatic stress disorder. *Progress in Neuro-Psychopharmacology and Biological Psychiatry, 30,* 827–853.

Brass, M., Bekkering, H., Wohlschlager, A. and Prinz, W. (2000). Compatibility between observed and executed finger movements: Comparing symbolic, spatial, and imitative cues. *Brain and Cognition, 44,* 124–143.

Brennan, S.E. (1985). The caricature generator. *Leonardo, 18,* 170–178.

Brown, J.L. (1975). *The Evolution of Behavior*. New York: Norton.

Buccino, G., Sato, M., Cattaneo, L., Roda, F. and Riggio, L. (2009). Broken affordances, broken objects: A TMS study. *Neuropsychologia, 47*(14), 3074–3078.

Busch, N.A., Dubois, J. and VanRullen, R. (2009). The phase of ongoing EEG oscillations predicts visual perception. *Journal of Neuroscience, 29,* 7869–7876.

Campbell, F.W. and Kulikowski, J.J. (1972). The visual evoked potential as a function of contrast of a grating pattern. *Journal of Physiology, 222,* 345–356.

Carlson, T., Alink, A., Tovar, D. and Kriegeskorte, N. (2012). The evolving representation of objects in the human brain. *Journal of Vision, 12*(9), 272.

Castelli, F., Happe, F., Frith, U. and Frith, C. (2000). Movement and mind: A functional imaging study of perception and interpretation of complex intentional movement patterns. *NeuroImage, 12*(3), 314–325.

Cervero, F. and Tattersall, J.E.H. (1987). Somatic and visceral sensory integration in the thoracic spinal cord. *Progress in Brain Research, 67,* 189–205.

Chao, L.L., Haxby, J.V. and Martin, A. (1999). Attribute-based neural substrates in temporal cortex for perceiving and knowing about objects. *Nature Neuroscience, 2,* 913–919.

Connolly, A.C., Guntupalli, S., Gors, J., Hanke, M., Halchenko, Y.O., Wu, Y.C., Abdi, H. and Haxby, J.V. (2012). The representation of biological classes in the human brain. *Journal of Neuroscience, 32*(8), 2608–2618.

Cook, M. and Mineka, S. (1989). Observational conditioning of fear to fear-relevant versus fear-irrelevant stimuli in rhesus monkeys. *Journal of Abnormal Psychology, 98,* 448–459.

Cook, M. and Mineka, S. (1990). Selective associations in the observational conditioning of fear in rhesus monkeys. *Journal of Experimental Psychology, Animal Behavior Processes, 16,* 372–389.

Costantini, M., Ambrosini, E., Scorolli, C. and Borghi, A.M. (2011). When objects are close to me: Affordances in the peripersonal space. *Psychonomic Bulletin and Review, 18*(2), 302–308.

Darwin, C. (1872). *The Expression of Emotion in Man and Animals*. London: Murray.

Department of Defense. (2012). Department of Defense Design Criteria Standard: Human Engineering, MIL STD 1472G.

Desimone, R. and Ungerleider, L.G. (1986). Multiple visual areas in the caudal superior temporal sulcus of the *macaque. Journal of Comparative Neurology, 248,* 164–189.

Dewdney, A.K. (1986). Computer recreations: The computer caricaturist and a whimsical tour of face space. *Scientific American, 255,* 20–28.

Dhamija, R., Tygar, J.D. and Hearst, M. (2006). Why phishing works. In *Proceedings of the Computer-Human Interactions Conference*, April 22–27, Montreal, Canada.

Di Pellegrino, G., Fadiga, L., Fogassi, L., Gallese, V. and Rizzolatti, G. (1992). Understanding motor events: A neurophysiological study. *Experimental Brain Research, 91*, 176–180.

Ekman, P. (1993). Facial expression and emotion. *American Psychologist, 48*(4), 384–392.

Enquist, M. and Arak, A. (1998). Neural representation and the evolution of signal form. In R. Dukus (ed.), *Cognitive Ecology: The Evolutionary Ecology of Information Processing and Decision Making*, pp. 21–87. Chicago IL: University of Chicago Press.

Ettlinger, G. (1990). Object vision and spatial vision: The neuropsychological evidence for the distinction. *Cortex, 26*, 319–341.

Falchier, A., Clavagnier, S., Barone, P. and Kennedy, H. (2000). Anatomical evidence of multimodal integration in primate striate cortex. *Journal of Neuroscience, 22*, 5749–5759.

Finney, E.M., Fine, I. and Dobkins, K.R. (2001). Visual stimuli activate auditory cortex in the deaf. *Nature Neuroscience, 4*(12), 1171–1173.

Fischer, M.H. and Dahl, C.D. (2007). The time course of visuo-motor affordances. *Experimental Brain Research, 176*, 519–524.

Fisher, H.E., Aron, A., Mashek, D., Li, H. and Brown, L.L. (2002). Defining the brain systems of lust, romantic attraction and attachment. *Archives of Sexual Behavior, 31*(5), 413–419.

Fowler, J.H. and Christakis, N.A. (2008). Dynamic spread of happiness in a large social network: Longitudinal analysis over 20 years in the Farmington Heart Study. *British Medical Journal, 337*, a2338.

Frassinetti, F., Pavani, F. and Ladavas, E. (2002). Acoustical vision of neglected stimuli: Interaction between spatially converging audiovisual inputs in neglect patients. *Journal of Cognitive Neuroscience, 14*(1), 62–69.

Gangitano, M., Mottaghy, F.M. and Pascual-Leone, A. (2001). Phase specific modulation of cortical motor output during movement observation. *NeuroReport, 12*, 1489–1492.

Ganis, G., Thompson, W.L. and Kosslyn, S.M. (2004). Brain areas underlying visual imagery and visual perception. An fMRI study. *Cognitive Brain Research, 20*, 226–241.

Gaser, C. and Schlaug, G. (2001). Brain structures differ between musicians and non-musicians. *NeuroImage, 13*, 1168.

Gibson, E.J. and Walk, R.D. (1960). The visual cliff. *Scientific American, 202*, 64–71.

Gibson, J.J. (1979). *The Ecological Approach to Visual Perception*. Boston: Houghton Mifflin.

Grunwald, T., Boutros, N.N., Pezer, N., von Oertzen, J., Fernandez, G., Schaller, C. and Elger, C.E. (2003). Neural substrates of sensory gating within the human brain. *Biological Psychiatry, 53*(6), 511–519.

Hakan, F., Tomas, F., Gustav, W. and Mats, F. (2000). Brain representation of habituation to repeated complex visual stimulation studied with PET. *NeuroReport, 11*(1), 123–126.

Hermann, C.S. and Bosch, V. (2001). Gestalt perception modulates early visual processing. *NeuroReport, 12*(5), 901–904.

Hickok, G. (2009). Eight problems for the mirror neuron theory of action understanding in monkeys and humans. *Journal of Cognitive Neuroscience, 21*(7), 1229–1243.

Hodos, W. and Butler, A.B. (1997). Evolution of sensory pathways in vertebrates. *Brain, Behavior and Evolution, 50*(4), 189–197.

Hubel, D.H. and Wiesel, T.N. (1959). Receptive fields of single neurons in the cat's striate cortex. *Journal of Physiology*, *148*(3), 574–591.

Hubel, D.H. and Wiesel, T.N. (1962). Receptive fields, binocular interaction and functional architecture in the cat's visual cortex. *Journal of Physiology*, *160*(1), 106–154.

Hugdahl, K., Berardi, A., Thompson, W.L., Kosslyn, S.M., Macy, R., Baker, D.P., Alpert, N.M. and LeDoux, J.E. (1995). Brain mechanisms in human classical conditioning: A PET blood flow study. *NeuroReport*, *6*, 1723–1728.

Hutt, C., von Bernuth, H., Lenard, H.G., Hutt, S.J. and Prechtl, H.E.R. (1968). Habituation in relation to state in the human neonate. *Nature*, *220*, 618–620.

Iacoboni, M., Woods, R.P., Brass, M., Bekkering, H., Mazziotta, J.C. and Rizzolatti, G. (1999). Cortical mechanisms of human imitation. *Science 286*(5449), 2526–2528.

Jagatic, T., Johnson, N. and Jakobsson, M. (2005). Phishing attacks using social networks. Indiana U. Human Subject Study 05-9892 and 05-9893.

James, K., James, T. and Swain, S. (2012). The neural correlates of object expertise in the young child. In *Annual Meeting of the Cognitive Neuroscience Society*, March 31–April 3, Chicago, IL.

Johansson, G. (1973). Visual perception of biological motion and a model for its analysis. *Perception and Psychophysics*, *14*, 201–211.

Jolla, C., Davis, A. and Haggard, P. (2011). Proprioceptive integration and body representation: Insights into dancers' expertise. *Experimental Brain Research*, *213*, 257–265.

Kadunce, D.C., Vaughan, J.W., Wallace, M.T., Benedek, G. and Stein, B.E. (1997). Mechanisms of within and cross-modality suppression in the superior colliculus. *Journal of Neurophysiology*, *78*(6), 2834–2847.

Kan, I.P., Barsalou, L.W., Solomon, K.O., Minor, J.K. and Thompson-Shill, S.L. (2003). Role of mental imagery in a property verification task: fMRI evidence for perceptual representations of conceptual knowledge. *Cognitive Neuropsychology*, *20*(3), 525–540.

Keil, A., Muller, M.M., Ray, W.J., Gruber, T. and Elbert, T. (1999). Human gamma band activity and the perception of a Gestalt. *Journal of Neuroscience*, *19*(16), 7152–7161.

Kendler, K.S., Myers, J., Prescott, C.A. and Neale, M.C. (2001). The genetic epidemiology of irrational fears and phobias in men. *Archives of General Psychiatry*, *58*, 257–265.

Krubizer, L. (2007). The magnificent compromise: Cortical field evolution in mammals. *Neuron*, *56*(2), 201–208.

LeBlanc, S.A. and Register, K.E. (2003). *Constant Battles: The Myth of the Peaceful, Noble Savage*. New York: St Marten's.

Lee, M.C., Zambreanu, L., Menon, D.K. and Tracey, I. (2008). Identifying brain activity specifically related to the maintenance and perceptual consequence of central sensitization in humans. *Journal of Neuroscience*, *28*(45), 11642–11649.

Lewis, J.W. and Van Essen, D.C. (2000). Corticocortical connections of visual sensorimotor and multimodal processing areas in the parietal lobe of the macaque monkey. *Journal of Comparative Neurology*, *428*, 112–137.

Linden, M.H., Turennout, M.I. and Fernandez, G.S.E. (2011). Category training induces cross-modal object representations in the adult human brain. *Journal of Cognitive Neuroscience*, *23*(6), 1315–1331.

Loveless, N.E., Brebner, J. and Hamilton, P. (1970). Bisensory presentation of information. *Psychological Bulletin*, *73*, 161–199.

Martin, A., Wiggs, C.L., Ungerleider, L.G. and Haxby, J.V. (1996). Neural correlates of category-specific knowledge. *Nature*, *379*, 649–652.

Massaro, D.W. and Stork, D.G. (1998). Speech recognition and sensory integration: A 240-year-old theorem helps explain how people and machines can integrate auditory and visual information to understand speech. *American Scientist*, *86*(3), 236–244.

Masterton, B., Heffner, H. and Ravizza, R. (1969). The evolution of human hearing. *Journal of the Acoustical Society of America*, *45*(4), 966–985.

Mathewson, K.E., Gratton, G., Fabiani, M., Beck, D.M. and Ro, T. (2009). To see or not to see: Prestimulus alpha phase predicts visual awareness. *Journal of Neuroscience*, *29*, 2725–2732.

McBride, D. and Schmorrow, D. (2005). *Quantifying Human Information Processing*. Oxford: Lexington.

McCarthy, G., Puce, A., Gore, J.C. and Allison, T. (1997). Face-specific processing in the human fusiform gyrus. *Journal of Cognitive Neuroscience*, *9*(5), 605–610.

McGurk, H. and MacDonald, J. (1976). Hearing lips and seeing voices. *Nature*, *264*, 746–748.

Mesulam, M. and Mufson, E.J. (1982). Insula of the old world monkey. III: Different cortical output and comments on function. *Journal of Comparative Neurology*, *212*, 38–52.

Meyer, K., Kaplan, J.T., Essex, R., Webber, C., Damasio, H. and Damasio, A. (2010). Predicting visual stimuli on the basis of activity in auditory cortices. *Nature Neuroscience*, *13*, 667–668.

Moutoussis, K. and Zeki, S. (2002). The relationship between cortical activation and perception investigated with invisible stimuli. *Proceedings of the National Academy of Science*, *99*(14), 9527–9532.

Mummery, C.J., Patterson, K., Hodges, J.R. and Wise, R.J. (1996). Generating "tiger" as an animal name or a word beginning with "t": Differences in brain activation. *Proceedings of the Royal Society of London—Series B: Biological Sciences*, *263*, 989–995.

Naatanen, R., Paavilainen, P., Alho, K., Reinikainen, K. and Sams, M. (1989). Do event-related potentials reveal the mechanisms for the auditory sensory memory in the human brain? *Neuroscience Letters*, *98*(2), 217–221.

Nauhaus, I., Busse, L., Carandini, M. and Ringach, D.L. (2008). Stimulus contrast modulates functional connectivity in the visual cortex. *Nature Neuroscience*, *12*, 70–76.

Neuling, T., Rach, S., Hermann, C. and von Ossietzky, C. (2012). Oscillatory phase shapes auditory perception. In *Annual Meeting of the Cognitive Neuroscience Society*, March 31–April 3, Chicago, IL.

Niven, J.E. and Laughlin, S.B. (2008). Energy limitation as a selective pressure on the evolution of sensory systems. *Journal of Experimental Biology*, *211*, 1792–1804.

O'Craven, K.M. and Kanwisher, N. (2000). Mental imagery of faces and places activates corresponding stimulus-specific brain regions. *Journal of Cognitive Neuroscience*, *12*(6), 1013–1023.

Orban, G.A., Kennedy, H. and Maes, H. (1981). Response to movement of neurons in areas 17 and 18 of the cat: Velocity sensitivity. *Journal of Neurophysiology*, *45*(6), 1043–1058.

Pasley, B.N., Mayes, L.C. and Schultz, R.T. (2004). Subcortical discrimination of unperceived objects during binocular rivalry. *Neuron*, *42*(1), 163–172.

Potts, R. (1998). Environmental hypotheses of *Hominin* evolution. *Yearbook of Physical Anthropology, 41,* 93–136.

Poulton, R., Davies, S., Menzies, R.G., Langley, R.D. and Silva, P.A. (1998). Evidence for a non-associative model of the acquisition of a fear of heights. *Behaviour Research and Therapy, 36*(5), 537–544.

Ress, D. and Heeger, D.J. (2003). Neural correlates of perception in early visual cortex. *Nature Neuroscience, 6*(4), 414–421.

Ridley, M. (1993). *The Red Queen, Sex and the Evolution of Human Nature.* London: Penguin.

Rizzolatti, G. and Craighero, L. (2004). The mirror neuron system. *Annual Review of Neuroscience, 27,* 169–192.

Robinson, T.E. and Berridge, K.C. (1993). The neural basis of drug craving: An incentive-sensitization theory of addiction. *Brain Research Reviews, 18*(3), 247–291.

Rochat, P., Morgan, R. and Carpenter, M. (1997). Young infants' sensitivity to movement information specifying social causality. *Cognitive Development, 12*(4), 537–561.

Russeler, J., Altenmüller, E., Nager, W., Kohlmetz, C. and Munte, T.F. (2001). Event-related brain potentials to sound omissions differ in musicians and non-musicians. *Neuroscience Letters, 308,* 33–36.

Sadato, N., Okada, T., Honda, M. and Yonekura, Y. (2002). Critical period for cross-modal plasticity in blind humans. A functional fMRI study. *NeuroImage, 16,* 389–400.

Salvendy, G. (1997). *Handbook of Human Factors and Ergonomics.* New York: Wiley.

Samuels, J., Bienvenu, O.J., Riddle, M.A., Cullen, B.A.M., Grados, M.A., Liang, K.Y., Hoehn-Saric, R. and Nestadt, G. (2002). Hoarding in obsessive compulsive disorder: Results from a case-control study. *Behaviour Research and Therapy, 40*(5), 517–528.

Schiff, W. (1965). The perception of impending collision: A study of visually directed avoidant behavior. *Psychological Monographs, 79,* 1–26.

Schroeder, C.E. and Foxe, J.J. (2002). The timing and laminar profile of converging inputs to multisensory areas of the macaque neocortex. *Cognitive Brain Research, 14,* 187–198.

Small, D.M., Voss, J., Mak, Y.E., Simmons, K.B., Parrish, T. and Gitelman, D. (2004). Experience-dependent neural integration of taste and smell in the human brain. *Journal of Neurophysiology, 92*(3), 1892–1903.

Spitzer, M., Kwong, K.K., Kennedy, W., Rosen, B.R. and Belliveau, J.W. (1995). Category-specific brain activation in fMRI during picture naming. *NeuroReport, 6*(16), 2109–2112.

Stam, R. (2007). PTSD and stress sensitization: A tale of brain and body: Part I: Human studies. *Neuroscience and Biobehavioral Reviews, 31*(4), 530–557.

Stein, B.E. and Meredith, M.A. (1993). *Merging of the Senses.* Cambridge, MA: MIT Press.

Stein, B.E., Meredith, M.A., Honeycutt, W.S. and McDade, L. (1989). Behavioral indices of multisensory integration: Orientation to visual cues is affected by auditory stimuli. *Journal of Cognitive Neuroscience, 1,* 12–24.

Talsma, D. and Woldorff, M.G. (2005). Selective attention and multisensory integration: Multiple phases of effects on the evoked brain activity. *Journal of Cognitive Neuroscience, 17*(7), 1098–1114.

Thompson-Schill, S.L. (2003). Neuroimaging studies of semantic memory: Inferring "how" from "where." *Neuropschologia, 41,* 280–292.

Todd, J.W. (1912). Reaction to multiple stimuli. *Archives of Psychology, 3*, 1–65.

Turner, B., Mishkin, M. and Knapp, M. (1980). Organization of the amygdalopetal projections from modality-specific cortical association areas in the monkey. *Journal of Comparative Neurology, 191*, 515–543.

van Dijk, H., Schoffelen, J.M., Oostenveld, R. and Jensen, O. (2008). Prestimulus oscillatory activity in the alpha band predicts visual discrimination ability. *Journal of Neuroscience, 28*, 1816–1823.

Vuillerme, N. and Nougier, V. (2004). Attentional demand for regulating postural sway: The effect of expertise in gymnastics. *Brain Research Bulletin, 63*(2), 161–165.

Vuillerme, N., Teasdale, N. and Nougier, V. (2001). The effect of expertise in gymnastics on proprioceptive sensory integration in human subjects. *Neuroscience Letters, 311*(2), 73–76.

Watson, J.D.G., Myers, R., Frackowiack, R.S.J., Hajnal, J.V., Woods, R.P., Mazziotta, J.C., Shipp, S. and Zeki, S. (1993). Area V5 of the human brain: Evidence from a combined study using positron emission tomography and magnetic resonance imaging. *Cerebral Cortex, 3*(2), 79–94.

Woods, A.T., Poliakoff, E., Lloyd, D., Kuenzel, J., Hodson, R., Gonda, H., Batchelor, J., Dijksterhuis, G. and Thomas, A. (2010). Effect of background noise on food perception. In *Proceedings of the 11th International Multisensory Research Forum*, June 16–19, Liverpool UK.

Wyart, V. and Sergent, C. (2009). The phase of ongoing EEG oscillations uncovers the fine temporal structure of conscious perception. *Journal of Neuroscience, 29*(41), 12839–12841.

5

Strengths and Weaknesses

You have just received a new board game. It is called The Mind Game. The instructions state that the objective of the game is quite simple. You must solve problems to allow you to get things and to do things that bring pleasure, while avoiding pain and discomfort. Reading further, you see that all work is done within a workspace that can hold seven items, although sometimes you can squeeze in one or two more items and at other times the workspace will hold only five or six items. It depends on the complexity of the items and other factors that might enhance or detract from your performance. Items come into the workspace one at a time and if you do not take steps to maintain them, they exit the workspace, generally without you knowing it. Most of the time, you can only do one operation at a time, although there are some occasions when you may be able to do a couple of operations simultaneously. In solving problems, you will use items stored in a warehouse. The warehouse has an infinite capacity for storing items, although when items come out of the warehouse, they are often not quite the same as when they went into the warehouse. Furthermore, your ability to find a specific item in the warehouse will vary. Sometimes, it is easy. Sometimes, it is hard. And at other times, if you wait a little while, an item you are currently unable to locate can be easily found.

The Mind Game reflects the daily challenges faced by all of us as we make our way through life. There are some things that brains do remarkably well, yet there are other ways in which brains are quite limited. The limitations of the brain are well illustrated by a study in which subjects were placed in a room with lights embedded in the floor and they were asked to find which of 20 lights was the target for that trial (Longstaffe et al., 2012). The subjects were given no clues as to which light was the target and they could move freely around the room selecting lights. In this case, the problem was to find which of the 20 lights was the target. After making an incorrect guess, the subjects had to remember their selection so that they did not choose the same light again. Consequently, their performance depended on their ability to remember which lights had and had not been selected. However, two other factors were introduced that affected their performance. First, some of the lights flashed on and off, making them more salient. The subjects were attracted to the flashing lights and tended to choose them, even though the likelihood of a light being the target was the same for flashing and nonflashing lights. Furthermore, on some trials, subjects were given a five-digit number to remember. The five-digit number would have consumed much of their workspace. Likewise, to the extent that the flashing lights captured the subjects' attention, this would have consumed more of their available workspace. The results showed that when the subjects had to remember the five-digit number, they were much more susceptible to the allure of the flashing lights. Yet, the allure of the flashing lights vanished when the subjects either did not need to remember the five-digit number or did not need to remember which lights they had already selected (i.e., lights were no longer illuminated after being selected).

This study illustrates the limitations of the brain's workspace and how our susceptibility to external factors (i.e., the flashing lights) varies with the demands that are being placed on the workspace. The demands that the experimenters imposed on the subjects in this study are analogous to those faced by individuals working in many occupations. This could be radar operators who must allocate their attention to different contacts or forensic analysts who must divvy up their time as they investigate different cases or instructors who must decide which of their students gets their assistance. In any of these situations, there is a need to remember how one's attention has been distributed and where it may be needed. However, the equivalent of the flashing lights may also be faced. Some items may have a natural tendency to attract one's attention, whereas other items may tend to drift into the shadows. For example, in a classroom, some students may be naturally gregarious, drawing much of the instructor's attention; being charismatic, they may also be favored, with the additional attention coming at the expense of more reserved students. Furthermore, there may be additional demands that have the effect of making the flashing lights more difficult to resist. When struggling with a malfunctioning piece of classroom equipment, it is likely that the gregarious student is the only one who will receive any of the instructor's attention. In each of these situations, individuals must struggle to cope with their ability to only focus on a few items at any given time, while contending with various extraneous factors that make it even more challenging.

The strengths and weaknesses of the human brain are most apparent in the conscious thought processes that underlie everyday problem solving. It may be argued that the greatest strength of the human brain is its seemingly endless capacity for storing information within memory. This applies to our capacity for remembering factual knowledge, or what is sometimes referred to as declarative knowledge. This capacity is evidenced when playing games of trivia that call on players to recall obscure facts, many of which they have not thought about for years. With respect to life experiences, or our episodic memory, we do not retain a perfect record, but we do retain enough information from our everyday experiences that we can easily reconstruct countless episodes from our past. We are constantly acquiring new skills as we engage in activities or familiarize ourselves with new devices. On average, a 5-year-old, English-speaking child has a vocabulary of approximately 1,500 words that by adulthood will balloon to around 10,000 words and continue to grow as he or she grows older. Finally, our perceptual knowledge encompasses all the various objects, people, places, and so on that one can distinguish, whether one has had direct perceptual experience or the experience has occurred secondhand (e.g., books, television, and movies). Each of these examples illustrates the seemingly endless capacity of the human brain to store information it has attained during a lifetime that, while often not perfect, can be later retrieved and applied in solving current problems.

The inverse or most prominent weakness of the human brain is its limited capacity for conscious awareness. Granted, the vast majority of information processing occurs at an unconscious level within the brain; however, this is largely inaccessible. Unconscious processes may impact our decisions and affect our reactions to different situations, but we generally have no awareness of what information has been processed or how that information has influenced our conscious thought processes. Our capacity for conscious thought, whether this involves our attention to the world around us, our deliberative problem solving, or our voluntary control of bodily activities, is severely limited. We can closely attend to only one thing at a time and our attention quickly wavers when there are distractions. Likewise, we can only keep a limited number of items immediately accessible in our memory, and some level of effort is necessary to sustain the immediacy of items within our memory for more than a few seconds. The effort required to retain items in working memory increases as one attempts to retain more items, with this increased effort evidenced in the increased activation of the prefrontal executive regions of the brain (Rypma and D'Esposito, 1999).

Unless an activity is well practiced (e.g., driving an automobile), it is difficult to do more than one thing at a time. While our brains are constantly active in responding to a broad range of stimuli, we have an extremely limited capacity to voluntarily engage and intentionally direct our brain processes, whether the goals involve mental or physical activities. It is difficult for our brains to do more than one thing at a time, and we sometimes struggle to do one thing when it is complex and we are distracted.

How to Cope with the Inherent Weaknesses of the Human Brain

Consider what happens when we call on our memory. The areas engaged when recalling information from memory are distributed across many different regions of the brain. A given memory may encompass different elements that include location, people, time, activities, and perceptual and emotional experiences, with each element of the memory associated with neural processes that are distributed across different areas of the brain. These localized neural processes involve the synchronous oscillations of brain cells within a given area of the brain. Our experience of a memory in which all the various elements are integrated into a coherent recollection requires that the different regions of the brain oscillate in a coordinated fashion (Watrous et al., 2013). The extent to which there is coordinated activity of the different brain regions appears to underlie whether or not we are able to successfully recall what we are trying to remember. A successful recollection corresponds to the activity of assemblies of brain cells within diverse brain regions oscillating at approximately the same frequency, or some harmonic of one another, with the transfer and integration of information facilitated by the coherence of the oscillations. The successful operation of the brain requires that many different elements operate in coordination with one another. Consequently, it is easy to imagine how the slightest disturbance (e.g., an emotionally significant event) can upset the balance, rendering ineffective our capacity to access our memory stores. Many people have had the experience of going blank when faced with the stress of taking an important test or presenting in front of a large audience. Yet, generally, the brain is remarkably robust, successfully calling on memory on a moment-to-moment basis as we accomplish various activities. More often than not, the brain gets it right and does so in an efficient manner, making human memory the envy of scientists and engineers who long for the capacity to duplicate its capabilities in similarly compact computer hardware.

How do we cope with the inherent weaknesses of the brain and, in particular, our inability to attend to more than a slender slice of the world around us at any given moment? In general, we play to our strengths, with perhaps our greatest strength being our seemingly endless capacity for memory. There are many mechanisms, most of which we rarely think about due to the extent to which they are embedded in our everyday behavior and, in some cases, institutionalized within the cultures in which we live. The following sections describe some of these mechanisms.

Routines or Habits

Often without realizing it, our lives can become so routinized that we hardly have to think about what we are doing. It is not until something breaks our routines that we can truly appreciate the extent to which our lives consist of a series of well-learned patterns of behavior. The neural circuits that underlie the ritualistic behavioral routines seen in many animal species (e.g., the courtship dance of a bird or the depositing and fertilization of eggs seen in fish) reside within a region of the brain known as the basal ganglia. In humans, these same circuits are co-opted in the formation of habits (Graybiel, 2008). Except that, in humans, routines arise and adapt to ongoing circumstances with tremendous fluidity. Furthermore, in humans, routines can go beyond simple motor routines to include habits of thought or the tendency to gravitate toward a certain cognitive perspective or problem-solving strategy. For example, within engineering domains, one regularly encounters the habit of thought characterized by the expression, "a hammer looking for a nail." This expression describes the tendency that once one has a clever technical solution to one problem, there is an inclination to overgeneralize and apply the same solution to other less applicable problems. Here, a pattern of thought has become a routine, not unlike the route taken when driving to work each morning, and the individual applies that same pattern of thought, regardless of its appropriateness to the immediate situation.

The link between the expression of habits and the basal ganglia lies in the specialization of these neural circuits for iteratively evaluating situations and matching situations to known sequences of actions or cognitive operations (Graybiel, 2008). I once worked with a subject-matter expert with many years of experience in assault teams with the military and law enforcement, who used the analogy of a Rolodex (i.e., a cardholder where one can rotate through a series of cards to find the one with the desired information). He said that when he was presented with a situation, he quickly surveyed it to gain a general sense of the environment, characters, and events that had transpired, and once he had seen a pattern, it was like flipping through a rolodex to find the card that contained the instructions for what to do in that situation. This analogy offers a nice depiction of how the basal ganglia operates, with our everyday lives consisting of a series of situational appraisals occurring both consciously and unconsciously. Our reliance on routines leverages the capacity of our brains to store vast collections of routines, with many continually evolving to become increasingly more elaborate over time. This relieves us from the in-depth, moment-to-moment analysis that would otherwise be required. The result is that our brains are free to attend to other considerations, or perhaps to merely daydream. It is through our basal ganglia and its capacity for quickly sizing up a situation and identifying the appropriate learned behavior, that routines and habits offer a mechanism by which we play to the strength of our brains to learn and retain a seemingly limitless collection of behavioral sequences and cognitive operations.

Conventions

When presented with a new device or placed in an unfamiliar situation, the conscious effort that is required to recognize and learn the appropriate behavior, whether sequences for activating controls or expected or generally agreed on activities, can be all-consuming, preventing one from doing anything else or sometimes even enjoying the experience. Within nearly every human endeavor, there are conventions that serve to ensure consistency of expectations and behavior. Depending on the country, everyone travels on either the right or the left side of the roadway, with this convention extending to pathways, stairways, and escalators. With devices, one expects that turning a control knob to the right will increase whatever feature the knob controls. Within the home, there may be conventions such as where different items are placed within the refrigerator or how to make a certain type of sandwich. As with routines, our brains have an unlimited capacity to learn various conventions, and often do so implicitly with little conscious effort. Then, once one has learned the conventions, there is little need to devote much thought to what to do. The conventions become deeply engrained and are exercised almost reflexively. Conventions not only free cognitive resources, they also create efficiencies and enable possibilities that would not be possible otherwise. I believe that the power of conventions is perhaps best illustrated by the German autobahn. German drivers seem naturally inclined to rigorously adhere to the rules of the road. It is through this compliance with agreed on conventions that I believe it becomes possible to have roadways where there can be a 40–50 mph difference in the speeds of vehicles driving in adjacent lanes, with surprisingly few accidents.

Vocabulary

Whenever one must operate within a new domain, for example, an occupation, sport, or academic discipline, one cannot hope to be effective until the vocabulary or jargon of the domain has been learned. Jargon has the capacity to capture complex ideas within a single word or phrase. This can be similarly seen with acronyms, where a complex title or phrase is reduced to letters spelling a word that can be easily recalled. The chunking that occurs with both jargon and acronyms serves to allow individuals to communicate, as well as to think, using units that have a much greater information content or density. As a result, those familiar with the jargon of a given domain are able to communicate more efficiently. I have observed this in research where we found that experts in a given domain tend to communicate substantially less (i.e., number of utterances and duration of utterances) than novices (Lakkaraju et al., 2011). Communication generally consumes much of our conscious awareness, making it difficult to do anything else effectively. In achieving more efficient communication through the use of jargon, which relies on the capacity to learn and retain an extensive vocabulary, one lessens the demands imposed by communication, freeing resources to focus on other activities.

Symbols and Icons

Pictorial representations, such as the icons that are used to depict the location of a restroom or a computer's trash folder, operate similar to jargon in that they allow complex information to be engrained within a simple image. Similarly, the result is to achieve a relatively high level of information density. Symbols and icons also benefit from their familiarity, especially those that attain some degree of universality such that people from different backgrounds can look at them and recognize their meaning. With a familiar icon, once one has learned the symbol, this knowledge translates across situations, devices, and, often, cultures, with the associated conceptual knowledge becoming engrained within the perceptual representation (Barsalou et al., 2003).

Retrace Steps

In getting around the world, people can often be creatures of habit. Once individuals have found a route that takes them to a destination, it is not uncommon that they will continually retrace their steps, following the same route on subsequent journeys, without considering whether there is a more practical option. Interestingly, in navigating the Internet, as well as computer software interfaces, the same behavior occurs. A person will follow the same sequence of links that he or she followed when first finding a webpage, as opposed to taking advantage of the ability to go directly to the webpage by bookmarking it or using the automatic fill-in feature of the browser's address bar. Similarly, once a person has found a useful feature within a software user interface that is several layers below the surface, often, he or she will continue to navigate through the menu layers to find it, instead of using shortcuts to directly access the feature.

When navigating physical or virtual space, our brains construct a map with the route and the various landmarks that are encountered along the way (Ekstrom et al., 2003). It can be demanding to contemplate the physical layout of a city, park, or building to identify and assess alternative routes for traveling from one location to another. Then, once you have set out on an unfamiliar path, there is the need to confirm that the route that is being taken corresponds to the intended route. Furthermore, there may be unexpected obstacles along the way, forcing you to rethink your route. In contrast, while perhaps not optimal, by retracing your steps, there is the opportunity to rely on your memory of a given path. Thus, there is no need to devote resources to route planning, and since you have seen everything along the way at least once, the presence of familiar landmarks and surroundings serves to verify that you are on the intended route. By taking a familiar path, one is freed of the cognitive demands of tracing a new path, and the uncertainty of an unknown route with the accompanying need to monitor progress along the way and potentially reassess the route if faced with unexpected obstructions.

Favor the Familiar

While stimulating, novelty can be demanding, particularly when one must make a choice. Furthermore, with novel selections, one inevitably incurs some risk. Thus, it is not surprising that people adopt routines in which they return to the same restaurants or stores, and are often reluctant to venture out to try new establishments. With any business or product, one of the greatest challenges involves inducing potential customers to come in for the first time or to make their first purchase. Most of us are quite familiar with the experience of driving by a restaurant that seems interesting from its external appearance, yet never actually stopping to try the restaurant. People naturally favor the familiar, often accepting suboptimal returns to avoid the risk of the unknown. While favoring the familiar allows one to avert risks, it also lessens the cognitive demands associated with an activity. When one visits a familiar restaurant, skims the menu, and selects a favorite dish, one is freed from the demands associated with studying an unfamiliar list of options and weighing these options to make one's selection. When one shops for groceries in another country where there are the same products but few of the same brands, it can be like going grocery shopping for the first time. You may know what you want, yet it takes some mental effort to match these wants with an array of unfamiliar products. In our everyday lives, we are constantly drawn to familiar products, establishments, people, and so on, and in doing so, we rely on our memory of past experiences to make our choices easy and to allow us to focus our cognitive resources on other facets of our lives.

Infer Rules

With most endeavors, there are simple rules or heuristics that one may learn to make one's experience more efficient and productive. For example, by leaving 30 min later, one may encounter substantially less traffic on the way to work. By delaying one's purchase of a new product, one may avoid many of the defects that will be discovered and corrected during the first few months after the product's release. We are constantly assessing situations to try and deduce rules of this nature. The result is that once an effective rule has been identified, thereafter it may be applied without much further thought. While the optimal solution may be to assess situations anew on each occasion, having a rule that regularly provides a satisfactory solution, although perhaps not the best solution, frees one from the demands of considering the unique circumstances of each occurrence and the subsequent demands of coordinating a strategy that is tailored to the immediate circumstances.

Chunking

In transporting apples, one could handle one apple at a time or put them in cases and move them one case at a time. Similarly, much of the information that people contend with on a day-to-day basis can be processed one item at a time or in larger chunks. A familiar example occurs with counting. It is much more efficient to count by fives or tens than to count one item at a time. With various activities, opportunities exist to process information in chunks, with individual chunks involving some level of abstraction or casting aside unnecessary details. One relies on memory for knowledge that each chunk represents a certain set of individual items, with it being much less demanding to operate with chunks than to individually process each item.

Designating to Our Strengths

These are only a few of the mechanism that people regularly employ to minimize the demands for real-time cognitive processing. In each case, there is a reliance on memory. The primary mechanism by which people cope with their limited ability for real-time cognitive operations is to play to their strengths, with their primary strength being an essentially boundless capacity to store information in their memory.

In the design of systems, through careful analysis of the tasks to be performed, situations may be identified that impose demands on real-time cognitive processes. Left to their own devices, operators will devise their own mechanisms for coping with these demands, with it likely that these coping strategies will involve derivatives of the mechanisms described in the preceding sections. Some of these solutions may be quite awkward. For example, a control room may be littered with ancillary electronic devices (e.g., handheld calculators) that allow operators to perform tasks using equipment and software products with which they are familiar. Within the design of any relatively complex system, there will be points that exceed the capacity for operators, users, or customers to cope through real-time processing. Thoughtful design acknowledges this reality and accommodates the mechanisms that people commonly employ to cope with demanding situations.

The majority of the activities that a person engages in may be organized into a few categories, and systems designed around these categories. This provides opportunities for the formation of a basic set of routines that encompasses most activities. For example, clerical workers may repeatedly receive the same requests. Consequently, routines may be facilitated through forms that capture the essential information for each requester in a common format, procedures that allow common requests to be similarly processed, and the layout of offices to accommodate sequential activities and segregate unrelated activities. Invariably, people will establish routines to aid them in performing frequent activities. Recognizing this fact, designers may incorporate mechanisms to accommodate and facilitate these routines.

Most designers are attentive to common conventions (e.g., controls should rotate clockwise to increase a quantity and people walk and drive on the right in the United States and many other nations). However, within the home and the workplace, people regularly adopt idiosyncratic conventions that represent their own preferred organization of objects and activities.

One of the insights that arose during my personal experience in designing and assessing systems for which there exist the potential for critical, high-consequence events is that not all activities are created equally or should be treated equally. For some activities, there is no tolerance for variability from one instance to another. In these cases, it is important that the activity be performed in the same way every time. Often, through various engineering design solutions, the opportunity for deviations in the performance of these activities can be essentially eliminated, with written procedures and training used to further ensure compliance. For example, a mechanical stop may be inserted to reduce the potential for overtightening bolts and crushing critical components.

With most actions, there is tremendous tolerance for variability. It may not matter if workers perform a set of steps in varied sequences, if people layout items differently, or if each individual uses his or her own unique vocabulary. In these cases, no matter how a competent person conducts the activity, it is unlikely that the outcome will differ in any significant way. Where there is tolerance for variability, it can be assumed that people and often teams will develop their own idiosyncratic conventions. For example, workers may carry their own preferred set of tools in their work belt and organize them in a way that makes most sense or is most comfortable for them. For these situations, where safety and operational performance do not depend on conformity, design may accommodate individual variability. Shelves, storage containers, workbenches, and so on may be made adjustable or perhaps portable. Within software, users may be allowed to arrange their desktop how they wish and create their own shortcuts. Businesses may allow customers to wander freely and check out at a time and a location that is most convenient for them. People will expect adherence to certain conventions, but where there is tolerance for variability, there is an opportunity to allow individuals to experiment and to adopt the conventions that make most sense to them.

Design features that allow or encourage personalization enable idiosyncratic conventions. This can be seen with music playlists that allow users to select the songs that they want to hear in combination with one another and in the order in which they want to hear them. It suits the taste of the individual who created the playlist and perhaps others who share the individual's musical preferences, but it may not generalize beyond a relatively small group of individuals. Many activities occur within social contexts that vary in their acceptance of idiosyncratic conventions and, particularly, idiosyncrasies that deviate from the norm. For many activities that occur within a social context, effective communication is vital to their success. Idiosyncratic conventions often occur in the vocabulary and symbology that are adopted by individuals and teams, which may directly affect communication. An individual may refer to a certain operation or activity that is unpleasant but necessary as "taking out the trash," with this reference subsequently adopted by other members of his or her team. However, others will not understand and may misinterpret the expression. In fact, learning the idiosyncratic vocabulary and symbology (e.g., hand gestures) of a team may serve as a barrier to newcomers, delaying their effective integration into the group.

Vocabulary and symbology both serve communicative functions. As discussed earlier with respect to conventions, within a given operation there will be varying tolerance for variability in vocabulary and symbology. There will be points where effective communication requires that there is essentially no variability, with everyone using exactly the same vocabulary and perhaps even verbal inflection, and the same symbology. Likewise, there will be other points where there is tolerance for variability and little or no loss of efficiency associated with the idiosyncratic use of terms and symbols. As with routines and conventions, a vocabulary and symbology will naturally emerge. It is important for the designer to recognize those points where there is little or no tolerance for variability and those points where individuals and teams may develop their own terms and symbols. Where there is no tolerance, the vocabulary and symbology should be consistent throughout every facet of the operation (i.e., labeling, written procedures, and training). In contrast, where there is tolerance for variability, it may be desirable for the material elements of the system to be consistent so that there is a common reference (e.g., physical labels), yet adherence to a common vocabulary or symbology should not be a requirement for the system to function effectively. For example, the software algorithms that are used with search engines often employ some degree of fuzziness so that when a user enters one term (e.g., home repair businesses), the search returns results for related terms (e.g., plumbers and electricians).

Similarly, fuzziness may be incorporated into the design of organizations. Several years ago, I read a story about a company in Silicon Valley where the president had instituted a policy whereby the employees were expected to create their own job titles. While some chose titles that were silly, even narcissistic, most of the job titles described meaningful roles and responsibilities that also corresponded to the culture and the unique ways in which the company operated. Here, the system could tolerate individual variability and the company used this opportunity to allow its employees to create a vocabulary that was meaningful to them.

While it may not be optimal for people to retrace their steps, they will inevitably do so and there are measures that designers can take to facilitate retracing a previous path. This is true whether one is traveling through physical space or the virtual space of the Internet or software products. One approach is to capture a history of traversals through a system, with this history then serving as a reference when later retracing one's path. This occurs within Internet browsers that highlight links that have previously been selected. While the highlighting does not explicitly map the path that was previously taken, it does offer landmarks that can be used to reconstruct the path. The designer has fewer opportunities within physical space. However, useful landmarks may be provided by placing distinct, memorable features at key junctions and locations. This is done in the parking lots at theme parks, such as Disneyland, where otherwise indistinguishable sections of the lots are named after memorable characters from Disney movies. In buildings, hallways may be painted different colors. Within buildings, parks, and cities, signs may be regularly placed along frequented corridors that indicate one's current location and the direction of other recognizable destinations. It is assumed that when a person initially travels from one location to another, he or she will construct a mental map that contains information concerning the path taken and key landmarks along the way. The designer can facilitate the construction of a meaningful map and the later use of that map to retrace one's path by situating distinct, memorable landmarks at key locations.

In some circumstances, the designer will want to create a sense of familiarity and take advantage of the tendency to favor the familiar. In other cases, the designer may be concerned that if allowed to follow familiar routines, people will become complacent or bored, with there being the need to encourage people to explore new ideas and consider different choices. People will not only favor the familiar, but if asked to rate alternatives on some valued attribute (e.g., which chocolate bar is tastier or which city has the most people), they will select the most familiar option (Gigerenzer and Todd, 1999). Where it is advantageous for people to favor the familiar, the designer must ensure that his or her product is recognized and associated with familiar experiences. This can be accomplished through distinguishable packaging and placement; the use of memorable names and slogans; and recognizable features such as layouts, menus, uniforms, and procedures. With popular fast-food restaurants, a comfortable familiarity is created through a distinct yet consistent exterior and interior design; menus that look similar and contain the same selections; and procedures for ordering, receiving, and paying for an order that are the same from one location to another. On many occasions, I have personally made the decision to eat at a restaurant knowing that I would not get a great meal, but having some certainty that my meal would be satisfactory. The end result may have been less optimal, but by favoring the familiar, I assured myself of some degree of predictability and incurred less mental effort.

However, with predictability there can also be complacency. This is particularly worrisome where safety is an issue. When activities become too familiar, there is a tendency to consciously disengage, resulting in a failure to recognize signs of impending dangers. For example, the ferry operator who makes the same routine transit on numerous occasions every day, may fail to recognize a gradually worsening fuel leak or may fail to adjust his or her speed in response to reduced visibility on a hazy or stormy day. There is an analogy to skiing or sledding. Going down a snow-covered hill, ruts will begin to form and one will naturally be drawn to those ruts. While the snow is plentiful, these can be ideal for a fast, effortless glide down the hill. But as the snow thins, rocks or other hazards may become exposed within the ruts, yet until one makes an effort to carve out a new path, one will be continually drawn to the path with the ruts and the accompanying hazards. A familiar operation is analogous to ruts in the snow. Once learned, it may be the easiest and most effective way to do things. However, because of this familiarity, one may ignore developing hazards or even disregard them as one enjoys the mental disengagement that comes with familiarity.

It is a challenge for the designer to balance the trade-off between the efficiencies that come with a familiar routine and the risk of complacency. With facility security, this is often accomplished by regularly rotating assignments. An individual may often work at a given checkpoint, but rotate between different checkpoints on a daily basis. Consequently, the experiences of security personnel vary somewhat from one day to the next. While care must be taken to avoid incurring undue risks, in general it can be beneficial to occasionally introduce circumstances that force workers or operators to step outside their daily routines. The logic for accomplishing key tasks may be essentially the same, but altering the surrounding circumstances removes the elements of familiarity that make it easy to disengage.

Through their experiences of using a product, users will infer certain rules for achieving effective or satisfying outcomes. These rules may not correspond to the optimal solution for achieving a given objective, but if they are good enough, users will come to rely on them. In system design, it is important to facilitate users as they infer the rules that they will rely on to accomplish their objectives, by masking nonessential complexity while exposing users to the essential logic underlying the operation of the system. For example, an electronic device may offer users a relatively straightforward set of functional capabilities. However, the same device may also contain the logic for various specialized operations, personalizing the device along different dimensions and performing trouble-shooting operations to diagnose malfunctions. Exposure to the latter functions makes the users' experience unnecessarily complex, interfering with their ability to infer a basic set of rules for achieving their objectives. Ideally, a user would be provided with immediate access to essential functions, while nonessential functions would be available, yet somewhat below the surface. Analogously, in architectural design, there may be many paths for traveling from one point to another, yet if these paths mask the essential spatial layout of a facility, individuals may find themselves continually disoriented.

If users and operators are going to infer rules, a system must operate in a consistent manner. Unpredictable behavior, or at least, seemingly unpredictable behavior will be disregarded and dismissed as bugginess. Rules will be learned based on those facets of a system that appear to operate consistently from one occasion to the next and from one situation to the next. Consequently, if a designer wants to facilitate acquiring a set of rules for achieving various objectives, the system behavior on which this learning will be based must be consistent. I have observed this while working with children and teaching them robotics. Often, the simplest solution for programming a robot will involve basic dead reckoning where the program tells the robot to go a certain distance at a certain speed and turn a certain amount to reach the intended destination. However, the children have been frequently confounded because a program that works one day does not work another day or a program that works on one robot does not work on another robot. These difficulties are rooted in less power being delivered to the motors as the charge on the batteries diminishes and subtle differences in the motors. These inconsistencies serve to complicate the basic programming rules that the children are trying to learn and as a result, they often become frustrated, assuming that there is no rhyme or reason to the behavior of the robot, when they had actually inferred a reasonably good working knowledge of the logic of the robot programming. In this case, the rules are straightforward and not hard to infer, but due to the inconsistent behavior of the system, the children give up, concluding that the system is buggy and incapable of consistently achieving their objectives.

Our daily lives are filled with examples of chunking. A six-pack container for carrying beverages allows us to operate in units of six as opposed to one. The combination meal at a fast-food restaurant allows us to combine an entrée, side dish, and drink in one unit. Music playlists allow us to create different mixes of songs, each being a separate unit. It is common practice for retailers to analyze the purchase behavior of their customers to identify patterns in which the same items tend to be purchased in combination. These data afford chunking, allowing items that are frequently purchased together to be placed in proximity to one another or even sold as a package. Using existing systems and behavioral data collection, opportunities may be identified to employ various mechanisms to effectively chunk individual items or activities. In system design, some patterns of behavior may be anticipated, but often users and operators will adopt patterns that cannot be anticipated. Consequently, once recurring patterns of behavior have been identified, there is a need to build flexibility into the design to later accommodate chunking. For example, the design of a facility may emphasize modular construction that provides flexibility in the physical layout, and multiuse components such as work surfaces and storage areas that can be assigned a variety of purposes. In contrast to dedicated spaces that cannot be readily adapted for alternative purposes, these design features enable the facility to be adapted in various ways to accommodate recurrent patterns, or chunks, of behavior.

Earlier, it was stated that the brain compensates for its limited capacity for real-time processing by relying on its seemingly endless capacity for memory storage and retrieval. The preceding sections have discussed the mechanisms by which this occurs and the various design approaches that facilitate this process. Within the design process, at any given point, it is pertinent to ask what activities should occupy the limited capacity for real-time processing of users and operators. Once this question has been answered, the designer may consider what mechanisms may be introduced to facilitate the formation of memory representations and the subsequent reliance on these memory representations. These may consist of procedures that promote the formation of routines, conventions that encourage consistency, vocabulary that captures complexity within jargon, or other approaches. Furthermore, as a user or operator gains experience, these same mechanisms provide opportunities to translate experience into improved efficiency, whether the mechanisms focus on primary, secondary, or other activities. Accordingly, through experience, individuals should amass more and more knowledge within their memory, allowing them to function at increasing levels of abstraction, while freeing resources for real-time processing to better focus on the most essential aspects of the activity.

The Google Effect and the Symbiosis between Brain and Technology

A prominent trend throughout much of human history has been the increasing reliance on physical artifacts to enable us to exceed the inherent limitations of our brains. Perhaps the most pervasive example is the accumulation of knowledge in books. But, there are countless other examples, including devices for counting and numerical operations, calendars, and maps. In each case, the demands that would otherwise be placed on the brain (e.g., memory for events, mathematical operations) are off-loaded to an external object, freeing the brain to focus on other activities. Where these artifacts have been widely adopted (e.g., books), a symbiosis may be observed between the brain and the artifact. For example, with reading, functional circuits within the brain provide the basic capability to interpret text. Then, through extensive practice, these circuits are refined and expanded to enable greater efficiency and sophistication. A symbiosis arises where the technology allows the brain to accomplish more than it ever could in its absence while the brain adapts to become better equipped to realize the benefits afforded by the technology.

A recent illustration of this trend can be observed with the vast stores of knowledge that are available through the Internet and its associated software products for locating and retrieving specific information. Sparrow et al. (2011) first described what has been termed *the Google effect*. These researchers conducted a series of studies in which they presented subjects with questions that they might ordinarily turn to an Internet search engine to answer (see figures 1 and 2 in Sparrow et al., 2011). In one study, they presented subjects with either easy or difficult trivia questions. For example, a difficult trivia question might be, "How many countries have only one color in their flag?" They then measured the reaction time to various words, some of which were related to computers and Internet searches. After getting a difficult question, compared with general words, the subjects showed a faster reaction time to the computer-related words. This suggests that when posed with a difficult question for which the subjects did not know the answer, they were primed to think about computer technology.

In a second study by Sparrow et al. (2011), subjects were given facts such as, "An ostrich egg is as big as its brain." The subjects were asked to type the facts into a computer, with half the subjects told that the computer would retain this information and half told that the information would be erased. The subjects were then asked to write down as many of the facts as they could recall. The subjects who were told that the computer would retain the information recalled fewer facts than the subjects who believed that the information would be erased. This suggests that when there is a belief that information will be available later, there is less inclination to process the information in a manner that would facilitate its later recall. In a third study, subjects were given a series of statements and after each statement, a message appeared indicating that the statement had either been saved on the computer, saved to a specific folder on the computer, or erased. Afterward, the subjects were presented with the statements, but the wording of some of the statements had been altered. When the subjects were asked if the statements were the same as those presented originally, they were more accurate in recognizing the statements they believed had been erased than the statements they believed had been saved on the computer. In contrast, when they were presented with statements and asked if the statements had been saved, saved to a certain folder, or erased, they were more accurate about statements that they believed had been saved or saved to a certain folder. This suggests that when there is a belief that information will be retained, there is a shift in emphasis from remembering the information *per se* to remembering that the information has been saved and will be available later. Finally, the subjects were tested on their recollection of the statements as compared with their recollection of the name of the folder where the statements had been stored. It was found that when the subjects believed that the information had been stored in a specific folder, they exhibited better recollection of the name of the folder than of the statement itself.

In combination, these findings illustrate how experience with Internet technology has shaped the manner in which information is processed and memory is utilized. When we believe that technology will be there to support our memory processes, the emphasis shifts from the specifics of the information to the specifics of how to retrieve the information. In this case, brain processes have adapted to the affordances of the technology, and it may be conjectured that with extensive experience, those brain processes that are engaged by the technology will become increasingly efficient and effective at carrying out these operations.

Once a Task Has Become Automated, Conscious Control Can Be Surprisingly Effortful

In almost any domain where an individual repeatedly performs an activity, over time, the activity becomes increasingly automated. This automation involves establishing routines within memory such that once the routine is triggered, it will then be executed without the need for much, if any, conscious attention. The propensity for the automation of routine activities is a key mechanism whereby the brain copes with its limited capacity for real-time processing. By relying on learned actions stored in memory (i.e., automated routines), conscious attention may be turned to other activities as the unconscious brain carries out various automated routines.

While beneficial and perhaps necessary for many of our daily activities, this propensity for the automation of routine activities carries a cost. Specifically, once an activity has become automated, it becomes less accessible to conscious attention. A common example involves familiar songs where the words and melodies are stored in memory as a sequential unit, and when recalled, we replay the elements in sequential order. Consequently, if asked to recall the words of a familiar song, it is easy to start from the beginning, but very difficult if you are asked to start from a point midway through the song.

When learning a sequence of actions, there is a differential engagement of the brain regions as one progresses from initial exposure to intermediate and proficient levels of performance. Initially, there is involvement of the cortical regions associated with the executive control of movement (i.e., prefrontal cortex and supplementary motor area), and the cerebellum, which is associated with the detailed timing of activities in relation to movement kinematics (Hikosaka, 2002; Penhune and Doyon, 2002). During the intermediate stages, cortical mappings between the motor and sensory representations develop and these mappings serve as the substrate for recalling and executing the routine. Then, with more practice, there is a migration from cortical control to control by circuits within the striatum. This migration involves a shift from cortical circuits that are readily accessible to conscious awareness to subcortical circuits that are largely inaccessible to conscious awareness. In practice, the learning of sequences can occur either explicitly where there is a conscious intention to learn the activity or implicitly through casual exposure to repeated sequences of actions or sensorimotor experiences. While explicit learning tends to rely on cortical processes, implicit learning has been attributed to the activity of the subcortical basal ganglia (Destrebecqz et al., 2005). Furthermore, the extent of implicit learning has been correlated with the level of activity in the basal ganglia and related striatal regions of the brain (Rauch et al., 1997).

A key implication of automation, and the underlying brain processes, is that once an activity is automated, it can become largely inaccessible to conscious thought processes. This can often be seen in experts within a given domain. While experts can perform tasks at a performance level that is clearly superior to less capable individuals, it may be difficult for them to explain exactly how they do it. When conducting expert elicitation, one must be aware that many of the activities of interest have become automated to the point that the experts no longer think about what they are doing, and may not really be cognizant of how they do it. Consequently, expert accounts may often consist of accounts of what they consider best practices and retrospective interpretations of past events, and may say very little about the mechanics that underlie their ability to outperform those with less experience.

A second downside of automation is that once a routine has become automated, it is often less malleable to corrections and refinements, or adaptation to unexpected situational factors. Trainers and educators are frequently confronted with the challenge of how to get someone to unlearn an inefficient or ineffective behavior. I have found a useful measure of the extent to which a behavior has become automated to the point of it being outside the realm of conscious control is to try and perform the activity in mirror-reversed conditions. Anyone who has spent most of his or her life driving on the right side of the road and is placed in the situation of driving on the left side can appreciate how foreign it can seem to perform an otherwise well-learned behavior. For myself, after having driven on the right side of the road for 16 years, the first time I drove a car in Australia it felt like I was driving for the first time.

With automated routines, to restore conscious awareness, one must intentionally focus one's attention on one's performance, or modify situational factors in some way that either interferes with the automated routine or provides cues to deviate from the established routine. For me, driving on the left side of the road meant that I had to take a moment prior to every turn to think about which lane I should steer the vehicle.

To illustrate how cues might be used to interrupt an automated routine, on my way to work in the morning, I occasionally need to leave mail at the mailbox about half a mile from our home. My routine for going to work in the morning is so deeply engrained that without taking special measures, it is unlikely that I will remember to stop at the mailbox. My solution has been to place the mail on top of the steering column of my truck, making it awkward to drive and serving as a continuous reminder.

In system design, one must be aware of how elements of design promote the development of automated routines, and the need to sometimes interrupt this automaticity. One example occurs with routine checklists where an individual must go through a series of identical checks repeatedly in the same order. Such an activity is highly conducive to automation with the individual carrying out a behavioral routine without much conscious attention to what he or she is doing. A hallmark of automaticity is the act of looking without seeing. One may follow through with the behavioral act of looking at the item to be inspected, but this does not mean that one sees it. Input enters the brain and activates visual circuits, yet there is little or no conscious attention to the visual input. One way to reengage conscious attention is to alter the structure of the activity in a manner that does not fundamentally change the task, but forces the individual to think about what he or she is doing. For example, a series of visual inspections may be performed in reverse, or in an otherwise altered order. Another approach would be to periodically request that some additional information be recorded with every visual observation. Another effective means to reengage conscious attention is to take advantage of circuits within the brain that naturally respond to stimuli that are surprising or in some way out of context. For instance, stimuli that are unexpected or in some way out of the ordinary may be occasionally inserted. A tag might be placed adjacent to a part that is being inspected or an unexpected item might be inserted into a series of identical pieces. The basic point with each of these approaches is to introduce a stimulus that captures the person's attention while minimally interfering with his or her productivity and, as a result, pull the person out of the inattentive state into which he or she may have lapsed.

Are We Multitaskers or Merely Good Task Switchers?

We commonly engage in multiple simultaneous activities. For instance, I frequently talk on the phone while doing the dishes or folding the laundry.

Often, multitasking involves the introduction of some form of stimulation (e.g., music or television) to keep our mind engaged as we perform a mundane, otherwise boring activity. Multitasking becomes a concern when there is a risk associated with individuals having their attention split between a critical primary task and one or more noncritical secondary tasks. For example, great concern has been expressed about the dangers of talking on a cell phone while driving. Yet, multitasking is common, and it is difficult to say that any greater risk is incurred by talking on a cell phone while driving than adjusting the radio dial or engaging in a spirited discussion with other occupants of the vehicle. Furthermore, it is unrealistic to believe that attention is regularly focused solely on driving given the routine and often monotonous nature of most automotive excursions. Driving is highly prone to automaticity, as well as mind wandering, and one might question whether a cell phone discussion is any riskier than daydreaming. The point is that multitasking is a regular part of our day-to-day lives and if it is broadly defined to include activities such as listening to music while running or walking, combining a business discussion with lunch, rehearsing a presentation while waiting one's turn to speak, and so on, we may spend as much or more of our waking hours multitasking as we spend committed to a single activity.

Charron and Koechlin (2010) devised an experimental method to assess how the brain copes with multitasking situations. In their studies, subjects were presented with two series of letters. Each time a letter appeared, their task was to indicate if the current letter was the same or different from the last letter in its respective series. In essence, the subjects were asked to simultaneously perform two tasks, although the tasks were identical. This activity was challenging, but the subjects had little difficulty coping with the demands and performed the task with reasonable levels of success. As the subjects performed the task, functional magnetic resonance imaging (fMRI) recordings provided an indication of their ongoing brain activity. When the two tasks were equivalent, there were relatively equal levels of activity in the left and right hemispheres of the subjects' brains. Next, the experimenters introduced a differential monetary reward such that each successful performance of one task produced a substantially greater reward than the other. With the differential reward, activity in one hemisphere increased, while activity in the opposite hemisphere decreased. Then, when the differential reward was reversed so that a large reward was received for the successful performance of the task that had previously produced a small reward, and the task that had produced the large reward gave a small reward, the differential activity of the two hemispheres reversed. These findings suggest that the subjects coped with the two tasks by devoting one hemisphere of the brain to one task and the other hemisphere of the brain to the accompanying task. It was particularly interesting to see what happened when a third task was introduced. In this condition, the subjects performed at chance levels for the third task. These findings imply that the brain is quite capable of performing two simultaneous tasks and accomplishes this feat by allocating one hemisphere of the brain to one task and the other hemisphere to the other task. However, there are no further resources available when there is a need to perform a third task.

The findings of Charron and Koechlin (2010) suggest that our brains are well equipped to perform two tasks, although it may be noted that the experimental tasks used in these experiments are not very demanding, nor do they pose a risk to the well-being of the individual. Today, with the proliferation of electronic gadgets, it is common to see multitasking go well beyond a pair of simultaneous tasks to involve numerous simultaneous tasks. Ophir et al. (2009) reported that among the students at Stanford University, on average, their subjects simultaneously used three devices. A typical scenario might involve a student working on a computer, periodically shifting his or her attention to a cell phone for messaging, while playing music in the background. To study the effects of chronic multitasking, students were identified who were categorized as either high multitaskers, meaning that they regularly combined four or more tasks, and light multitaskers, who, on average, only combined two tasks. In one study, subjects were presented with an array of blue and red rectangles. Their instructions were to focus on the red rectangles, with the blue rectangles being distractors. An array was shown to the subjects and then, after a brief pause, a second array was shown in which one of the red rectangles may or may not have been rotated. The subjects' task was to say if any of the red rectangles had changed orientation. As the number of distractors increased from 0 to 2, 4, or 6, there was no drop-off in performance for the light multitaskers, but there was a substantial drop-off in performance for the high multitaskers (see Figure 5.1). This finding was interpreted as evidence that the high multitaskers were less effective in ignoring the distractors, with the result being that they performed less well on the primary task.

Ophir et al. (2009) extended this research to consider the effects on memory. They used a procedure known as the N-back, where subjects are presented with a series of letters and their task is to say if each letter is the same as or different from a previous letter. The difficulty of the task can be varied by requesting that subjects compare the current letter with the letters that preceded the current letter by one, two, or three positions. To successfully perform this task, a subject must be able to retain the immediate sequence of letters in his or her memory without becoming distracted by intervening letters. The researchers found that the high multitaskers performed less well than the light multitaskers. Interestingly, the high multitaskers' performance was highly sensitive to both the frequency of occurrence for a given letter and the number of different letters used. As the frequency with which a given letter appeared increased, the letter became a greater source of distraction. The researchers concluded that in the high multitaskers, their capacity for managing their memory resources had been lessened. As new information came into their memory, they had a diminished capacity to clear old information that was no longer needed from their memory and, consequently, the old information became a distraction.

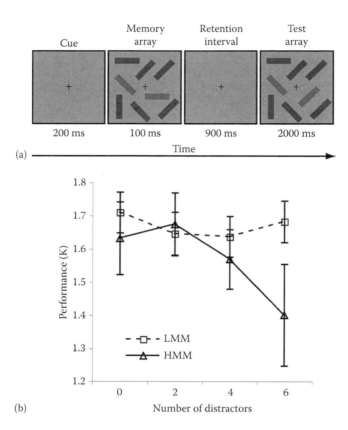

FIGURE 5.1

(a,b) Subjects were required to recall the orientation of the center rectangles with a varying numbers of distractors in the periphery. As the number of distractors increased, there was a reduction in the performance of the high multitaskers. HMM, heavy media multitaskers; LMM, light media multitaskers. (From Ophir, E., Nass, C., and Wagner, A.D., *Proceedings of the National Academy of Sciences*, 106, 15583–15587, 2009. With permission.)

In another study, these researchers considered the performance of high and light multitaskers with regard to their ability to effectively switch from one task to another. It was presumed that if there was any skill for which the high multitaskers would exhibit an advantage, it would be one that required an individual to frequently shift between different tasks. For this task, the subjects were presented with a combination consisting of a letter and a number. Prior to seeing the letter–number pair, they were presented with a cue that indicated if they should focus on the letter or the number. If the cue was for letters, their task was to say if the letter in the letter–number pair was a vowel. If the cue was for numbers, their task was to say if the number was even. On successive trials, the high multitaskers were significantly less accurate than the light multitaskers when there was a transition from letter to number or from number to letter. This indicated that the high multitaskers had a harder time discontinuing one task and switching to the other. However, the high multitaskers were also slower in responding on trials in which the task did not switch (i.e., a letter trial was followed by another letter trial or a number trial was followed by another number trial). This implies that even on the nonswitch trials, the high multitaskers had a difficult time not thinking about the other task.

Finally, the researchers replicated the classic study discussed in a preceding chapter in which subjects are shown a video of several people passing a ball and are asked to count the number of passes. In this study, at some point, a person dressed in a gorilla suit steps into the scene, does a few distinct movements, such as chest pounding, and steps out of the scene. Most people viewing this film for the first time do not see the gorilla because their attention is focused on counting the number of times that the individuals in the film pass the ball back and forth. This was true for the light multitaskers, who, on average, did quite well at counting the number of passes, but generally failed to see the gorilla. In contrast, the high multitaskers performed poorly on counting the passes, yet were more likely to say that they saw the gorilla. In this case, the inability of the high multitaskers to filter out the irrelevant stimuli (i.e., the gorilla) allowed them to avoid the inattentional blindness that characterizes the performance of most of the people who perform this task. In short, if the objective is to detect irrelevant, yet critical stimuli, high multitaskers are likely to be quite effective. However, this will come at the cost of diminished performance on almost every other activity.

The researchers point out that many organizations have adopted policies that either explicitly or implicitly establish the expectation that employees will multitask. For example, companies may require that employees keep a chat window open continuously on their computer with the implication that they will regularly interrupt their work to respond to messages from their coworkers. Similarly, policies have been implemented that require employees to respond to all emails within a certain time period. These policies demand that employees regularly shift their attention from one task to another, with the potential outcome that they will become increasingly susceptible to distractions, similar to the high multitaskers in the studies of Ophir et al. (2009). Whereas these examples involve obvious interruptions to ongoing activities, in many systems, similar but not as obvious interruptions occur, forcing individuals to continually shift their attention. This may occur with open office spaces where workers are surrounded by activities such as conversations, phones ringing, people coming and going, and so on. Whether workers actively or passively attend to these activities, the distraction draws their attention away from their primary task, forcing them to continuously task switch. The same situation may arise where workers are exposed to periodic announcements, or warnings and alarms. Each instance forces workers to suspend their attention to their primary task and afterward, return their attention.

In system design, it is important to be aware of the moment-to-moment allocation of attention, whether shifts in attention occur as a part of normal operations or they are due to periodic disturbances. Where task switching is essential, mechanisms may be employed to facilitate the shift in context from one task to another. For example, this might involve capturing and possibly providing playback of the sequence of activities that occurred immediately prior to an interruption. Another mechanism might entail capturing cues concerning one's activities that may be carried from one context to another. The level of multitasking that occurs with different individuals may vary, as well as their susceptibility to distractions. Consequently, design should accommodate individual differences, allowing users to control the extent to which they must cope with interruptions and distractions. Likewise, over the course of a day, there may be periods when there is a desire for uninterrupted solitude, and other periods when disruptions are welcomed as a source of stimulation, when activities have grown monotonous or frustrating. In summary, with system design, one should be aware of the potential effects of multitasking, understanding that interruptions and distractions are implicit forms of multitasking. Furthermore, while individuals may choose deleterious levels of multitasking, the designer should be careful not to impose unfavorable multitasking conditions on individuals.

Brains Reflexively Respond to Exceptions

Imagine you are gazing at a large screen on which a large circular disc flashes briefly every second. You are instructed to tap your finger on the table in front of you each time the disc flashes. After several flashes, your tapping is in time with the rate at which the disc is being flashed and you have begun to anticipate the flashes. In fact, if the activity of the motor cortex of your brain was being recorded, a readiness potential would be evident. This is indicative of preparatory processes whereby given awareness of an impending action, the brain readies its response. Then, when the sequence of flashes is interrupted by an unexpectedly long delay, for instance, the 1 s delay between flashes is extended to 3 s, there is a momentary surprise, with a heightened attention to the task. Similarly, many of us have participated in the group activity where the leader claps his or her hands at a constant rate and you are asked to clap in rhythm with the leader. Then, unexpectedly, the leader does not clap. Invariably, a few in the group will be unable to suppress their response and will clap. Yet, everyone experiences the same sense of surprise in response to his or her expectations having been violated.

Both of the examples in the previous paragraph illustrate the basic capacity of the brain to infer patterns within everyday events and based on these patterns, establish predictions or expectations of forthcoming events. In a classic series of studies, Emanuel Donchin and Michael Coles (e.g., Coles et al., 1985) established that there were distinct physiological responses within the brain associated with anticipation and violations of expectations, which occur within specific time frames relative to the presentation of a stimulus. For instance, in a reaction time study, different letters were presented that served to prime an impending response (Gratton et al., 1990). However, the letters varied with respect to the probability that the stimulus would immediately follow (i.e., for a given letter, there was a 20%, 50%, or 80% likelihood that the stimulus would follow the prime). Electrophysiological recordings of brain activity revealed that a wave of activity peaked approximately 300 ms following the letters that served to prime the impending stimulus, with the amplitude of this activity correlated with the probability that the stimulus would follow the prime. Furthermore, there was a recognizable readiness potential in anticipation of an impending stimulus with there being a correlation between the probability of the stimulus occurrence and the magnitude of the readiness potential. These studies demonstrated that the brain anticipates the relative likelihood of forthcoming events and not only generates a preparatory response, but also modulates this preparatory response in regard to the likelihood that the anticipated response will actually occur.

Whereas the P300 described by Donchin and Coles is indicative of anticipation and response preparation, a second distinct pattern of activity occurs in response to an unexpected stimulus. This activity, referred to as *mismatch negativity*, consists of a wave of activity that is present when a predictable series of stimuli is interrupted by an unexpected stimulus (Naatanen, 1992). The unexpected stimulus has been referred to as an *oddball*. A typical research paradigm might involve an auditory presentation of a series of letters such as "s,s,s,s,s,s,s,s,s,s,s,s,d,s,s,s,s,s,s,…," with the "d" serving as the oddball. The electrophysiological response occurs whether or not a person is paying attention to the stimulus and it has been demonstrated for both auditory and visual stimuli. Furthermore, the mismatch can involve the physical characteristics of a stimuli (e.g., loudness and color), as well as the identity of the stimulus. It has been suggested that the P300 and mismatch negativity reflect two distinct functional circuits with the P300 emanating from higher-level cognitive control functions and the mismatch negativity arising from bottom-up perceptual processes (Ritter et al., 1999).

At an unconscious level, our brains are continually processing the array of sensory input that is received from the environment, comparing ongoing events with known patterns of events, and piecing together and inferring new patterns. Then, when events diverge from the patterns that we have come to expect, a response is triggered that has the effect of capturing our conscious awareness and directing our attention to the anomaly. We experience this process as the surprise that occurs when something deviates from our expectations. The surprise is generally mild, as occurs when we hear someone use a word in an unusual fashion or when we notice that a friend has rearranged his or her furniture. However, on occasion, surprise can overwhelm our thoughts and emotions, as occurs when we receive unexpectedly good news or an unexpected but much appreciated gift. It can be argued that surprise is what makes life interesting. For instance, a basic mechanism by which jokes make us laugh is through shifting from one context to another in a surprising manner (Coulson and Kutas, 2001). Consider the joke, "When he told his mother about having gone to a topless bar, she asked, 'What do they do when it rains?'" Much of the humor we enjoy, as well as popular fiction, builds on unexpected shifts or mixing of contexts that evoke surprise. Similarly, the aesthetic quality of music has been linked to the extent to which it establishes and diverges from predictable patterns (Abdallah and Plumbley, 2008). This accounts for the appeal of live music (Sloboda, 2000). The adept live musician will perform a familiar song, but with each performance, he or she will introduce slight, unexpected variations within the overall structure of the song, creating a sensation that combines a sense of familiarity with a few surprises here and there.

There is an important distinction to be made. It is not novelty that elicits a response from the brain, but instead it is the violation of expectations. For instance, Vachon et al. (2012) showed that as subjects listened to voice narrations, variations in the information content did not evoke surprise, yet an unexpected change in speakers did so. However, this response diminished as the listeners learned what to expect. Thus, in general, random comments are not funny and disjointed stories are not entertaining. Likewise, the joke that elicits a laugh the first time you hear it, does not do so the second time and the drama that is shocking the first time loses its impact after watching it once or twice.

Within the foregoing, there are lessons for engineering entertaining or aesthetically pleasing experiences. First, there is the need to provide a recognizable structure. This may involve evoking a familiar storyline (e.g., the downtrodden individual who is having bad luck). The structure may arise from the process or procedures involved in carrying out a common activity (e.g., going to a restaurant and ordering a meal). Likewise, structure may be created through physical properties such as the spatial layout of a building or an outdoor facility. Next, there must be elements that, given the structure, are readily predicted. The downtrodden individual may experience a series of disappointments or indignities. On entering a restaurant, there may be a waiting area where the hostess greets diners at a podium and there are benches to sit on while waiting to be seated at a table. The passageways of a building may be orderly and symmetrical. Much of the art in designing experience lies in attaining the appropriate degree of predictable regularity. There must be enough to not just create expectations, but to leave little doubt that anything is going to be any different from what would be predicted on the basis of those expectations. However, one must also know when enough is enough so that the experience does not become monotonous. Finally, one must introduce the unexpected. Again, it cannot merely be random. The unexpected element of the experience must be reasonable given the structure that has been created, yet unpredicted given associated expectations. Within the story of the downtrodden individual, it would seem weird if he or she inexplicably got into a luxury car and drove away. However, the story might work if someone recognized that the downtrodden individual possessed a hidden talent and through this unappreciated talent, the individual was able to change his or her fortunes. In the restaurant, it would merely seem strange if one was handed a toolbox and told to assemble one's table. Yet, one might find it a curious change of pace if one was handed a spatula and led to an open grill to cook one's own meal. Within a building, one would find it odd if a hallway widened and narrowed for no apparent reason, yet be pleasantly surprised if a long hallway opened into a spacious atrium. In each of these examples, the designer has taken advantage of basic brain circuitry whereby we unconsciously recognize structure and predictable patterns within our environment, and then assess ongoing experiences with regard to these predictions, experiencing surprise, perhaps even wonder or fascination, when our expectations are violated.

There is a related facet of the brain's reflexive response to violations of expectations that is worth mentioning. It occurs for activities where there is a relationship between certain actions and the expected results. For instance, when dialing a friend's phone number, we know the series of actions that will produce the response of ringing his or her phone. Similarly, when someone asks a question, we know the sequence of verbalizations that will give the person the desired answer. Yet, we have all had the experience of thinking one thing and then witnessing ourselves doing something different. We intend to call our friend, but catch ourselves dialing another familiar number. We open our mouth to answer a question, but catch ourselves saying something unintended. In the same way that the brain senses environmental events that violate expectations, the brain monitors our actions and responds when our actions differ from our intentions. There is a measurable electrophysiological signal that takes the form of a wave of activity, which travels over much of the brain and has been referred to as *error-related* or *conflict-related negativity*. This signal emanates from a structure known as the anterior cingulate cortex and is generated when one's actions deviate from the expectations for a given situation or one's intentions (van Veen et al., 2001).

A Huge Relief

For an American who experienced the height of the Cold War, Russia can seem like a forbidding destination, one that conjures fearful images of totalitarianism and repression. From my childhood, I recall the drills during which we practiced how we would respond if there was an imminent nuclear attack, hiding underneath our desks at school. Since those days, such images have been replaced with an impression of Russia as being relatively lawless, where criminal organizations operate with impunity. With the totalitarianism of the 1950s and 1960s and the criminal threats of the 2000s in mind, as an American making his first trip to Russia, some caution seemed reasonable.

My first trip to Russia was for business meetings in Moscow in 2006. I was warned of the tactics that are commonly used by criminals to take advantage of unsuspecting foreigners. As in most large cities, I was told that there were many pickpockets and to be wary of crowded locations. I was told about how thieves had masterfully used a razor knife to slice open a traveler's back pocket and steal his wallet without him knowing about it. I was also warned of more sophisticated ruses. For instance, there is the pigeon drop in which the trickster drops money, jewelry, or some other valuable in clear sight of the traveler, appearing unaware of having done so. When the helpful traveler picks up the valuable to try and return it, the scammer acts alarmed and accuses the traveler of having stolen it from him or her. Conveniently, the scammer has one or more accomplices nearby. One may be dressed in plain clothes and step in to reinforce the accusations. Another may be dressed in the uniform of a police officer or security personnel who attempts to adjudicate the situation, taking the perspective of the accuser. The ultimate objective is to pressure the traveler into giving them money to resolve the matter. With three or more agitated foreigners angrily confronting the traveler with threats and verbal assaults, a payoff becomes a convenient means to bring the matter to a conclusion.

However, the warning that was particularly poignant involved a scam attributed to members of the police force. It was explained that the typical police officer was very poorly paid and many supplemented their income with bribes and payoffs. In this scam, the police officer approaches the traveler and asks to see his or her papers. These would consist of both a passport and a visa. When the traveler does so, the police officer looks over the documents and insists that there is a problem. Then, the police officer asserts that the traveler will need to come with him or her to the station to resolve the matter. However, at this point, the traveler is offered an option. For a relatively small sum of cash, the police officer will forget the matter and let the traveler go. I was told that this was the point where you can negotiate and that generally they would accept a much smaller sum than originally requested. It was emphasized that these incidents are primarily an inconvenience and that the traveler is rarely in any danger. Yet, they can be extremely stressful, ruining an otherwise pleasant experience.

It was the third or fourth day of my trip and I was walking back to my hotel after having had dinner with a couple of colleagues. All the while, wary of any uniformed official, I had been trying to keep a low profile and not draw any attention to myself. However, on this evening, as I walked down the street alone, there was no escaping as two men in uniform approached. They stopped and said something in Russian that I did not understand. I immediately assumed that this was the scenario about which I had been warned. There seemed to be no other option so I asked in English if they wanted to see my documents and started to reach for my passport. However, hearing my English, one of the men replied in his own broken English, "We are Russian soldiers. Can you give us money for food?" I was immediately overcome with an enormous sense of relief. In my mind, I had prepared myself for the worst. Reaching into my pocket, I pulled out a bill and without paying much attention to the denomination, I handed it to the man and quickly continued on my way. I had still given up some money, but strangely, under those circumstances, I was happy to do so.

In this situation, not knowing one uniform from another, my brain put the pieces together to recognize a pattern that was consistent with the scam for which I had been warned. I had had a set of expectations and based on those expectations, I had processed the available cues, filled in the missing pieces, and confidently concluded that the two men were police officers intent on placing me in an unpleasant situation. Then, when one of the men announced that they were soldiers and asked for a donation, my expectations were drastically violated. Instantly, my brain transitioned from one state in which I was wary of an unpleasant interaction with Russian authorities to another situation where I was being humbly asked for assistance. My brain made this transition in an instant and I knew exactly what to do. Notably, it is this violation of expectations that makes the story interesting.

Since this first experience, I have made many trips to Russia and have gotten past my initial trepidation. While I have always exercised caution and have been the target of thieves on a couple of occasions, I do not consider traveling in Russia to be any more dangerous than visiting certain large cities in the United States. Furthermore, I have had the opportunity to meet and work with many Russians who have proven to be respectable, caring, and considerate, and outstanding colleagues and friends.

As "Pattern-Seeking Primates," the Default Condition Is to Believe

In one of my favorite Technology, Entertainment, Design (TED) talks, delivered by Michael Shermer, who edits a journal known as *The Skeptic*, Shermer introduces the term *patternicity* to describe our tendency to find meaningful patterns within our everyday experiences. As previously noted, the brain is constantly recognizing and often differentially responding to patterns, with these often occurring at an unconscious level. However, Shermer primarily concerns himself with the conscious willingness to believe that patterns are real and meaningful. He asserts that by default, our tendency is to believe that patterns are meaningful whenever the cost of making a false alarm is less than that of a false rejection. For instance, most superstitious behavior is harmless, with there being little cost in believing that the associated ritualistic behavior has a real effect on the outcome of everyday events. The basketball player who insists on wearing a new pair of socks for every game suffers little for this belief. Likewise, the individual who readily accepts outlandish conspiracy theories may seem odd to many, but can endure without realizing any significant consequences for these beliefs. Furthermore, Shermer emphasizes that patternicity is particularly prevalent when it is difficult to assess the truth. In the case of conspiracy theories, the theories generally involve covert activities for which evidence has been hidden or destroyed, and powerful individuals or groups who have an express interest in concealing the truth. This creates conditions that are ripe for those who are inclined to believe in such theories to see connections between seemingly unrelated events and infer patterns for which there is little or no substantiation.

The propensity to recognize and believe in patterns varies in response to our life experiences. In research by Whitson and Galinsky (2008), they hypothesized that there would be a heightened willingness to see patterns within otherwise meaningless stimuli when individuals are feeling frustrated or out of control. In such situations, the recognition of patterns serves to impose some order on events at a time when one may feel somewhat helpless to affect critical aspects of the world around oneself. Whitson and Galinsky presented their subjects with images that consisted of numerous black lines of various lengths and orientations against a white background. For some trials, the image consisted of nothing more than randomly placed lines. However, on other trials, there was a line drawing of an actual object embedded within the image. For example, there might be a distinguishable outline of the planet Saturn or an airplane, with randomly placed lines surrounding and intersecting the outline of the object. The subjects were asked to indicate whether or not they believed that the images contained an embedded object. On 95% of the trials in which the image actually contained an object, the subjects responded correctly, saying that there was an object within the image. However, the researchers were primarily interested in those trials in which images did not contain an embedded object, yet the subjects responded that an object was present.

In one study, prior to viewing the images, some of the subjects were assigned a frustrating task in which there was no clear relationship between the rewards and punishments, and their performance. The subjects who had undergone the frustrating experience were more likely to respond that the images contained objects when there was no embedded object. Similarly, in a second study, prior to viewing the images, some of the subjects were asked to recall an experience from their lives in which they had experienced a loss of control. These subjects were more prone to false alarms, saying that objects were present when they were not. Finally, a similar result was obtained with business people who reported that they were currently experiencing a stressful situation where they felt that they had little control over events.

Together, these findings suggest that when people are placed in frustrating situations where they feel that events are outside their control or that they are being affected by events over which they have no influence, they will be more prone to see associations between otherwise unrelated events, and assume and behave as if patterns exist that may be largely constructions of their own mind.

This is important to system design because it is common for individuals to experience frustration within the course of everyday transactions, both frustrations that are a direct product of the system and those that merely coincide with their interactions with the system. Most of us are familiar with this experience during our everyday computer use. For some reason, the system may be unresponsive or behave oddly, and having no obvious explanation, we may link these experiences with unrelated events. For example, observing telephone technicians nearby with a cabinet open, one might presume that the problems with one's computer are associated with the telecommunications network. Having just had new software installed, one may blame the problem on the new software. Those using Windows-based systems that receive automated software updates are quite familiar with the experience where their computer behaves oddly at either startup or shutdown. Then, they realize that there are new software updates and that the anomalous behavior may be attributed to the installation and configuration of these updates. In fact, an expert in cybersecurity once commented to me that a substantial portion of the everyday reports of suspected computer viruses is attributable to unexpected system behavior resulting from Windows updates.

The first lesson for the system designer is to appreciate that from the perspective of a user or an operator, the patterns that he or she infers to exist are real, whether or not they do actually exist. In a study by Ress and Heeger (2003), subjects were shown a pattern and were then shown blurred images that either did or did not contain the pattern, with the subjects' task being to indicate whether or not the pattern was present within the blurred images. Brain imaging data were recorded from the subjects as they performed this task. It was observed that whether or not the pattern was present, on trials in which the subjects indicated that the pattern was present, the activity of their brains was comparable to that when viewing an image with the pattern. This suggests that when the brain believes a pattern exists, regardless of the sensory inputs to the perceptual system, it responds as if the pattern is actually there. A designer cannot dismiss the inferences of users because from the users' perspective, these patterns are real. Furthermore, users may change their behavior or do things that are counterproductive as a result of these beliefs. For example, if users falsely believe that the sluggishness of their computer may be attributed to new software, they may uninstall the software. If users falsely believe that the anomalous behavior caused by a system upgrade is due to a hacker having compromised their system or their having downloaded a virus, they may unnecessarily have their system wiped clean and rebuilt. These actions are unnecessary, but from the perspective of the users, given their beliefs, they seem logical and necessary.

Obviously, the best way to avoid situations of this type in which users or operators attribute system malfunction or lack of reliability to unrelated factors, and consequently behave in a manner that is counterproductive based on these beliefs, is to design systems that are extremely robust. However, given that this may not always be possible, there are steps that can be taken to minimize the tendency to make erroneous associations. First, to the extent that anomalous system behavior can be anticipated, there is value in warning the user or operator. Such warnings provide an immediate link between the anomalous behavior and normal operational routines so that there is less of an inclination to search for alternative explanations. Where practical, another approach is to shield the user or operator from the anomalous behavior. For example, an alternative workspace may be supplied that while it does not offer full functionality, will behave in a reliable manner. Frustration will only heighten the tendency to infer extraneous causes for anomalous system behavior. Thus, steps may be taken to minimize frustration. For instance, the user or operator may be allowed to control when the system operations producing the anomalous behavior occur so that while being unable to avoid the experience, at least the user or operator can control when it happens. Likewise, steps should be taken to avoid the potential loss of ongoing work or data so that once the system operations causing the anomalous behavior are complete, at a minimum, the operator can resume his or her activities without having lost anything. All these measures serve to establish valid connections between the normal operations of a system and the occasional anomalous behavior of the system, and by establishing these connections, minimize the opportunity for users and operators to form spurious connections. Furthermore, these methods serve to transfer some sense of control to the user or operator as a mechanism to avoid the frustration and stress that result when one is negatively impacted by events beyond one's control.

While everyone is susceptible to "patternicity," as described by Shermer, and this susceptibility varies in response to ongoing circumstances, it has been observed that there are individual differences in this susceptibility (Krummenacher et al., 2010). Krummenacher and colleagues have equated the propensity to see patterns with the concept of a signal-to-noise ratio (see figure 2 in Krummenacher et al., 2010). Those with a greater propensity to report patterns, with a corresponding higher incidence of false alarms, would be considered to have a low signal-to-noise threshold (i.e., more likely to report the presence of a signal and likewise, more likely to mistake noise for a valid signal). In contrast, those who are less likely to report patterns, with a corresponding higher incidence of false rejections, would be considered to have a high signal-to-noise threshold, being more likely to reject valid signals as noise.

A collection of traits that characterize those with a greater propensity to see patterns includes being more creative, more willing to believe in the paranormal, more prone to psychotic illnesses, and having a lower sensitivity to negative feedback. In contrast, an opposite collection of traits associated with those who are less prone to see patterns includes being more analytic, more skeptical, and having a greater susceptibility to depression and a greater sensitivity to negative feedback. Interestingly, these traits seem to be linked to either intrinsic levels or sensitivity to the neurochemical transmitter dopamine. Dopamine is a primary substrate mediating the reward systems within the brain such that increased dopamine is associated with positive, rewarding experiences. In the research reported by Krummenacher et al. (2010), it was shown that by manipulating the level of dopamine, the experimenters could shift individual subjects' signal-to-noise thresholds (i.e., propensity to see patterns). This led the researchers to conclude that the opposing traits were linked to the differential functioning of the dopamine-mediated reward circuits of the brain. Thus, those with an intrinsically high dopamine response are more prone to see patterns, whereas those with an intrinsically lower level of dopamine response are less likely to see patterns.

In applied settings, these findings have important ramifications. First, it can be assumed that the members of a workforce will vary in their intrinsic responses to dopamine and show varying propensities to see patterns. Furthermore, some professions are likely to attract those with a lower signal-to-noise threshold (i.e., greater intrinsic dopamine response). In particular, these are likely to be professions that hinge on creative processes (e.g., concept design, marketing, and various arts). These are occupations that demand a willingness to suspend concern for critical judgment and explore unproven ideas. However, in these situations, the associated insensitivity to negative feedback could promote the pursuit of unproductive paths and an unwillingness to accept critical appraisal. In contrast, professions attracting those with higher signal-to-noise thresholds would include those involving intense analytic analysis (e.g., engineering analysis, hazard and risk assessment, and accounting). These are positions where one must be wary of unproven ideas and keen to explore the various ways in which things can go wrong. However, in these professions, one must be concerned with the tendency to be excessively skeptical and the stagnation that can result when one is overly sensitive to potential negative outcomes. Within an organizational setting, these opposing forces may sometimes collide. Conflict can result due to those who are blind to risks wanting to move forward while others resist and find it difficult to accept anything but incremental steps due to the potential risks. This is a perpetual conflict that exists within many organizations and I do not believe that there is a remedy, with the conflict reflecting a healthy balance of opposing traits deeply rooted in the basic circuitry of the brain. Perhaps, the primary point is that these traits may not be particularly malleable and represent manifestations of fundamental mechanisms underlying the operations of our brains, contributing to an overall healthy range of individual differences.

Acknowledgments

Sandia National Laboratories is a multiprogram laboratory managed and operated by Sandia Corporation, a wholly owned subsidiary of Lockheed Martin Corporation, for the US Department of Energy's National Nuclear Security Administration under contract DE-AC04-94AL85000.

References

Abdallah, S. and Plumbley, M. (2008). Information dynamics: Patterns of expectation and surprise in the perception of music. *Connection Science, 2008*, 1–32.

Barsalou, L.W., Simmons, W.K., Barbey, A.K. and Wilson, C.D. (2003). Grounding conceptual knowledge in modality-specific systems. *Trends in Cognitive Sciences, 7*(2), 84–91.

Charron, S. and Koechlin, E. (2010). Divided representation of concurrent goals in the human frontal lobes. *Science, 328*(5978), 360–363.

Coles, M.G.H., Gratton, G., Bashore, T.R., Erikson, C.W. and Donchin, E. (1985). A psychophysiological investigation of the continuous flow model of human information processing. *Journal of Experimental Psychology: Human Perception and Performance, 11*, 529–553.

Coulson, S. and Kutas, M. (2001). Getting it: Human event-related brain response to jokes in good and poor comprehenders. *Neuroscience Letters, 316*, 71–74.

Destrebecqz, A., Peigneux, P., Laureys, S., Degueldre, C., Del Fiore, G., Aerts, J., Luxen, A., van der Linden, M., Cleeremans, A. and Maquet, P. (2005). The neural correlates of explicit and implicit sequence learning: Interacting networks revealed by the process dissociation procedure. *Learning and Memory, 12*, 480–490.

Ekstrom, A.D., Kahana, M.J., Caplan, J.B., Fields, T.A., Isham, A., Newman, E.L. and Fried, I. (2003). Cellular networks underlying human spatial navigation. *Nature, 425*, 184–188.

Gigerenzer, G. and Todd, P.M. (1999). *Simple Heuristics that Make Us Smart*. Oxford: Oxford University Press.

Gratton, G., Bosco, C.M., Kramer, A.F., Coles, M.G.H., Wickens, C.D. and Donchin, E. (1990). Event-related brain potentials as indices of information extraction and response priming. *Electroencephalography and Clinical Neurophysiology, 75*(5), 419–432.

Graybiel, A.M. (2008). Habits, rituals and the evaluative brain. *Annual Review of Neuroscience, 31*, 359–387.

Hikosaka, O. (2002). A new approach to the functional systems of the brain. *Epilepsia, 43*(Supplement 9), 9–15.

Krummenacher, P., Mohr, C., Haker, H. and Brugger, P. (2010). Dopamine, paranormal belief, and the detection of meaningful stimuli. *Journal of Cognitive Neuroscience, 22*(8), 1670–1681.

Lakkaraju, K., Stevens-Adams, S., Abbott, R.G. and Forsythe, C. (2011). Communications-based automated assessment of team cognitive performance. In D. Schmorrow and L. Reeves (eds) *Foundations of Augmented Cognition. Directing the Future of Adaptive Systems*, pp. 325–334. Berlin: Springer.

Longstaffe, K.A., Hood, B.M. and Gilchrist, I.D. (2012). Executive function in large scale search. In *Proceedings of Annual Meeting of the Cognitive Neuroscience Society*, March 31–April 3, Chicago, IL.

Naatanen, R. (1992). *Attention and Brain Function*. Hillsdale, NJ: Earlbaum.

Ophir, E., Nass, C. and Wagner, A.D. (2009). Cognitive control in media multitaskers. *Proceedings of the National Academy of Sciences*, 106(37), 15583–15587.

Penhune, V.B. and Doyon, J. (2002). Dynamic cortical and subcortical networks in learning and delayed recall of timed motor sequences. *Journal of Neuroscience*, 22(4), 1397–1406.

Rauch, S.L., Whalen, P.J., Savage, C.R., Curran, T., Kendrick, A., Brown, H.D., Bush, G., Breiter, H.C. and Rosen, B.R. (1997). Striatal recruitment during an implicit sequence learning task as measured by functional magnetic resonance imaging. *Human Brain Mapping*, 5, 124–132.

Ress, D. and Heeger, D.J. (2003). Neural correlates of perception in early visual cortex. *Nature Neuroscience*, 6, 414–420.

Ritter, W., Sussman, E., Deacon, D., Cowan, N. and Vaughan Jr., H.G. (1999). Two cognitive systems simultaneously prepared for opposite events. *Psychophysiology*, 36, 835–838.

Rypma, B. and D'Esposito, M. (1999). The roles of prefrontal brain regions in components of working memory: Effects of memory load on individual differences. *Proceedings of the National Academy of Sciences*, 96(11), 6558–6563.

Sloboda, J.A. (2000). Individual differences in musical performance. *Trends in Cognitive Sciences*, 4(10), 397–403.

Sparrow, B., Liu, J. and Wegner, D.M. (2011). Google effects on memory: Cognitive consequences of having information at our fingertips. *Science Express*, 333, 776–778.

Vachon, F., Hughes, R.W. and Jones, D.M. (2012). Broken expectations: Violations of expectations, not novelty, captures auditory attention. *Journal of Experimental Psychology: Learning, Memory and Cognition*, 38(1), 164–177.

van Veen, V., Cohen, J.D., Botvinick, M.M., Stenger, V.A. and Carter, C.C. (2001). Anterior cingulate cortex, conflict monitoring and levels of processing. *NeuroImage*, 14, 1302–1308.

Watrous, A., Tandon, N., Conner, C.R., Pieters, T. and Ekstrom, A.D. (2013). Frequency-specific network connectivity increases underlie accurate spatiotemporal memory retrieval. *Nature Neuroscience*, 16(3), 349–356.

Whitson, J.A. and Galinsky, A.D. (2008). Lacking control increases illusory pattern perception. *Science*, 322(5898), 115–117.

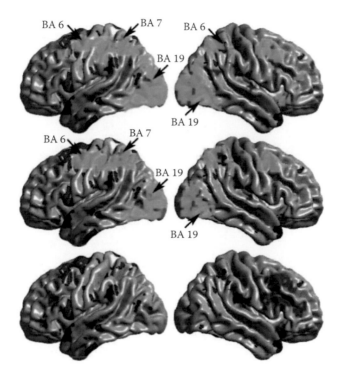

FIGURE 2.1

Areas in *red* indicate regions in which there is increased cortical thickness following practice playing the game Tetris. Areas in *green* exhibit increased activation and areas in *blue* exhibit decreased activation while playing the game. The top panel represents baseline recordings, the middle panel represents recordings at follow-up, and the bottom panel represents the follow-up recordings minus the baseline recordings. (From Haier, R.J., Karama, S., Leyba, L., and Jung, R.E., *BMC Research Notes*, 2, 174, 2009. With permission.)

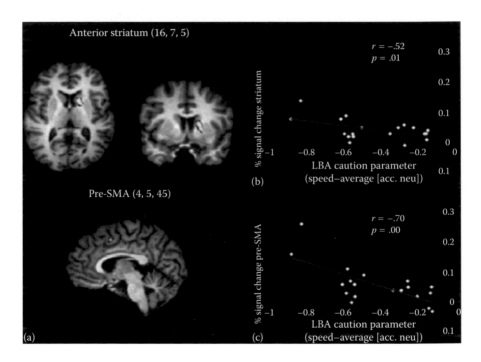

FIGURE 3.1
(a–c) Trials in which subjects were cued to try and produce a speeded response resulted in elevated levels of activity in the striatum and the presupplementary motor areas. LBA, linear ballistic accumulator. (From Forstmann, B.U., Dutilh, G., Brown, S., Neumann, J., von Cramon, D.Y., Ridderinkhof, K.R., and Wagenmakers, E.J., *Proceedings of the National Academy of Science,* 105, 17538–17542, 2008. With permission.)

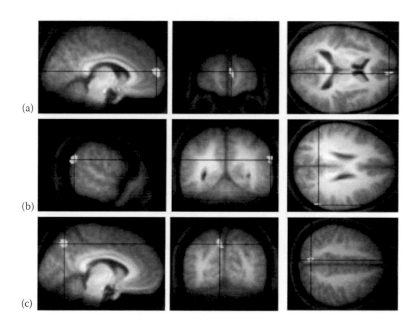

FIGURE 3.2
When subjects heard their own name, the corresponding electrophysiological response was correlated with increased activation of the right medial prefrontal cortex (a), right superior temporal sulcus (b), and left precuneus (c). (From Perrin, F., Maquet, P., Peigneux, P., Ruby, P., Degueldre, C., Balteau, E., Del Fiore, G., Moonen, G., Luxen, A., and Laureys, S., *Neuropsychologia*, 43, 12–19, 2005. With permission.)

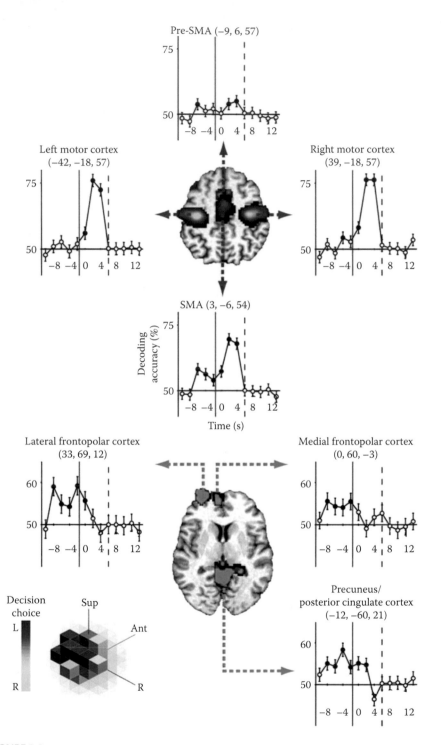

FIGURE 3.3
Brain regions are highlighted for which patterns of activity predicted forthcoming behavioral responses, with the activity in these areas several seconds prior to conscious awareness of a decision being predictive of the eventual response decision. (From Soon, C.S., Brass, M., Heinze, H.J., and Haynes, J.D., *Nature Neuroscience*, 11, 543–545, 2008. With permission.)

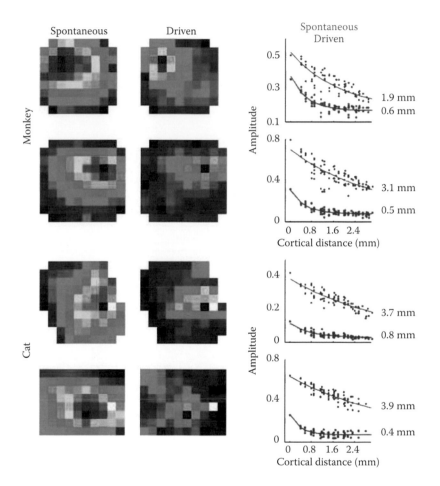

FIGURE 4.1
The differential trajectory of the spread of cortical neural activation in response to visual stimulation is depicted with regard to spike-driven versus spontaneous activity. (From Nauhaus, I., Busse, L., Carandini, M., and Ringach, D.L., *Nature Neuroscience*, 12, 70–76, 2008. With permission.)

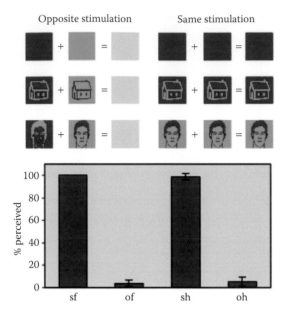

FIGURE 4.5
Simultaneous stimuli used by Moutoussis and Zeki (2002) in their study illustrating brain activation in response to stimuli that are not perceived at a conscious level. sf, same faces; of, opposite faces; sh, same houses; oh, opposite houses. (From Moutoussis, K. and Zeki, S., *Proceedings of the National Academy of Science*, 99, 9527–9532, 2002.)

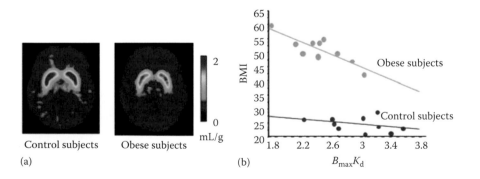

FIGURE 7.1
(a,b) Differential presence of dopamine receptors in obese subjects as compared with controls and the relationship between dopamine receptor density and body mass index. (From Volkow, N.D. and Wise, R.A., *Nature Neuroscience*, 8, 555–560, 2005. With permission.)

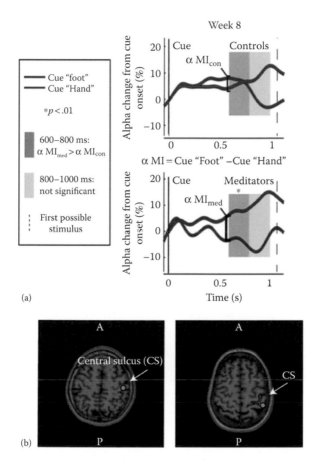

(a)

(b)

FIGURE 7.3
(a,b) Peak alpha frequency for meditators and nonmeditators during sustained attention to body and breath-related sensations. (From Kerr, C.E., Sacchet, M.D., Lazar, S.W., Moore, C.I. and Jones, S.R., *Frontiers in Human Neuroscience*, 7, 1–15, 2013. With permission.)

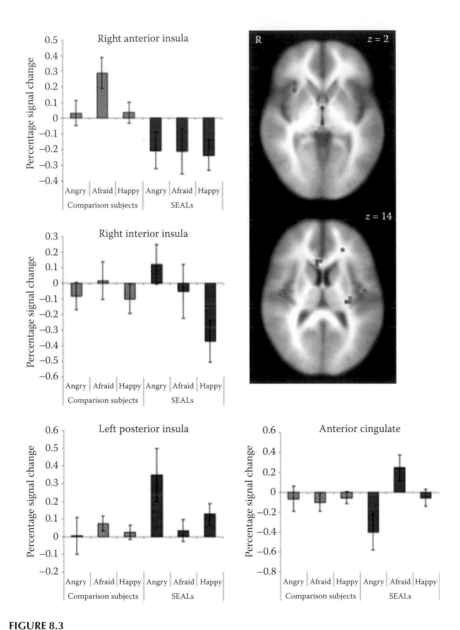

FIGURE 8.3
US Navy SEALs showed greater activation of the right insula in response to angry faces than control subjects did, suggesting greater sensitivity and awareness of potential threats. (From Paulus, M.P., Simmons, A.N., Fitzpatrick, S.N., Potterat, E.G., Van Orden, K.F., Bauman, J., and Swain, J.L., *PLoS ONE*, 5, e10096, 2010.)

6

Error

Fallibility is intrinsic to human behavior. As Alexander Pope (1688–1744) put it, "to err is human." That might explain why there are many terms (e.g., errors, mistakes, failures, blunders, faults, slips, and lapses) to describe situations where things do not happen as we expect. Regardless of what we call them, human error is pervasive. Just like gravity and weather, it is an unavoidable fact of life that occurs every day and every hour—as we speak, as we drive, and as we do other daily routines.

The innate fallibilities of people are built into every system that involves human beings, making those systems vulnerable to flawed human actions. As increased complexity becomes a crucial feature of contemporary human–technical systems involving mechanization, computerization, and automation, it increases the prospects of human error and makes such failures increasingly dangerous. Statistics show that human errors are implicated in over 90% of failures in the nuclear industry, over 80% of adverse events in health-care systems, over 80% of failures in the chemical and petrochemical industries, over 75% of marine casualties, and over 70% of aviation accidents. The potentially devastating consequences of erroneous human actions are exemplified by catastrophic disasters such as Chernobyl, Bhopal, Challenger, and Air Florida Flight 737. All these names are etched in our consciousness because of the deaths, injuries, and substantial property damage that have occurred over extended periods of time and across large geographic spaces, and have received extensive public, political, and scholarly attention. The human contributions to economic loss were illustrated in a study conducted by The National Institute of Standards and Technology (NIST) (Tassey, 2002) that considered major US software development firms. It was reported that software engineers spend an average of 70%–80% of their time testing and debugging, and it takes them an average of 17.4 h to fix a bug, costing the US economy over $50 billion annually.

Error from the Brain's Perspective

From the perspective of the brain, you are right all the way up until the point that you realize that you are wrong. This expression captures the common experience that accompanies our committing errors during everyday activities. We place the kettle on the stove, turn on the burner and walk away, waiting for the water to boil. Everything we have done seems fine and we continue with our morning routine of fixing breakfast. From the brain's perspective, everything we have done is correct, we have no reasons for concern, and we are making progress toward our goal of having breakfast and getting ready to start our day. Then, for some reason, we realize that we forgot to put water in the kettle. In a momentary realization, everything we had previously taken for granted when carrying out our morning routine is called into question as we berate ourselves for being so absentminded and putting our family and home in danger. This is our common experience of having committed an error. Everything is fine all the way up to the point that it becomes apparent that everything is not fine.

Within experimental research studies, this common experience of realizing that one has committed an error has been studied and the underlying brain mechanisms have been elucidated. A typical experimental paradigm presents a test participant with two buttons and an indicator that informs the subject which of the two buttons to press. The objective is to press the correct button as fast as possible once the indicator appears. In this paradigm, known as a *choice reaction time* study, subjects usually commit numerous errors as they attempt to maximize the speed of their response. On those trials in which the subject commits an error, there is a distinct neurophysiological signal that accompanies this realization (Holroyd and Coles, 2002). Specifically, a wave of activity, which is measurable using an electroencephalogram (EEG), emerges at the point where the motor response commences, peaking at about 80 ms afterward, and spreading across a broad swath of the brain (i.e., error-related negativity). This signal has been attributed to a general-purpose system within the brain that functions to detect the occurrence of errors and prompt a reorientation of attention in response to an error. The system is differentially responsive to motivational considerations and it has been demonstrated that when rewards are provided for a successful performance, the magnitude of the signal varies in accordance with the corresponding payoff (Gehring et al., 1993). Furthermore, the magnitude of the error signal varies in response to the magnitude of the error. For example, in a four-choice reaction time task where subjects responded using both hands and two different fingers on each hand, the more the errors diverged from the correct response, the greater the magnitude of the error-related response (Bernstein et al., 1995). For example, there would be a larger amplitude response when the subject used the wrong finger on the wrong hand, as opposed to merely responding with the wrong finger or the wrong hand.

The brain's realization that an error has occurred provides the basis for the brain's response to errors. A study was conducted in which subjects were presented with an indicator light and asked to wait 1 s before they pressed a button (Miltner et al., 1997). Following the button press, the subjects were given no feedback concerning their performance. At the end of a trial, the subjects were told whether their performance on the trial had fallen within the criteria. An error-related electrophysiological response was seen when the subjects received the feedback, suggesting that it was the knowledge of how well they had performed, which had been dissociated from the actual performance, which elicited the brain response. The error response emanates from a region of the brain known as the anterior cingulate cortex (Dehaene et al., 1994). It has been suggested that this region serves as a comparator. For a given response, there is an intended outcome and the anterior cingulate cortex compares the actual outcome with the expected outcome. When there is a discrepancy, a response is emitted that then orients attention to the discrepancy. Furthermore, Holroyd and Coles (2002) have proposed that there is a link between the anterior cingulate cortex and the reward circuits of the brain such that the comparative function of the anterior cingulate cortex serves to modulate the level of reward (i.e., dopamine release in association with the response). Thus, through an ongoing comparison of actual and intended outcomes by a generic and highly flexible response monitoring circuit, the error response of the anterior cingulate cortex provides the basis for continually refining behavioral performance.

Organizational Approach to Human Error

Since human fallibility is inevitable, within the context of an organization it is counterproductive to attempt to completely eliminate errors or establish goals such as a flawless performance, which is often advocated by engineering system designers and management. Rather, we first need to adopt a perspective that recognizes the existence and potential occurrence of human errors, and then focus on the goals of developing a means to prevent errors from occurring and minimizing the consequences of errors when they do occur. This approach mirrors the functional organization of the brain where a premium is placed on the detection of errors and error monitoring provides a basis for continual refinement of performance. Within organizations, continuous efforts are needed. As emphasized by Weick and Sutcliffe (2001), in contrast to the pervasive nature of error, what is not pervasive are well-developed systems, processes, and skills to detect and contain errors at their early stages. Echoing this perspective, there is a long tradition of research and practice in the disciplines of human factors, safety management, and risk analysis focused on the development of approaches to assess system reliability, evaluate potential risks of errors, identify error causes, and minimize error occurrence.

Given their potential costs and adverse effects, we normally ascribe errors a negative role in our lives, with a deeply ingrained aversion. Compared with the extensive efforts that are devoted to preventing errors, the potential benefits of errors have been largely overlooked. The history of human civilization provides numerous examples of innovations and discoveries that have been inspired by errors. As James Joyce noted, "mistakes are our portals of discovery." Errors can provide insights, stimulate creativity, and invite us to explore new paths to "success on the far side of failure" (Thomas J. Watson, Sr., 1874–1956). We owe thanks to errors for many major inventions and discoveries, including antibiotic penicillin, smallpox vaccine, pacemakers, dynamite, plastic, and radioactivity. These inventions and discoveries have fundamentally changed our lives, while inspiring the emergence and transformation of major industries. Furthermore, as a natural part of learning, errors indicate performance deficiencies and, under some circumstances, provide informative feedback about where knowledge and skills need further improvement (Keith, 2010). Therefore, at an organizational and societal level, understanding how to learn from errors, as naturally occurs with the brain, is as important as preventing errors. This is not to say that we should forego the prevention of errors. Rather, we should foster a positive attitude toward errors when they occur by recognizing their potential instructive value in germinating new insights. Scott Adams expressed this sentiment in his famous line, "Creativity is allowing yourself to make mistakes. Art is knowing which ones to keep." Errors will cause losses, but they are like bitter medicine, of which we need to take a few gulps to spark the creative genius inside us.

   Although human error is a concept rooted in the discipline of psychology that describes an aspect or phenomenon of human behavior, it has increasingly drawn attention and interest from a wide range of domains outside psychology, including engineering, medicine, and social science. This is not a coincidence, but a consequence of the paramount importance of understanding and managing human error in the safety of sociotechnical systems and our desire to avoid disasters. The past several decades have seen a multitude of developments made through cross-disciplinary efforts, with an impetus to understand the human contribution to safety in complex systems from individual, organizational, social, and design perspectives.

Confusion Regarding the Term *Human Error*

Throughout history, the term *human error* has been used in our daily language as if the term were well understood and defined. On the contrary, although many working definitions have been proposed, the term is difficult to define. Here, the term is used to refer to an activity that (1) was not intended by the actor; (2) is undesirable with respect to relevant rules or an external observer; or (3) resulted in a task or system diverging from its acceptable limits (Senders and Moray, 1991). As noted by Hollnagel and Amalberti (2001), while the term has the connotation of something that should be avoided, it is used with many denotations, each of which can be misleading in understanding the nature of error.

Human Error as Judgment

To understand the term human error, it is important for us to realize that when we say that an error has occurred, we are making a judgment by comparing, either explicitly or implicitly, the so-called error with some performance standard or criterion. That is, without a comparison it is not meaningful to say that an error has been made, even though the outcome is undesirable; an error can only be said to exist if there is a clear performance standard to define the criterion for an acceptable response or outcome.

Judgments regarding error imply that human performance is either correct or incorrect—a binary distinction. In some circumstances, the distinction can be made rather easily and objectively with a clear performance criterion. For example, for tasks that require a discrete action, such as turning on a pump, the correctness of the action can be easily specified. However, the binary distinction between right and wrong is not always justifiable for human performance. For instance, when there are multiple alternative strategies to achieve a goal, even though some strategies may be less optimal, they cannot be considered erroneous if the outcome is acceptable. Furthermore, even for the optimal strategy, the outcome may vary as a product of the natural and irreducible variability in human performance. Under these circumstances, it is difficult to define what is meant by incorrect performance, except for situations where human actions are clearly inappropriate or beyond the acceptable limits of a specific task. That is, the defining qualities of the judgment may be unclear and thus may be prone to interpretation, especially when the criterion involves human internal, unobservable cognitive constructs such as intentions and purposes. Hence, the term human error, to some extent, is relative and subjective. What one person considers an error may not be what another person considers an error, depending on his or her perspectives. There is a range of possibilities from the entirely correct to the totally incorrect, and the distinction between right and wrong is normally a matter of degree, rather than absolutes (Hollnagel, 2007).

Hollnagel and Amalberti (2001) present an interesting example that illustrates the subjectivity in judgment regarding human error. In a study analyzing air traffic controller (ATCO) errors, two observers watched a controller's training performance on a full-scale simulator and took note of all the errors that they observed. Although the observers witnessed the same performance, there were substantial differences in the number of errors that they noted. More importantly, only a small number of errors were noted by both observers.

From the brain's perspective, the subjectivity in judgment regarding human error is evident in the physiological response accompanying an erroneous performance. For example, it has been demonstrated that there are multiple components to the error-related electrophysiological response of the brain. There is an initial component that has a negative polarity that is present whether or not an individual is aware of having made an error (Nieuwenhuis et al., 2001). In contrast, there is a second, later component with a positive polarity that is generally absent in conditions where a subject commits an error, but is unaware of having done so. When subjects are asked to evaluate their own performance and estimate the magnitude of their errors, there is a correlation between the magnitude of the electrophysiological response and the individual's subjective appraisal regarding the extent to which he or she has erred (Scheffers and Coles, 2000). Furthermore, when faced with an erroneous outcome, the brain responds differently depending on whether an individual perceives that he or she is the source of the error, as opposed to believing that he or she had no role in causing the error (Knoblich and Sebanz, 2005). These findings point to the subjectivity inherent in human error. From the brain's perspective, error is not absolute, and one's response to an error differs in regard to whether one perceives that one is the cause of the error.

Human Error as Cause

In our daily language, we often say that an undesirable event occurred because of human error. In this context, the term human error is used with a denotation of being the cause of an event. Logically and philosophically, such a denotation represents a reverse causality (i.e., reasoning from effect to cause). Hence, the use of the term human error risks falsely associating an observed effect with a presumed cause (Hollnagel and Amalberti, 2001).

Human error may be one of multiple possible causes for an observed outcome or one variable in a complex process leading to an outcome. Therefore, the denotation is misleading in that it reduces all the possible causes and the associated complexity to a simple explanation labeled "human error." This attribution often occurs when an analysis of events is carried just far enough that there is insufficient evidence to "blame" technological systems, such that human error constitutes a catch-all satisfactory explanation (Hollnagel and Amalberti, 2001; Woods et al., 2010). Such an explanation is often convenient, as well as sufficient, in accident investigations, because, as Perrow (1986, p. 146) noted, "Finding that faulty designs were responsible would entail enormous shutdown and retrofitting costs; finding that management was responsible would threaten those in charge, but finding that operators were responsible preserves the system, with some soporific injunctions about better training."

Since the denotation suggests that a meaningful cause has been identified, namely, the human, it stifles search for a systematic explanation and paints a partial picture of the undesirable event. The misleading implications of this denotation are that (1) the problem originated with humans;

(2) humans are responsible for the problem; and (3) error prevention can be achieved by changing humans or reducing their role in complex systems (Woods et al., 2010). As emphasized by Woods et al. (2010), error is a symptom rather than a cause and should serve as a call for further probing and investigation.

Human Error as Consequence

When we conclude that an error was caused by human action, the term human error is used to characterize the observable outcome of the action. Such a denotation is commonly used in the probabilistic risk analysis (PRA) community to refer to human-caused failures of a system. One problem with this detonation is that it does not provide insight concerning potential errors, except for stating that the planned action fails to achieve its desired goal.

Another problem is that judgments concerning error, in this case the consequence of an action, can only be made after the error has occurred. Such judgments represent after-the-fact inferences based on observations of unsatisfactory results and, consequently, are prone to hindsight bias. As Woods et al. (2010) expressed, with the benefit of hindsight, we know what factors were critical to the results and tend to assume that knowledge of these factors was available before the results were known. Consequently, we tend to oversimplify or trivialize situations, as well as the mechanisms that could have affected the results, exaggerating what could have been known in foresight.

Human Error as Action, Event, or Process

When we say an error has occurred, or an event or a process has gone wrong, we address the manifestation of the error without consideration of the cause. One problem with this denotation is that, to some extent, it implies that human error is intentional, an observable human function, or an observable category of human performance. As discussed earlier, human error is inferred from observations and involves judgments made in hindsight (Hollnagel, 1983; Woods et al., 1994).

There is no good reason to suppose a close coupling between an action, event, or process and the subsequent outcome or consequence (Woods et al., 1994). A slip may cause momentary embarrassment and trifling inconvenience in a forgiving circumstance, but could lead to a catastrophic accident in a safety-critical system such as a nuclear power plant. As Reason and Mycielska (1982) stated, the difference lies not in the nature of the action, event, or process, but the extent to which its circumstances will produce penalties. Furthermore, "incorrect" actions do not necessarily lead to failures, and actions or processes can be corrected before they generate an undesirable outcome. Likewise, there may be good reasons for performing some actions, yet they still lead to unwanted consequences.

Interactive Nature and Complexity of Human Error

Error is the product of the dynamic interaction between a human and the system or task to achieve a specific goal in a specified context. This section discusses three elements in the processes underlying error: *intention, cognitive and neurophysiological mechanisms*, and *context*.

Intention

Intention includes the motivation to interact with a system or perform a task, and the goal(s) of the interaction. The notions of error and intention are inseparable (Reason, 1990, p. 5). Error is not a human function. We do not *commit* an error intentionally; however, error is only applicable to intentional acts where there was *prior intention*, meaning the intention was formed prior to performing the act (Searle, 1980). Some intentional actions, such as spontaneous behavior, are carried out without plans. In such cases, no mismatch between the achieved results and goals is present to evaluate whether a specific action is correct or not (i.e., whether the action deviates from intention). Hence, it is only meaningful to talk of error when we act on a prior intention.

According to Reason (1990), prior intention is comprised of two elements: (1) the end-state to be attained; and (2) the means to achieve the end-state. Based on these two elements, error can be classified into two forms (Norman, 1983):

- *Slips* (or *lapses*) are unintended actions (i.e., actions that deviate from prior intention) that do not achieve the intended end-state.
- *Mistakes* are intended actions that do not achieve the intended end-state because of the mismatch between the prior intention and the intended consequences.

Discussion of intent generally presumes some degree of conscious awareness. However, in research summarized in Chapter 2, it has been demonstrated that activity is present within the brain that is predictive of the intent to act and the specific nature of the action several seconds prior to the subject becoming consciously aware of his or her intent to act (Soon et al., 2008). Furthermore, conditions may be distinguished in which conscious awareness is focused on the intent to execute a specific action, as opposed to consciously focusing on the actual execution of the action, based on activity occurring in a region of the brain known as the presupplementary motor area (Lau et al., 2004). In a typical experimental paradigm, subjects are asked to choose between one or more actions and then hold this intent in mind for some period of time until cued to execute their response (see figures 1 and 2 in Lau et al., 2004). Based on activity observed within the brain, the specific choice may be reliably predicted. Once the action begins, activity shifts to other regions of the brain as the subject executes the action and monitors his or her performance (Haynes et al., 2007). Brain processes underlying the intention and execution of an action are in play, whether or not one is consciously aware of one's intentions or consciously attends to the action. Notably, conscious awareness is not essential, and an intent may exist within the brain to carry out a specific act without conscious awareness of this intention. These observations confuse our common conceptions of intentionality and error. Conscious awareness of the act, including the erroneous nature of the act, may not occur until the act is either underway or an individual has reached a point of no return, with the erroneous act being unstoppable.

Cognitive and Neurophysiological Mechanisms

While information-processing models based on analogy between human brain processes and the operations of a digital computer have been extremely influential in analyzing and interpreting human error (e.g., Ivergard and Hunt, 2008), their depictions of brain processes are questionable. At best, the functioning of the human brain is weakly analogous to the functions of a digital computer. Consequently, adherence to an information-processing model may prompt erroneous conclusions regarding the basis of human error. A consideration of the key differences between the brain and a digital computer elucidate several sources of human error within brain functions.

Whereas computers involve digital information processing, the brain is largely analog, with its operations being continuous and often nonlinear. The rate of firing and the synchronization of firing across neural circuits are essential to information processing within the brain. Consequently, performance can be variable depending on the relative timing of events. For example, visual perception is characterized by synchronous activity in the 8–13 Hz (alpha) bandwidth. It has been shown that the likelihood of the detection of a visual stimulus varies in accordance with the phase of these cycles such that a stimulus presented during the ascending portion of the cycle is more likely to be detected than a stimulus presented during the descending phase (Busch et al., 2009). Similarly, variability in trial-to-trial performance has been linked to spontaneous fluctuations in the oscillatory activity of neural circuits (Fox et al., 2005). Thus, it is misleading to think of the brain as a digital processor carrying out a sequence of instructions. Instead, the brain is more appropriately conceptualized as a collection of oscillating neural assemblies that are capable of processing information through the phase and harmonic synchronization of oscillatory processes (Singer, 1993). Accordingly, human error may arise as a product of the inherent variability in these processes, including factors that accentuate the variability inherent to these processes (e.g., fatigue, age), or as a result of perturbations affecting these processes (e.g., emotional responses).

With a computer, memory is accessed through reference to a precise address corresponding to its location on the memory drive mechanism (i.e., byte-addressable memory). This design allows for great precision in recalling specific memory records. In contrast, memory within the brain is content-addressable, meaning that recall is based on reference to the content of the memory. Thus, when recalling a specific memory, various cues to the memory contents serve as the basis for accessing and activating patterns of neural activation corresponding to the memory. Furthermore, within the brain, memory is subject to spreading activation. Through spreading activation, recalling a given item from memory primes other related items and, as a result of this priming, recall of related items is facilitated, with related items often consciously recalled.

Compared with a digital computer, memory processes within the brain are imprecise and subject to interference. Consequently, errors may arise due to erroneous recall. For example, with routine activities that have become highly automated, an irrelevant cue is often sufficient to trigger activation of an incorrect sequence of actions. This can be seen during daily routines when you lose track of where you are in the routine and repeat a step (e.g., brush your teeth twice or put the milk away before pouring some on your cereal). Likewise, interference attributable to spreading activation can impair accurate memory recall. For example, when trying to recall the name of someone who you have not seen in a long time, it is easy to mistakenly retrieve the wrong name based on the names of other people who you had known around the same time being more accessible within memory. In this situation, memory is accessed on the basis of the context in which you had known the person, but there were other people associated with this same context and in recalling the context, the wrong name is triggered. Yet, while the memory mechanisms of the brain are prone to error, the brain is often capable of retrieving memories given scant cues or, at the least, recalling a partial memory. In contrast, computers are generally incapable of retrieving items from memory without specific reference to the memory address, with memory retrieval being all or none.

Whereas computers are modular and carry out serial operations, the brain operates in a manner that is massively parallel. During everyday experiences, the entire brain is active in processing and integrating sensory inputs, interpreting events, and coordinating responses. This includes processes occurring at both the conscious and unconscious levels. All these processes are interwoven to create our memories. Consequently, activities are context sensitive. This means that given appropriate contextual cues, memories may be retrieved that would otherwise be inaccessible. However, it also means that placed in the wrong context, memory retrieval may fail or inappropriate memories may be retrieved. Likewise, misinterpretation of the context can lead to the retrieval of inappropriate routines. For example, an examination of accidents often reveals that the operators misinterpreted the situation and given their interpretation of the situation, the seemingly erroneous actions were actually quite appropriate. The parallel nature of the brain lends itself to operational processes that are contextually based, meaning that the brain creates an integrated representation of events. Then, as one moves between contexts, the brain shifts from one contextually linked collection of memory representations to another. This implies that for effective performance, there must be an accurate interpretation of contexts, with the failure to accurately interpret contexts leading to the retrieval of erroneous and inappropriate memory representations.

As a result of the parallel manner in which the brain operates, its operations tend to be nondiscrete. In contrast, the operations of a computer are serial and discrete. Consequently, with the brain, there is potential for interference between related operations. When there is activation of a given operation, this activation produces spreading activation to other related operations. For example, while fixing breakfast, the act of pouring a bowl of cereal produces spreading activation to the act of pouring milk onto the cereal. As a result, if the next step is to take orange juice from the refrigerator, it is not unlikely that one will erroneously pour the orange juice onto the cereal. While specific steps may be carried out one at a time, spreading activation and the resulting priming of memory representations, with multiple representations being simultaneously activated, creates an operational environment where individual actions overlap with one another and can interfere with one another, and occasionally, actions may be performed out of sequence.

Whereas computers have a system clock and their operations are precisely timed relative to this clock, the timing of brain processes is variable. The extent of this variability can differ with there being associated effects on performance. For example, as one gains proficiency with a motor task, there is a reduction in the variability of the neural processes involved in performing the task. This was demonstrated in a go/no-go paradigm in which subjects were presented with an initial cue to warn them that the cue prompting their response was impending (Churchland et al., 2006). During the interval, there is activation of the premotor regions of the cortex that corresponds to the preparation to respond. With practice, there is reduced variability in neural activation during this interval and with this reduced variability, there is a reduction in the response time.

In other research, it has been shown that variability in neural responses impacts perceptual experience. A study was conducted using Rubin's vase-faces picture for which subjects viewing the figure from one perspective report seeing a vase and from an alternative perspective report seeing two faces (Hesselmann et al., 2008). The researchers noted that there were ongoing fluctuations in neural activity and when presentation of the figure corresponded to elevated activity in the fusiform gyrus, which is a region of the brain associated with recognizing faces, there was a greater tendency to report seeing two faces, as opposed to seeing a vase. This finding suggests that our propensity to interpret sensory information one way or another is a product of the relative timing of ongoing fluctuations of neural activity. The operation of the brain involves the coordination, or synchronization, of neural activity, both at a local level corresponding to specific functional circuits, as well as at distributed levels for producing a response that integrates the activity of various functional circuits. The capacity to achieve the synchronization of neural circuits can vary with the result being variability in behavioral performance. Furthermore, individual differences in intrinsic levels of neural variability have been linked to the level of connectivity within the prefrontal cortex (Ullen et al., 2008). Thus, there appears to be a neural substrate underlying individual differences in the ability to generate coordinated neural activity, with associated impacts on cognitive performance.

Macrocognition

Macrocognition is a term originally coined by Cacciabue and Hollnagel (1995) to describe cognition in real-world settings. It focuses on the nature of the human performance in "the field," where decisions are often very complex and must be made quickly by domain experts in risky or high-stakes situations (Klein et al., 2003). According to macrocognition theory, a macrocognitive function is the high-level mental activities that must be successfully accomplished to perform a task or achieve a goal in a naturalistic environment (Letsky, 2007). Although there are a number of different macrocognition models, the general consensus is that there are five macrocognitive functions: (1) detecting and noticing, (2) understanding and sensemaking, (3) decision making, (4) action, and (5) team coordination (US NRC, 2012; Whaley et al., 2012). As an illustration, Whaley et al. (2012) adapted the macrocognition concept to operator behavior in nuclear power plants. They identified the cognitive mechanisms underlying work in this environment. The operation of these mechanisms is considered crucial to a successful performance. If part of the process fails (either internal or external to the human), the failure may manifest itself as a *macrocognitive function failure*.

Over 300 mechanisms have been identified along with the associated boundary conditions that can lead to the failure of the macrocognitive functions. The mechanisms are then clustered into categories (i.e., *proximate* causes) based on the effects of the failures. A proximate cause reflects the failure of a mechanism. For example, one cognitive mechanism states that, "important sensory cues must be sufficiently salient to be easily detected by higher cognitive functions." The failure of this mechanisms results in the cue not being perceived. Thus, "cue/info not perceived" is an identifiable cause (i.e., a proximate cause) for failing to detect a cue (i.e., the detecting and noticing macrocognitive function). The proximate causes for the failure of the five macrocognitive functions are listed in Table 6.1.

By establishing direct linkages (i.e., causal relationships) between cognitive mechanisms and observed outcomes, the macrocognitive model provides an analytical approach to address different classes of errors (e.g., errors of commission [ECOs] and errors of omission [EOOs]), using a common set of cognitive mechanisms. Furthermore, since the model addresses failures

TABLE 6.1

Proximate Causes for the Failure of Macrocognitive Functions

Macrocognitive Functions	Proximate Causes
Failure of detecting and noticing	• Cues/information not perceived • Cues/information not attended to • Cues/information misperceived
Failure of understanding and sensemaking	• Incorrect data • Incorrect integration of data, frames, or data with a frame • Incorrect frame
Failure of decision making	• Incorrect goals or priorities set • Incorrect pattern matching • Incorrect mental simulation or evaluation of options
Failure of action	• Failure to execute desired action • Execute desired action incorrectly
Failure of team coordination	• Failure of team communication • Error in leadership/supervision

at the level of cognitive mechanisms, it can be readily extended to various domains.

Context

All human actions are performed within a specific context and are subject to a complex range of situational or environmental influences that bear on our ability to accomplish a task, such as training, procedures, human–system interfaces, communication standards, and so forth. The relevance and importance of contextual elements may vary with the situation, with contextual elements often difficult to identify and measure.

Retrospective analyses of actual operational events in industrial complexes (e.g., nuclear power plants) show that human operators generally perform routine tasks well with reasonable, natural variability. Human performance problems often arise in unusual circumstances, where operators perform actions that are not required and may worsen conditions during an accident. An isolated analysis of individual operational events may leave an impression that failures are caused by operators' illogical actions under system- or event-specific circumstances. However, a deeper scrutiny from a holistic perspective suggests this impression is a biased and simplified explanation for the undesired performance. Such unusual circumstances involve a combination of the following complicating factors that are relevant to all events:

- Multiple equipment failures and unavailabilities
- Deviations from operators' expectations, beyond their training and experience

- System conditions not addressed by procedures
- Time pressure
- Uncertainty and limited information
- Conflicting goals and shifting priorities

These complicating factors frequently result in a significant mismatch between system behavior and operators' expectations; a mismatch that frequently creates the need for operator actions. In retrospect, it may be quite obvious that the situational appraisals, goals, and action plans that operators exhibited were inappropriate given the circumstances of the accident. Furthermore, it may be difficult to understand the tendency of operators to persist in implementing action plans given ineffective results. However, if we consider the seemingly illogical actions in the context of corresponding complicating factors, the actions often make sense given the engineered and operational conditions.

The Three Mile Island (TMI) accident offers an example of how operators can be "made to fail" by combinations of operator mindset and unexpected, confusing conditions (see Kemeny 1979). The accident occurred in Pennsylvania in March 1979, and has been the most serious commercial nuclear power plant accident to occur in the United States, with significant reactor core damage and a small release of radioactivity. The accident started with a loss of heat sink (i.e., all secondary cooling), due to the loss of feedwater systems. The factors contributing to the unavailability of the systems included preexisting misaligned valves and a maintenance tag that obstructed the position indicator of the valves. A pilot-operated relief valve (PORV) was then lifted automatically to relieve the pressure caused by the lost heat sink, releasing steam to a pressure relief tank (PRT). When the PORV failed to reclose as designed, the following factors acted together to complicate the situation and eventually lead to the accident.

- The actual position of the PORV was not displayed in the main control room. Although the valve was stuck open, after the operators had sent a close signal to the valve, they assumed that the valve was completely shut. As a result, the valve was open for more than 2 h, causing water loss from the reactor vessel.
- The steam released from the PORV was dumped into a PRT; however, the indicator for the tank water level, which could have shown an improperly functioning PORV, was on the back panel of the control room. The operators did not check the indication partly because they were overloaded. The workload and cognitive noise during the early and middle stages of the accident were excessive. For example, there were 7 significant alerts in the first 28 s following the unknown opening of the PORV.

- The rising water level in the pressurizer resulting from the loss of heat sink was unanticipated. The operators' understanding and responses to the phenomenon were conditioned by their naval submarine training, in which the dangers of a rising water level in the pressurizer were emphasized as it was indeed of more consequence and importance to operating a nuclear submarine than a nuclear power plant. This partly caused the operators to fixate on the water level and overlook cues that could have indicated an ongoing loss of coolant accident (LOCA). More importantly, driven by training that emphasized the need to respond to the rising water level in the pressurizer, the operators switched off a safety system to avoid increasing the reactor pressure, which caused the reactor to overheat and guaranteed that there would be a meltdown of the reactor core.

The discussion above indicates that the cause of the accident was not simple and cannot be solely attributed to the operators. From the perspective of phenotype (i.e., what happened), the accident was a consequence of the operators' inappropriate decisions and their overlooking cues that could have helped their diagnosis. From the perspective of genotype (i.e., why it happened), the operators' inappropriate decisions and actions were a result of their effort to create success, cope with complexity, and bridge the gap between their expectations and the evolving conditions by adapting their training and experience to the ongoing challenges. Their training and experience allowed them to perform skilled and speedy operations under normal circumstances; however, when applied in the wrong context, they led to inappropriate behavior with unsafe consequences. The operators did not knowingly commit an error; they were performing actions that seemed "correct" at the time. In general, this observation is consistent with those derived from other incident analyses. That is, human error is not random and is conditioned by a conjunction of system conditions (e.g., equipment failures) and contextual factors, which in combination may be referred to as an *error-forcing context* (EFC; Nuclear Regulatory Commission, 2000). The EFC can lead to a refusal to believe evidence that runs counter to an initial misdiagnosis, or failure to recognize evidence, which can result in subsequent mistakes and, ultimately, a catastrophic accident. This echoes the earlier discussion that attributing failures to humans is an over-simplified explanation. A proper understanding of human error requires a systematic and holistic point of view that accounts for the context.

An Error in Judgment

The radio industry was changing and ST had been unusually effective in adapting to these changes. Since assuming an executive position working out of the corporate headquarters, he had overseen the transformation of numerous stations in cities across the country. In many cases, this had come with the dismissal of key personnel, including station managers and their staff. It was never pleasant, but ST believed that he was a decisive leader and took pride in his willingness to make tough decisions.

It was a radio station in a large city in the southern United States, which the corporation considered to be a valuable market. Yet, holding on to the same format it had used since the 1960s, its audience had dwindled to the point that the station was no longer profitable. The station was in desperate need of a major change and ST had no remorse when he fired the station manager of 15 years and replaced him with an individual who had been enormously successful at a small station in Southern California. The first step was to change the format from pop to talk radio to capitalize on the growing audience for this format at the time. While several key staff were retained, there was a tremendous turnover with new personalities brought in to appear on the air and many of the support staff replaced with individuals who had more experience working with the new format.

ST believed that he had a thorough understanding of the situation. However, working in corporate headquarters a thousand miles away, he had little appreciation of the day-to-day dynamics within the station. Most prominently, the sales manager, who ST had retained, was close friends with the former station manager and had been assured that he would soon become station manager when the former manager retired. The sales manager wanted this position and had proudly proclaimed on many occasions that his ascent to the top job was inevitable. He had planned accordingly, purchasing a second home and assuming a lifestyle consistent with the income and perks typically given to station managers.

The sales manager was shocked when the announcement was made that the former station manager had been fired and a new manager was being brought in to the station from outside. He felt angry and betrayed. He went to the former manager, but there was nothing that could be done. It was humiliating to have to explain that he had been passed over. Fueled by his outrage, he declared that he was not going to let this happen and dedicated himself to undoing what had been done.

His scheme began with the recruitment of a key ally. He turned to the chief engineer who had openly expressed his discontent with having lost a couple of staff and cuts to the budget that he needed to make technical upgrades. They had never been great friends, but they quickly found a common cause in their animosity toward everyone involved in the shake-up.

As with any new manager taking over a troubled radio station in an unfamiliar city, the first few months were rough going. The change in format did not go smoothly and many of their customers either quit buying commercial time or significantly reduced their purchases. This was accompanied by an economic downturn that impacted many of the station's traditional advertisers. There were technical problems that caused unplanned expenses and it proved difficult to operate the station with a smaller staff. The sales manager waited a couple of months during which he documented every negative event and once sufficient time had passed that he could claim to have been open-minded and given the new station manager a fair chance, he reached out to ST. His initial inquiry was modest, asking if ST might have time to speak to him about the situation at the station following the change in format. Having been taught that executives should have an open door, ST agreed to talk with the sales manager. Their first discussion over the phone was tame. The sales manager expressed that it had been difficult since the change in formats and asked if headquarters could contribute to the station's advertising budget. The goal had been to establish a rapport and to seem reasonable and constructive.

ST had never worked with the new station manager before and their initial interactions did not go well. Reports from the station were bad and there was an immediate tension between ST and the station manager due partly to the challenging circumstances and partly to a differences between East Coast and West Coast personalities. Events continually placed ST and the station manager in conflict with one another. An animosity rooted in incompatible priorities began to develop. Consequently, ST was primed when the sales manager began his assault on the station manager. It started with a series of reports that chronicled and exaggerated the station's misfortunes. Over the next few months, this escalated to direct attributions to the station manager, impugning his intelligence, and his managerial and personal skills. At this point, the sales manager brought his ally, the chief engineer, into the discussions to reinforce his assertions and contribute his own criticisms. They presented a situation in which the station was falling apart and the staff was ready to mutiny. Next, the sales manager turned to several friends whose companies advertised with the station and recruited them to express their discontent with the station.

From ST's perspective, he was receiving a constant litany of the failings of the station manager as he developed a personal distaste for the manager due to their constant conflicts. His decision seemed obvious. The station manager would have to go and ST commenced the process for his dismissal. It was another 4 months before the firing was announced, coming 15 months after the initial hiring. The sales manager was not promoted to the station manager's job, but instead, another new manager was hired. Within 3 months, both the sales manager and the chief engineer had left the station and taken new jobs. In retrospect, a careful analysis of the situation would have revealed that the station manager had been effective in turning the station around after the format change. Revenues had initially dipped, but were on the rise and the station had returned to profitability after several years of losses. It would also become apparent that the sales manager had been carrying out an elaborate scheme in which he reported sales of commercial time at a discount rate, yet he had sold the time at standard rates and pocketed the difference. While illegal, he was never indicted and he had left the station before the discrepancy was discovered. The station manager was out of work for 9 months before he was hired to manage a small station in Texas where he resumed his success and was soon recognized within the radio industry for his talents. ST continued in his job for the next year and following a buyout of the company, was dismissed and left the radio industry.

Most discussions of error are focused on operators, line workers, and other low-level personnel. However, as this story illustrates, errors can occur at any level of an organization, with impacts that reverberate throughout an organization. At every step of the way, ST believed that he was making the correct decision and to this day would likely assert that he had not erred in his appraisal of the station manager and his decision to dismiss him. This is the nature of human error. From the perspective of the individual caught up in day-to-day events, the situation may seem clear and the appropriate course of action obvious. However, when viewing the events in retrospect and knowing what could not be known at the time, the nature and magnitude of the error is clear.

Error Classifications

A large number of taxonomies or classification schemes have been developed to describe error. For example, Meister (1971) divided human errors into four types based on where they originate: (1) operating errors, (2) design errors, (3) manufacturing errors, and (4) installation and maintenance errors. In probabilistic safety assessment (PSA) and human reliability analysis (HRA) for high-consequence industries (e.g., the nuclear and aviation industries), human errors are often classified into three categories based on the relative timing of the errors and the accident sequence. The first category is *preinitiator human errors*, which are faults that occur before the beginning of an accident sequence. The second category is *initiator human errors*, which are human actions that contribute to the initiating event of an accident sequence. The third category is *postinitiator human errors*, which are faults that occur after an incident that aggravate the incident (IAEA, 1996).

The error taxonomies vary with respect to their theoretical orientations and practical concerns. Due to the complex nature of human error, it is difficult for a taxonomy to be comprehensive and reconcile specific contextual triggers with general error tendencies (Reason, 1990). That is, there is more than one way to classify an error, depending on the nature of the error and the tasks of interest. With a given application, a particular taxonomy may be preferred over others. The taxonomies range from simple binary classifications to complex hierarchical structures (Groth and Mosleh, 2012), and can be distinguished with respect to the following three levels at which the taxonomies approach the problem of classifying errors (Reason, 1990; Senders and Moray, 1991).

- *Phenomenological or behavioral level.* Taxonomies at this level classify errors in terms of observable features. Although they can effectively describe *what* errors occurred at the superficial level of human behavior, these taxonomies do not provide insights with regard to *why* and *how* errors occurred.
- *Contextual level.* Taxonomies at this level emphasize the observable contextual triggering factors that prompted an error; however, like phenomenological taxonomies, they provide limited insights as to why and how errors occurred.
- *Conceptual level.* Taxonomies at this level are based on conceptual considerations of the cognitive mechanisms involved in error production, and provide the greatest insight into the nature of errors.

Most of the available error taxonomies are useful only for retrospective error analysis, and few can be used to predict the imminent occurrence of errors (Senders and Moray, 1991). This is in contrast to the error classification schemes described in the following sections.

Errors of Omission and Errors of Commission

One frequently used scheme classifies human errors into EOOs, which are instances in which actions that are necessary for a particular circumstance are not performed, and EOCs, which refers to errors in which incorrect actions are performed or an intended action is performed incorrectly (Swain and Guttman, 1983; Wickens et al., 1998). EOOs are often caused by distraction or diverted attention and are particularly prevalent in maintenance tasks. Generally, EOOs do not alter the trajectory of events and are correctable in that they merely result in time delays. In contrast, EOCs are often caused by inadequate training, poor instruction, or unrecognized hazards. Although the scheme was expanded by Swain and Guttman (1983) with two additional categories (*sequential errors*, which are actions performed out of the correct order, and *time errors*, which are actions performed too slow, too fast, or too late), only the first two categories have been widely used in HRA methods, such as the technique for human error rate prediction (THERP) (Swain and Guttman, 1983).

EOOs, where an operator fails to perform some action, may be attributed to multiple causes. In an earlier chapter, there was discussion of mental lapses and the relationship between lapses and the brain's default network. A lapse refers to states in which an individual's conscious awareness is turned inward and, as a result, he or she is less attentive and responsive to events occurring within the surrounding environment. Cheyne et al. (2009) have linked EOOs to mind wandering, attributing omissions to either momentary or prolonged lapses in attention. For instance, those exhibiting attentional deficits linked to attention deficit hyperactivity disorder (ADHD) show a greater incidence of EOOs (Johnson et al., 2007).

Certain conditions make disengagement more likely, with some individuals more prone to disengagement than others. EOOs can be expected to occur when disengagement results in either a failure to recognize cues prompting certain actions or there is a failure in task monitoring such that one loses track of what has and has not been done. Sustained task attention hinges on the integrity of the brain circuits associated with executive functions and contextual awareness, and conditions disrupting the integrity of these interrelated circuits increase the propensity for lapses and the associated EOOs (Uddin et al., 2008). It has also been suggested that lapses may involve interference resulting from a failure to suppress task-irrelevant, spontaneous activation of neural circuits (Helps, 2009). Thus, there is competition between task-oriented and task-irrelevant thoughts, causing one to occasionally lose track of one's ongoing activities. Taken together, it would appear that a primary source of EOOs lies within the capacity of the brain to maintain sustained attention to a task, suppressing the tendency to drift into conscious states dominated by the activity of the default mode network, with impediments to sustained attention (e.g., boredom, fatigue, distractions) increasing the likelihood of activities being omitted.

A second source of EOOs involves situations where a routine or a procedure has been learned, but there is a failure to adequately recall this knowledge from memory, resulting in one or more steps being omitted. This situation will be most prevalent with routines for which there have been limited opportunities for practice or there has been an extended duration during which there has been little or no practice. It has been demonstrated that the ability to accurately recall a procedural routine depends on the activity of a region of the brain known as the supplementary motor area (SMA), during the period immediately following practice sessions (Tanaka et al., 2010). When currents were applied to the brain to suppress SMA activity immediately following practice, there was little benefit to the practice, in comparison with a condition where currents were applied 6 h subsequent to the practice session. It has been suggested that the activity of the SMA serves to stabilize the memory representation within the primary motor area, and when this process is disrupted, the memory representation for a series of steps is more susceptible to decay. However, deficits in the ability to recall procedural routines have also been linked to disruptions in the dopamine input to a region of the brain known as the caudate (Carbon et al., 2004). Dopamine serves to reinforce patterns of neural activation and in the absence of dopamine, memory representations linking a series of steps could decay, leaving one more prone to omit steps or fail to complete a series of procedural steps. These findings suggest that the ability to accurately produce sequential patterns of behavior depends on the integrity of neural circuits that serve to establish and sustain the corresponding memory representations. When there is an inadequate opportunity to establish these routines or the routines are allowed to decay due to nonuse, one might expect an increase in the incidence of EOOs.

A third factor contributing to the occurrence of EOOs involves failures of prospective memory. Prospective memory refers to the capacity to remember an activity that is to be performed sometime in the future. For example, talking to friends one evening, one may agree to call one of them the next morning. Prospective memory would involve the processes whereby one forms a memory representation for the activity that is to be performed the next day and then recalls that memory the next day. When prospective memory fails, and one does not recall the intended activity, the resulting omission may be considered an EOO. Brain imaging studies suggest that there are two somewhat distinct functional circuits associated with prospective memory (Burgess et al., 2001). One serves to maintain an intention to perform the intended task, whereas the second provides the basis for realizing this intention. Consequently, activities that interfere with either function would be expected to produce prospective memory failures and associated EOOs. For example, there are cognitive demands associated with sustaining an intention to carry out a future activity. Intervening demands due to other tasks or activities will diminish the capacity to sustain the intention. It is a common experience to realize that once a demanding situation has reached a conclusion, one or more routine tasks that would have ordinarily been remembered, have been forgotten. Similarly, task demands at the time of the intended action can overshadow the intended activity. As a result, one may recall the intention, but being unable to carry out the intention, it is neglected and the corresponding actions are omitted.

Slips (or Lapses) and Mistakes

A second widely used binary classification scheme distinguishes between slips (or lapses) and mistakes (Norman, 1981; Reason, 1990). Slips (or lapses) are instances in which the intention is correct, but a failure occurs when carrying out the associated activities (Reason and Mycielska, 1982). Simply put, slips (or lapses) are low-level errors of execution. Generally, a slip refers to an unintended deviation from a correct plan of action due to suboptimal attention allocation, whereas a lapse involves omitting part of a plan of action. As noted previously, both slips and lapses are unintended actions. Unlike the terms *commission* and *omission*, which are descriptive and reflect the impact of the error, the terms *slip* (or *lapse*) and *mistake* imply a causal mechanism.

Studies of slips and lapses date back more than a century century when Freud (1901), started to record, classify, and analyze slips of the tongue and pen to understand the underlying mechanisms for language production. Recent research concerning slips of the tongue has shed light on the brain mechanisms underlying the occurrence of slips (Moller et al., 2007). In this research, subjects were exposed to an experimental procedure that is known to induce spoonerisms. A spoonerism is a slip of the tongue where the elements of a sentence are misplaced (e.g., instead of saying, "go and take a shower," one might say, "go and shake a tower"). On trials in which subjects slipped and produced a spoonerism, there was heightened activation in the SMA, a region of the brain associated with the preparation of motor acts. This suggests that multiple motor acts were simultaneously prepared, with the failure to inhibit the inappropriate act resulting in the spoonerism. Once the act, whether verbal or otherwise, has been initiated, there is often an almost immediate recognition of the slip, with a corresponding electrophysiological response within the brain (Hiroaki et al., 2001).

In recent decades, extensive efforts have been devoted to expanding the studies to slips of action with a broader scope—understanding the organization of human performance and the role of consciousness in guiding action. In these studies, different classification schemes have been proposed for action slips. For example, Norman (1981) categorized slips into three groups (i.e., intention formation, activation, and triggering) based on the sources of the slips.

Slips may be distinguished from other forms of error with respect to the nature of the tasks and the mental and physical conditions that promote the occurrence of slips (Reason and Mycielska, 1982; Reason, 1990, p. 8).

- Slips occur during the execution of highly skilled or habitual tasks that require little continuous conscious monitoring. The likelihood of committing a slip increases with proficiency at a particular task. This paradox can be explained by looking at the quantity and type of errors made by experts and novices. Most of the errors made by novices arise from a lack of competence and take unpredictable forms. As a novice becomes increasingly skilled at a task, the increased automaticity in carrying out the details of the task diminishes the demand on conscious attention. As a result, the novice begins to make fewer errors. However, their errors become more predictable in the sense that they tend to take the form of slips. That is, slips are the price we pay for the automaticity that allows us to perform routine tasks efficiently.

- Slips are most often triggered by the context. Routines are normally carried out in familiar environments where vigilance is at a minimum. Environmental cues, such as similarities in locations, actions, purposes, and expectations, can elicit well-organized sequences of skilled actions that are habitually performed in these circumstances.

The actions are suitable for the context most of the time, but not when changed circumstances require some alteration of normal practice, or when new goals demand the modification of existing routines.

- Slips may be induced by external distraction or internal preoccupation. Automaticity in performing routine tasks allows conscious attention to be directed to matters that are unrelated to the ongoing activity. Divided attention often occurs because the performance of routine tasks in familiar surroundings requires little vigilance. When inadequate attention is allocated to monitoring events, inappropriate interpretations of events may occur resulting in biased perceptions, which in turn, lead to actions that are clearly recognizable as belonging to a different context, but are inappropriate given the current conditions.

Slips and lapses may be detected and corrected at various stages, ranging from the initiation of the activity up to the point when the action departs from the plan. Many slips may be caught by the perpetrator or an observer. However, slips and lapses are often unrecognized, or in Reason's (1990) words, they remain "latent" for long periods of time, awaiting windows of accident opportunities (e.g., weaknesses in safety barriers) to reveal themselves. The misaligned valves and maintenance tag previously mentioned in the TMI scenario are good examples. When these chance events were combined with other operating circumstances, they had a significant impact, resulting in a system breakdown.

Mistakes arise from the formation of an incorrect intention, which leads to an incorrect action sequence, although the actions may be consistent with the wrong intention. Compared with slips, mistakes are high-level errors with a substantial cognitive component and are therefore more resistant to detection and correction. Mistakes often occur at Rasmussen's (1983) level of knowledge-based processing and result from a failure to formulate a correct decision due to human processing limitations, incorrect knowledge, inadequate analysis, or planning failures.

The neural mechanisms that may be implicated in mistakes are much broader than those for slips. Often, the origin of mistakes involves erroneous inferences concerning the current context, and while actions may be appropriate for the assumed context, they are not appropriate for the actual context. Brain imaging studies suggest that the recognition of context involves two distinct processes (Wan et al., 2011). One involves the perception of patterns within the environment and the mapping of these patterns to a known context, with these operations linked to the precuneus region of the brain's parietal lobe. The second involves the execution of actions based on the recognition of a context, with this operation linked to the caudate nucleus of the basal ganglia. Failures associated with either of these operations provide the basis for making a mistake. Yet, mistakes may arise from other mechanisms as well. For example, the formation of memory for past events involves a process of construction in which memory traces are organized within the framework of current knowledge (Addis et al., 2007). The same neural substrates that underlie the construction of memory for past events provide the basis for imaging and planning future events. Being a process of construction, memory is quite susceptible to erroneous formulations, with errors in memory construction providing a basis for actions later characterized as mistakes.

Skills, Rules, and Knowledge (SRK) Taxonomy

Rasmussen's SRK taxonomy (Rasmussen, 1983) provides another framework for human error classification based on the different types of information processing involved. According to the SRK taxonomy, operators' behavior can be classified into three categories based on the levels of cognitive control: (1) skill-based behavior (SBB), (2) rule-based behavior (RBB), and (3) knowledge-based behavior (KBB). SBB consists of smooth, automated, and highly integrated patterns of action that are performed without conscious attention. It is usually based on feedforward rather than feedback control. A typical example of SBB is typing on a keyboard without visual support. RBB consists of stored rules derived from procedures, experiences, instructions, or previous problem-solving activities. It is goal oriented, but does not require reasoning. Actions are directly triggered by familiar perceptual cues in the environment. KBB requires analytical reasoning based on an explicit representation of goals and a mental model of the functional properties of the environment. The SRK taxonomy–based scheme classifies human error into *skill-based*, *rule-based*, and *knowledge-based* errors. It should be noted that the slips/mistakes classification discussed earlier is closely related to the SRK classification. Slips are skill based because they occur with well-practiced activities and are caused by misapplied competence. Mistakes, in contrast, are largely confined to the rule- and knowledge-based domains.

Summary

Human error is the product of the dynamic interaction between human and systems or tasks to achieve a goal in a specified context. Therefore, to understand error, it is important to examine all the elements involved in the interaction. An analysis of error should take into consideration the relationships between error and environmental, contextual factors as well as the interactions among the contextual factors. With the benefit of hindsight, the right action or process may seem crystal clear. However, if we place seemingly illogical actions in the context of the surrounding, complicating factors, actions seem sensible given engineered and operational settings. The implication is that we can reduce the likelihood of error by improving the conditions under which people.

Both incorrect and correct performances result from the same cognitive and neurophysiological mechanisms, which underlie all human performance. Thus, the study of human error is actually the study of human performance. There is no need for theories or models specific to human error as an adequate model for correct human performance must be able to account for error; conversely, an adequate explanation of error must begin with some understanding of correct performance (Reason and Mycielska, 1982).

Acknowledgments

Sandia National Laboratories is a multiprogram laboratory managed and operated by Sandia Corporation, a wholly owned subsidiary of Lockheed Martin Corporation, for the US Department of Energy's National Nuclear Security Administration under contract DE-AC04-94AL85000.

References

Addis, D.R., Wong, A.T. and Schacter, D.L. (2007). Remembering the past and imaging the future: Common and distinct neural substrates during event construction and elaboration. *Neuropsychologia, 45*(7), 1363–1377.

Bernstein, P.S., Scheffers, M.K. and Coles, M.G.H. (1995). "Where did I go wrong?" A psychophysiological analysis of error detection. *Journal of Experimental Psychology: Human Perception and Performance, 21*, 1312–1322.

Burgess, P.W., Quayle, A. and Firth, C.D. (2001). Brain regions involved in prospective memory as determined by positron emission tomography. *Neuropsychologia, 39*(6), 545–555.

Busch, N.A., Dubois, J. and Van Rullen, R. (2009). The phase of ongoing EEG oscillations predicts visual perception. *Journal of Neuroscience, 29*(24), 7869–7876.

Cacciabue, P.C. and Hollnagel, E. (1995). Simulation of cognition: Applications. In J.M. Hoc, P.C. Cacciabue and E. Hollnagel (eds), *Expertise and Technology: Cognition and Human-Computer Cooperation*, pp. 55–73. Hillsdale, NJ: Lawrence Erlbaum Associates.

Carbon, M., Ma, Y., Barnes, A., Dhawan, V., Chaly, T., Ghilardi, M.F. and Eidelberg, D. (2004). Caidate nucleous: Influence of dopaminergic input on sequence learning and brain activation in Parkinsonism. *NeuroImage, 21*(4), 1497–1507.

Cheyne, J.A., Solman, G.J.F., Carriere, J.S.A. and Smilek, D. (2009). Anatomy of an error: A bidirectional state model of task engagement/disengagement and attention-related errors. *Cognition*, *111*, 98–113.

Churchland, M.M., Yu, B.M., Ryu, S.I., Santhanam, G. and Shenoy, K.V. (2006). Neural variability in premotor cortex provides a signature of motor prepration. *Journal of Neuroscience*, *26*(14), 3697–3712.

Dehaene, S., Posner, M.I. and Tucker, D.M. (1994). Localization of a neural system for error detection and compensation. *Psychological Science*, *5*, 303–305.

Fox, M.D., Snyder, A.Z., Zacks, J.M. and Raichle, M.E. (2005). Coherent spontaneous activity accounts for trial-to-trial variability in human evoked brain responses. *Nature Neuroscience*, *9*, 23–25.

Freud, S. (1901). *Psychopathology of Everyday Life*. London: Ernest Benn.

Gehring, W.J., Goss, B., Coles, M.G.H., Meyer, D.E. and Donchin, E. (1993). A neural system for error detection and compensation. *Psychological Science*, *4*, 385–390.

Groth, K.M. and Mosleh, A. (2012). A data-informed PIF hierarchy for model-based human reliability analysis. *Reliability Engineering and System Safety*, *108*, 154–174.

Haynes, J.D., Sakai, K., Rees, G., Gilbert, S., Firth, C. and Passingham, R.E. (2007). Reading hidden intentions in the brain. *Current Biology*, *17*(4), 323–328.

Helps, S.K. (2009). Response variability in ADHD: Exploring the possible role of spontaneous brain activity. Doctoral dissertation, University of Southampton.

Hesselmann, G., Kell, C.A., Eger, E. and Kleinschmidt, A. (2008). Spontaneous local variations in neural activity bias perceptual decisions. *Proceedings of the National Academy of Sciences*, *105*(31), 10984–10989.

Hiroaki, M., Hideaki, T., Noriyoshi, T. and Katuo, Y. (2001). Error-related brain potentials elicited by vocal errors. *NeuroReports*, *12*(9), 1851–1855.

Hollnagel, E. (1983). Position paper on human error. NATO Advanced Research Workshop on Human Error, Bellagio, Italy.

Hollnagel, E. (2007). Human error: Trick or treat. In F.T. Durso (ed.), *Handbook of Applied Cognition*, 2nd edn., pp. 219–238. Hoboken, NJ: Wiley.

Hollnagel, E. and Amalberti, R. (2001). The emperor's new clothes, or whatever happened to "human error"? In *Proceedings of the 4th International Workshop on Human Error, Safety and System Development*, June 11–12, Linköping, Sweden.

Holroyd, C.B. and Coles, M.G.H. (2002). The neural basis of human error processing: Reinforcement learning, dopamine, and its error-related negativity. *Psychological Reviews*, *109*(4), 679–709.

International Atomic Energy Agency (IAEA). (1996). *Human Reliability Analysis in Probabilistic Safety Assessment for Nuclear Power Plants: A Safety Practice* (IAEA Safety Series No. 50-P-10). Vienna: IAEA.

Ivergard, T. and Hunt, B. (2008). Models in process control. In T. Ivergard and B. Hunt (eds), *Handbook of Control Room Design and Ergonomics: A Perspective for the Future*, 2nd edn., pp. 11–42. Boca Raton, FL: CRC Press.

Johnson, K.A., Robertson, I.H., Kelly, S.P., Silk, T.J., Barry, E., Dáibhis, A., Watchorn, A., et al. (2007). Dissociation of performance of children with ADHD and high-functioning autism on a task of sustained attention. *Neuropsychologia*, *45*(10), 2234–2245.

Keith, N. (2010). Managing errors during training. In J. Bauer and C. Harteis (eds), *Human Fallibility: The Ambiguity of Errors for Work and Learning*, pp. 173–195. Dordrecht: Springer.

Kemeny, J.G. (1979). *The Need for Change: The Legacy of TMI—Report of the President's Commission on the Accident at Three Mile Island*. New York: Pergamon Press.

Klein, G.A., Ross, K.G., Moon, B.M., Klein, D.E., Hoffman, R.R. and Hollnagel, E. (2003). Macrocognition. *IEEE Intelligent Systems, 18*(3), 81–85.

Knoblich, G. and Sebanz, N. (2005). Agency in the face of error. *Trends in Cognitive Sciences, 9*(6), 259–261.

Lau, H.C., Rogers, R.D., Haggard, P. and Passingham, R.E. (2004). Attention to intention. *Science, 303*(5661), 1208–1210.

Letsky, M. (2007). Macrocognition in collaboration and knowledge interoperability. Paper presented at the *51st Annual Meeting of the Human Factors and Ergonomics Society*, pp. 544–548. 1–5 October, Baltimore, MD.

Meister, D. (1971). *Human Factors: Theory and Practice*. New York: Wiley.

Miltner, W.H.R., Braun, C.H. and Coles, M.G.H. (1997). Event-related brain potentials following incorrect feedback in a time-estimation task: Evidence for a generic neural system for error detection. *Journal of Cognitive Neuroscience, 9*, 788–789.

Moller, J., Jansma, B.M., Rodriguez-Fornells, A. and Munte, T.F. (2007). What the brain does before the tongue slips. *Cerebral Cortex, 17*(5), 1173–1178.

Nieuwenhuis, S., Ridderinkhof, K.R., Blom, J., Band, G.P.H. and Kok, A. (2001). Error-related brain potentials are differentially related to awareness of response errors: Evidence from an antisaccade task. *Psychophysiology, 38*(5), 752–760.

Norman, D.A. (1981). Categorization of action slips. *Psychological Review, 88*(1), 1–15.

Norman, D.A. (1983). Position paper on human error. NATO Advanced Research Workshop on Human Error, Bellagio, Italy.

Nuclear Regulatory Commission. (2000). *Technical Basis and Implementation Guidelines for a Technique for Human Event Analysis (ATHEANA)* (NUREG-1624, Rev. 1). Washington, DC: US Nuclear Regulatory Commission.

Perrow, C. (1986). *Complex Organizations: A Critical Essay*, 3rd edn. New York: Random House.

Rasmussen, J. (1983). Skills, rules, and knowledge: Signals, signs, and symbols, and other distinctions in human performance models. *IEEE Transactions on Systems, Man, and Cybernetics, SMC 13*, 257–266.

Reason, J. (1990). *Human Error*. New York: Cambridge University Press.

Reason, J. and Mycielska, K. (1982). *Absent-Minded?: The Psychology of Mental Lapses and Everyday Errors*. Englewood Cliffs, NJ: Prentice-Hall.

Scheffers, M.K. and Coles, M.G.H. (2000). Performance monitoring in a confusing world: Error-related brain activity, judgments of response accuracy, and types of errors. *Journal of Experimental Psychology Human Perception and Performance, 26*(1), 141–151.

Searle, J.R. (1980). The intentionality of intention and action. *Cognitive Science, 4*, 47–70.

Senders, J.W. and Moray, N.P. (1991). *Human Error: Cause, Prediction, and Reduction*. Hillsdale, NJ: Lawrence Erlbaum Associates.

Singer, W. (1993). Synchronization of cortical activity and its putative role in information processing and learning. *Annual Review of Physiology, 55*, 349–374.

Soon, C.S., Brass, M., Heinz, H.J. and Haynes, J.D. (2008). Unconscious determinants of free decisions in the human brain. *Nature Neuroscience, 11*, 543–545.

Swain, A.D. and Guttman, H.E. (1983). *Handbook of Human Reliability Analysis with Emphasis on Nuclear Power Plant Applications* (NUREG/CR-1278). Washington, DC: US Nuclear Regulatory Commission.

Tanaka, S., Honda, M., Hanakawa, T. and Cohen, L.G. (2010). Differential contribution of the supplementary motor area to stabilization of a procedural motor skill acquired through different practice schedules. *Cerebral Cortex, 20*(9), 2114–2121.

Tassey, G. (2002). *The Economic Impacts of Inadequate Infrastructure for Software Testing.* National Institute of Standards and Technology, RTI Project Number 7007.011.

Uddin, L.Q., Kelly, A.M.C., Biswal, B.B., Margulies, D.S., Shedzad, Z., Shaw, D., Ghaffari, M., et al. (2008). Network homogeneity reveals decreased integrity of default node network in ADHD. *Journal of Neuroscience Methods, 169*(1), 249–254.

Ullen, F., Forsman, L., Blom, O., Karabanov, A. and Madison, G. (2008). Intelligence and variability in a simple timing task share neural substrates in the prefrontal white matter. *Journal of Neuroscience, 28*(16), 4238–4243.

US Nuclear Regulatory Commission. (2012). *NRC/EPRI Draft Report on Integrated Decision-Tree Human Event Analysis System (IDHEAS).* Washington, DC: US Nuclear Regulatory Commission.

Wan, X., Nakatani, H., Ueno, K., Asamizuya, T., Cheng, K. and Tanaka, K. (2011). The neural basis for intuitive best next-move generation in board game experts. *Science, 331*(6015), 341–346.

Weick, K.E. and Sutcliffe, K.M. (2001). *Managing the Unexpected: Assuring High Performance in an Age of Complexity.* San Francisco: Jossey-Bass.

Whaley, A.M., Xing, J., Boring, R.L., Hendrickson, S.M.L., Joe, J.C., LeBlanc, K.L. and Lois, E. 2012. *Building a Psychological Foundation for Human Reliability Analysis* (NUREG-2114). Washington, DC: US Nuclear Regulatory Commission.

Wickens, C.D., Gordon, S.E. and Liu, Y. (1998). *An Introduction to Human Factors to Engineering.* New York: Addison-Wesley.

Woods, D.D., Dekker, S., Cook, R., Johannesen, L. and Sarter, N. (2010). *Behind Human Error*, 2nd edn. Aldershot: Ashgate Publishing Co.

Woods, D.D., Johannesen, L., Cook, R.I. and Sarter, N.B. (1994). *Behind Human Error: Cognitive Systems, Computers and Hindsight.* Dayton, OH: Crew Systems Ergonomic Information and Analysis Center, WPAFB.

7

Cognitive States

Cognition may be thought of as the processes that are utilized in organizing information, including perception, attention, memory, understanding, and learning (Bostrom and Sandberg, 2009). The "cognitive state" of an individual refers to the mental processes that modulate these core cognitive processes. Essentially, *cognitive state* refers to "state of mind," which encompasses factors that determine efficiency (e.g., sleepiness) or emotional state (e.g., agitated).

Most of us have attended a meeting or a class after a late night and have found it difficult to remain engaged in discussions. In this case, a cognitive state that we may describe as "sleepy" impacts the basic cognitive function of attention. This example illustrates the importance of cognitive states, since cognitive states affect basic cognitive processes, modulating our performance and coloring our experience of the world. Additionally, this example shows why we might want to alter our cognitive state (perhaps from "sleepy" to "alert" by drinking a cup of coffee). Doing so may have a beneficial impact on our academic or work performance. Any factor that affects our cognitive performance or our cognitive well-being may be thought of as impacting our cognitive state, and this impact can extend to virtually every facet of our conscious experience.

Stice et al. (2008) investigated the brain response of lean versus obese women during the consumption of a chocolate milkshake and found that, in response to the frozen chocolate treat, corpulent individuals experienced less activation of the dorsal striatum—an area associated with the reward centers of the brain. The overweight subjects derived less pleasure from the milkshake than the nonoverweight subjects—a situation that is reversed if the same brain areas are examined immediately prior to milkshake consumption. Obese individuals expect more reward, yet experience less; there is a greater craving, but less pleasure. This finding lends credence to the idea that compulsive eating is similar to other addictive behaviors—increased craving and blunted pleasure are commonly found in drug addiction (Volkow and Wise, 2005). But does hunger constitute a cognitive state? Researchers have demonstrated that hunger modulates attention to food, and this interacts with obesity. Hungry, obese individuals tend to focus more attention on food when compared with their similarly food-deprived, nonoverweight counterparts (Nijs et al., 2010). Therefore, since hunger impacts attention, it may be thought of as a cognitive state.

Cognitive emotional states may have substantial overlap with visceral changes within the body, which tend to be diffuse rather than specific (Cannon, 1927). For example, the same physiological arousal that occurs with fear or rage is also exhibited during periods of fever or exposure to cold. Simply identifying a physiological state may not enable an accurate determination of the emotion experienced by an individual. This is one reason that traditional lie detection tests have met with stiff criticism. Polygraphs tend to measure "arousal" (heartbeat, perspiration, respiration, blood pressure, etc.), which is assumed to increase as a physiological consequence of lying. However, it is difficult to distinguish this arousal from the arousal associated with anxiety or fear.

Artificially inducing the visceral changes associated with intense emotions (e.g., injecting adrenaline to elicit arousal) does not produce such emotions, though people are quick to recognize physiological arousal (Cannon, 1927). Individuals subjected to such injections may feel *as if* they are afraid, without actually *being* afraid. These observations demonstrate that physiology alone, without consideration of the environmental context, may be a misleading indication of cognitive state. To understand a cognitive state, it is important to consider the physiological circumstances (e.g., level of arousal, biochemical state of the brain), the content (i.e., what a person is thinking about, and any associated emotions), and the context (i.e., circumstances of the experience).

Slow and Surely

During my career, I have spent considerable time working with organizations that conduct high-consequence operations. Specifically, these are activities where there is the potential for negative events that could result in substantial loss of life and property, as well as other significant ramifications. Much of this work has involved operations with explosives associated with the assembly, disassembly, and disposition of bombs. In these cases, an accident could result in the immediate death of everyone in the vicinity, the destruction of multimillion-dollar facilities, substantial environmental harm, and other long-ranging consequences for the community, organization, and government sponsors. Consequently, a wide range of precautions are taken to understand the potential risks, apply measures to minimize these risks, and install mechanisms to mitigate the effects should there ever be an accident.

When observing these operations, one is immediately struck by the atmosphere that surrounds the operations and the nature in which the work is conducted. There is never a doubt that this is a serious business. Initially, one notes how sterile the facility seems. There is nothing in the facility that does not need to be there and everything in the facility has a place and is in its place. There is a continuous hum from the climate control system, but otherwise, there is no sound. It is cool, but not cold.

The centerpiece of the facility is generally the sophisticated equipment that has been uniquely designed for these operations.

The workers have a certain way of doing their job. Generally, one individual is assigned the role of reader and two or more others do the actual work. The reader stands at a music stand with the written procedures and reads the steps one by one. The other workers stand at attention as the reader reads a step and after the reader is done, they confirm that they have heard the step. Then, slowly and deliberately, they perform the step. Once completed, they announce that the step is done and the reader progresses to the next step. There are no extraneous activities. They do nothing that is not called out in the procedure. There is no extraneous conversation. All attention is focused on the step in the procedure being performed. Most strikingly, work proceeds at a slow and deliberate pace, with the ritualistic routine exercised flawlessly from one step to the next. For an observer, it is like watching paint dry. Everything is done so slowly and carefully that it becomes excruciatingly boring.

In this setting, the workers attain a certain cognitive state. This state represents one extreme of the speed–accuracy trade-off. The mind progresses at a slow deliberate pace, never hurrying or racing. This affords an opportunity for all attention to be focused entirely on the task and every minute detail associated with the task. Furthermore, through the structure provided in the written procedures and the ritualistic routines exercised in performing the procedures, the workers are not distracted by the need to think through how they are going to do the task or what might come next. Instead, they know exactly what needs to be done and all their attention is focused on carrying out these activities. If anything occurs that deviates from expectations (e.g., a bolt does not come loose), the whole operation comes to a halt as the engineers and technicians review the problem to determine how best to resolve it.

One might think that these operations are extremely boring and that there may be a risk associated with this boredom. Perhaps this is true, but I am also inclined to believe that for many of the workers, there is a sense of comfort that comes from the cognitive state that they must enter to perform their job. In some ways, it resembles a meditative state in that the workers' attention is focused on specific activities and they must clear their minds of distracting thoughts. From this perspective, it bears a strong resemblance to tai chi in that with tai chi, one seeks to clear one's mind of distractions and focus one's attention on slowly and deliberately carrying out a well-practiced series of actions. This represents a somewhat distinct cognitive state that most of us have probably experienced at some time. However, for the operations described here, the ability to attain this cognitive state and exercise the self-regulation that is essential to sustain this state is an essential element of these workers' ability to effectively carry out their jobs.

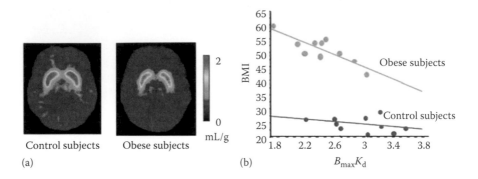

(a)   (b)

FIGURE 7.1   (See color insert)
(a,b) Differential presence of dopamine receptors in obese subjects as compared with controls
and the relationship between dopamine receptor density and body mass index. (From Volkow,
N.D. and Wise, R.A., *Nature Neuroscience*, 8, 555–560, 2005. With permission.)

Humans have a long history of manipulating their cognitive state in a
variety of ways for a variety of reasons. This extends from the time of the
ancient Sumerian use of opium (Brownstein, 1993) to the Irish consumption
of ether when traditional alcoholic beverages became taboo in the mid-1800s
(Strickland, 1996). These examples involve the use of psychoactive substances. While drug use is a common method of cognitive state manipulation, it is by no means the only mechanism. In fact, the same patterns of brain
activation thought to relate to the craving that can accompany drug use (i.e.,
the dopamine-mediated mesolimbic pathway) underlie a variety of cognitive state manipulations that occur with consuming certain foods such as
chocolate (Volkow and Wise, 2005) (see Figure 7.1), intense romantic love (Xu
et al., 2011), or contributing to social causes (Harbaugh et al., 2007). Countless
mechanisms have the effect of manipulating cognitive state. The following
sections describe two pharmacological approaches, caffeine and nicotine,
and two nonpharmacological approaches, physical exercise and meditation.
However, the range of mechanisms for manipulating cognitive state is much
broader, encompassing entertainment, education, play, and so on. In general,
any experience, whether self-administered or the product of the environment, that alters the brain mechanisms underlying cognitive processes may
be considered a cognitive state manipulation. Manipulations that result in
enhanced cognitive performance are emphasized here, with specific examples discussed in the remaining sections of this chapter.

Pharmacological Enhancement: Caffeine

There is probably no psychoactive substance that is used more broadly or
by more people to manipulate their cognitive state than caffeine (Gilbert,

1984). Aside from coffee, caffeine is present in significant quantities in tea, cocoa, soft drinks, chocolate, certain analgesics such as Excedrin, and over-the-counter stimulants such as No Doz. Caffeine has a wide variety of benefits in both the cognitive and affective domains, including increased alertness, decreased fatigue, improved performance on simple sustained vigilance tasks, elevated mood, and reduced depressive symptoms (Attwood et al., 2007; Glade, 2010; Lara, 2010), as well as enhanced control of attention (Brunyé et al., 2010), increased physical endurance (Costill et al., 1978), and improved logical reasoning and semantic memory (Smith et al., 1992). For instance, Smith et al. (1999) tested college students on a variety of performance and mood measures before administering either a caffeinated (40 mg of caffeine) or decaffeinated beverage. On subsequent testing, relative to the placebo group (decaffeinated), the students who ingested caffeine exhibited increased alertness, reduced tension, and faster reaction times.

While some of the effects of caffeine may result from peripheral physiological responses such as an increase in blood pressure and respiration rate, the major mechanism of action occurs in the brain. Caffeine has many effects on the body, including the inhibition of cyclic adenosine monophosphate phosphodiesterase (cAMP), an enzyme responsible for breaking down cAMP, thereby leading to a buildup of cAMP in the brain. Caffeine has also been found to block gamma-aminobutyric acid (GABA) receptors (associated with neural inhibition) and to stimulate calcium release within neurons. While these are likely contributing factors in explaining the effects of caffeine, the primary mechanism by which caffeine operates involves the blockade of adenosine receptors. In fact, the effects of the former mechanisms are only attainable with toxic concentrations of caffeine (Daly and Fredholm, 1998). Within the brain, adenosine functions as a neurotransmitter that binds to adenosine-specific neural receptors. During prolonged wakefulness, adenosine levels become elevated, which is believed to cause the feelings of drowsiness that occur after being awake for a prolonged period of time (Basheer et al., 2000). Given a link between adenosine levels and drowsiness, the blockage of adenosine receptors that occurs with caffeine explains the enhanced alertness that is experienced with caffeine.

While the half-life of caffeine may vary somewhat from person to person, it is generally around 4–6 h, meaning that 4–6 h after consumption, only half the caffeine will remain within the bloodstream. After another 4–6 h, only half of that caffeine will persist, and so on (Hammami et al., 2010). As the concentration of caffeine in the bloodstream lessens, there is a diminished effect on the brain. Additionally, as discussed in Chapter 2, the brain tends toward homeostasis and it will enact measures to counter perturbations to its normal functioning state, such as the perturbation resulting from caffeine consumption. These reactive countermeasures are imprecise and will sometimes overshoot when confronted with chronic or high doses of a substance. This has been termed the *rebound effect* (Julien, 2001). Consequently, following the enhanced alertness after initially ingesting caffeine, the positive effects will subside, often leaving an individual feeling sluggish and unfocused, despite continued caffeine consumption.

The regular consumption of caffeine leads to tolerance and the need for more and more caffeine in order to attain an effect (Evans and Griffiths, 1992). As a result, many individuals will consume caffeine throughout the day in order to stave off the withdrawal effects and the concomitant mental collapse. Griffiths et al. (1990) gave research participants 100 mg of caffeine per day in capsule form for 1 week. Afterward, without the subjects' knowledge, a placebo was substituted for the caffeine capsules. Almost immediately, caffeine withdrawal symptoms appeared as evidenced by headaches, lethargy, and a decreased ability to concentrate.

Caffeine intake may be timed to achieve optimal benefits—for instance, to ensure maximal alertness when it is most needed (Ritter and Yeh, 2011). An alternative strategy involves switching between methods of cognitive enhancement throughout the day (e.g., a morning cup of coffee followed by light exercise at lunch) to avoid the tolerance and rebound that occur with chronic caffeine consumption. Caffeine is best used sparingly and timed such that peak plasma concentration occurs during events that require an extra boost. Continuous ingestion, without regard to the context or timing, can lead to an eventual detriment, rather than an enhancement. Furthermore, with chronic use, the benefits of caffeine may primarily result from the alleviation of withdrawal symptoms (Rodgers and Dernoncourt, 1998). In contrast, used strategically, caffeine can provide a predictable enhancement of cognitive and physical performance.

Pharmacological Enhancement: Nicotine

Nicotine is a compound found in the leaves of the tobacco plant, of which there are two varieties—large leaf and small leaf. The large-leaf variety was domesticated in South America over 5000 years ago and currently serves as the principal source of tobacco. Inhaling nicotine via short, quick puffs produces a low level of blood nicotine, which generally produces a stimulant effect on nerve transmission. In contrast, deep, slow puffs produce a high level of nicotine in the blood, which causes more of a sedative effect (Gilbert, 1979). Smokers may be unaware of the different effects, yet learn these habits subconsciously over time and adjust their smoking to suit their desired outcome.

Nicotine was first isolated nearly 200 years ago (Posselt and Reimann, 1828). It is believed that the tobacco plant produces nicotine as a form of insecticide, as its toxic properties serve to paralyze insects when they absorb it through direct contact with the plant. These properties have been exploited in the manufacture of nicotine-based insecticides such as Black Leaf 40 (a 40%

water-based nicotine sulfate solution) and Nico-Fume liquid (a 40% solution of free nicotine). The manufacture of such insecticides has largely been discontinued due to safety concerns, but their prior existence underscores the point that nicotine is toxic to both humans and insects.

Nicotine enters the lungs on tiny particles referred to as *tar*, which is a complex mixture of hydrocarbons that gives cigarettes their distinctive taste and smell. This pulmonary delivery is quite efficient, with nicotine reaching the brain in approximately 7 s following inhalation (roughly twice as fast as an intravenous administration), due in large part to the roughly 100 m² surface area of the lungs (Newhouse, 1999). Each puff on a cigarette delivers a small burst of nicotine to the brain, and it is estimated that the typical smoker consumes approximately 30 cigarettes per day, taking 10 puffs from each cigarette (Moody et al., 1973). This represents a whopping 300 puffs of nicotine per day.

The half-life of nicotine varies depending on the individual, but it is typically around 2 h (Benowitz et al., 1982). If individuals wish to sustain their level of blood nicotine throughout the day, they must repeatedly smoke. This repeated intake leads to an increasing level of nicotine since each dose builds on previous doses. However, this does not lead to an increasing cognitive benefit, as acute tolerance develops, particularly in habitual smokers.

Once bursts of nicotine enter the body, they bind with nicotinic cholinergic receptors (nAChRs), which are one of the two basic subtypes of acetylcholine (ACh) receptors. Nicotinic receptors are noteworthy because they are present both within and outside the brain. In the peripheral nervous system, nicotinic receptors occur at neuromuscular junctions where ACh acts as a neurotransmitter, stimulating muscle fibers to imitate a muscular contraction. Nicotine also has effects on the autonomic nervous system, which include stimulation of the adrenal glands and concomitant release of norepinephrine and epinephrine (adrenaline). These cause an increased heart rate and blood pressure, as well as an increased metabolic rate.

In the brain, nicotine also binds to ACh receptors, although some ACh receptors bind nicotine with high affinity and others with low affinity. The high-affinity receptors are distributed throughout several areas of the brain, including the cerebral cortex, thalamus, striatum, hippocampus, substantia nigra, ventral tegmental area, locus coeruleus, and the raphe nuclei. As is the case at neuromuscular junctions, nicotine has a stimulating effect; the binding of nicotine to the receptor opens a channel allowing sodium ions to flow across the cell membrane resulting in an excitatory response. If the level of nicotine is high enough, leading to chronic activation of nicotinic ACh receptors, depolarization will eventually cause cells to become unable to fire until the nicotine is cleared, a response that may account for the biphasic effect of nicotine mentioned earlier (i.e., stimulation at low doses and sedation at high doses). Nicotine has been found to produce a variety of cognitive benefits, particularly with tasks that depend on attention (Sherwood, 1993). The beneficial effect of nicotine on attention has been supported by evidence from electroencephalogram (EEG) research in which transdermal administration of nicotine (i.e., a skin patch) resulted in changes in the EEG signal that are consistent with enhanced arousal and attention (e.g., lessening of alpha frequency activity and increased beta frequency activity). These effects have been demonstrated in nonsmokers (Griesar et al., 2002) as well as abstaining smokers (Knott et al., 1999).

One difficulty with this type of research is that it often utilizes current smokers and requires them to abstain from smoking for a period of time prior to the experiment in order to purge their systems of residual nicotine. This means that research on the cognitive impact of nicotine may often be examining the reversal of withdrawal symptoms in abstaining smokers, rather than demonstrating a boost above normal baseline performance. Foulds et al. (1996) compared abstinent smokers with nonsmokers on a visual attention task. The participants were shown a string of digits, and were tasked to respond when they detected three consecutive odd digits or three consecutive even digits. The reaction time of the abstinent smokers who were given 0.6 mg of nicotine was on par with the nonsmokers who were given a placebo, while the nonsmokers who were given 0.6 mg of nicotine responded substantially faster than their counterparts who smoked. This experiment supports the assertion that the cognitive benefit associated with nicotine administration in abstinent smokers is likely due to the alleviation of withdrawal-related deficits. While nicotine was effective in reducing the reaction time in both smokers and nonsmokers, the smokers responded more slowly overall, meaning that they needed nicotine just to respond at a level equivalent to the nonsmokers who were not given nicotine. Chronic nicotine consumption results in a cognitive deficit with continued smoking required to bring an individual back to baseline levels of performance.

A parallel situation may be found when considering the impact of nicotine on mood. Smokers often report that puffing on a cigarette leads to feelings of relaxation and the alleviation of stress, in addition to an increased clarity of thought. In reality, smokers become irritable and stressed (in addition to experiencing clouded concentration) due to nicotine withdrawal, and introducing nicotine to the bloodstream serves to alleviate these withdrawal symptoms, thereby reducing stress and facilitating concentration. For smokers, stress increases in the absence of nicotine in the bloodstream, and the reintroduction of nicotine alleviates these symptoms (Parrott, 1999; Parrott and Kaye, 1999). Similar to cognitive benefits, for smokers the enhanced mood following nicotine consumption is actually due to relief from a detrimental state, rather than a boost above baseline. Furthermore, for nonsmokers the benefits associated with nicotine consumption do not come without a cost. Whereas drinking coffee may be a pleasant experience, even for those who seldom partake in such an activity, the adverse effects of nicotine for nonsmokers are pronounced. A dose of 0.6 mg—the same dose that elicited a cognitive benefit for nonsmokers in the previously mentioned study—leads to relatively intense adverse reactions in nonsmokers, including cold hands, dizziness, headaches, heart palpitations, and sweating (Foulds et al., 1997).

Cognitive Enhancement through Physical Exercise

Over the past decade, evidence has accumulated suggesting a link between physical exercise and cognitive performance. Research was originally motivated by interest in the relationship between physical exertion and cognitive decline in old age. For instance, in 1995, Albert et al. (1995) demonstrated that for healthy 70- to 79-year-olds, the best predictor of cognitive decline, measured using a battery of tasks assessing language, verbal memory, nonverbal memory, conceptualization, and visuospatial ability, was strenuous physical activity. Other groups have found similar results in the elderly with follow-up periods ranging from 2 (Etgen et al., 2010) to 31 years (Andel et al., 2008). There is evidence that regular physical activity offers protection against dementia. Research participants who engaged in physical activities that lasted a minimum of 20–30 min resulting in breathlessness and sweating were 52% less likely than their more sedentary counterparts to have dementia 21 years later (Rovio et al., 2005). A number of studies have demonstrated similar findings (e.g., Abbott et al., 2004; Andel et al., 2008; Laurin et al., 2001). As a result of this research, physical activity has been recommended both as a preventative measure against dementia, and as a means of slowing memory decline in those individuals with dementia (Intlekofer and Cotman, 2013).

While numerous studies have addressed the impact of physical exertion on cognitive decline in old age, studies involving young participants are rare. The aging brain undergoes a number of changes, including deterioration of the frontal lobe structures (West, 1996) that relate to executive functioning (planning, organizing, managing time), and exercise is particularly suited to boosting these functions such that intervention may matter more for older individuals (Colcombe and Kramer, 2003). A recent study directly compared middle-aged adults (40–59 years of age) with older adults (60–82 years of age) to examine what has been referred to as the *age-dependence hypothesis*. It was found that physical exercise provided a greater benefit to the older individuals, supporting the idea that physical exercise has its greatest effect on cognitive functions during life stages at which these functions have begun to decline (Hötting and Röder, 2013).

In contrast, associations between physical activity and cognitive functioning in children have been the focus of recent research, with the finding that cardiovascular fitness is a strong predictor of performance on tasks that require significant cognitive control (Chaddock et al., 2012). Academic achievement (Donnelly et al., 2009) (see Figure 7.2), creativity (Tuckman and

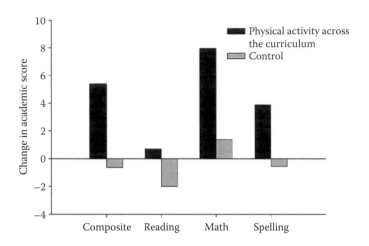

FIGURE 7.2

Changes in the academic performance of schoolchildren associated with a program of physical activity. (From Donnelly, J.E., Greene, J.L., Gibson, C.A., Smith, B.K., Washburn, R.A., Sullivan, D.K., DuBose, K. et al., *Preventative Medicine*, 49, 336–341, 2009. With permission.)

Hinkle, 1986), and planning ability (Davis et al., 2011) have been found to improve with physical exercise interventions in children. It is interesting that executive functioning seems to benefit from physical exercise in children (Barenberg et al., 2011; Best, 2010), just as in elderly individuals. While elderly individuals are experiencing a decline in the brain areas associated with executive functions, these same brain areas are only beginning to develop in children. Since executive functioning largely involves the frontal lobe structures that mature late in adolescence (Best and Miller, 2010), the nascent development of such circuitry may be more easily affected by physical exertion than the more developed brain structures (Best, 2010).

In addition to the ends of the age spectrum, the positive impact of physical exertion on cognitive functioning has also been shown for middle-aged individuals. Richards et al. (2003) collected measures of physical activity for 36-year-old men and women, and found that physical exercise at this age was predictive of higher memory scores during a follow-up session at 43 years of age, and was predictive of a slower rate of memory decline from ages 43 to 53. Interestingly, those individuals who ceased exercising after age 36 experienced more memory loss than participants who began an exercise regimen at age 36, while participants already active at age 36 and who remained active exhibited the least decay in memory function. This research suggests that starting exercise later in life still promotes the retention of cognitive faculties later on in life.

While all ages seem to benefit from exercise, there are many facets of exercise to consider, such as the type and intensity of exercise. The vast majority of research focuses on aerobic exercise (endurance programs such as running, walking, cycling, and swimming). This body of research indicates that aerobic exercise enhances a variety of cognitive functions, including auditory and visual attention, motor control, spatial cognition, and cognitive speed (Angevaren et al., 2008; Colcombe and Kramer, 2003). Recent research has addressed basic stretching activities and has found that both aerobic exercise and stretching/coordination training are effective in improving the cognitive functioning of participants (Hötting et al., 2012). Resistance training (e.g., weight lifting) in women aged 65 years or older improves executive functioning (Liu-Ambrose et al., 2010) and, in general, older individuals demonstrate enhanced short-term memory and attention following resistance training programs (Cassilhas et al., 2012). It is possible that different types of exercise enhance cognition via different mechanisms. For instance, cardiovascular training has been shown to improve episodic memory, while stretching/coordination training has been shown to improve attention (Hötting et al., 2012). Thus, a combination of training methods might be particularly effective in the overall improvement of cognitive function (Colcombe and Kramer, 2003). Regarding the intensity of exercise, research assessing the memory functions of older adults demonstrated that even low-intensity aerobic exercise leads to a significant enhancement of memory scores relative to a sedentary control group (Ruscheweyh et al., 2011).

In addition to the benefits derived from regular physical exercise that is sustained over months or years, exercise also provides a basis for the short-term enhancement of cognitive functioning. A recent meta-analysis found that exercise-induced arousal led to enhanced cognitive performance on tasks involving rapid decision making and memory storage and retrieval (Lambourne and Tomporowski, 2010), although prolonged exercise that resulted in dehydration tended to have a detrimental effect on cognitive performance (Tomporowski, 2003).

Exercise affects the brain via increased blood flow and vascularization. Physically active adults have been demonstrated to exhibit a greater number of small cerebral blood vessels relative to sedentary adults (Bullitt et al., 2009), which is thought to lead to a more efficient system of delivery of oxygen and nutrients to the brain. Given that the brain requires a disproportionate amount of oxygen and glucose compared with other parts of the body, the enhancement of the blood flow and the addition of blood vessels enable more efficient delivery of sugar and oxygen, thereby enhancing brain function. Exercise also reduces stress. There is a finite amount of blood in the brain, and if that blood supply, along with oxygen and nutrients, is being diverted to motor areas to facilitate intense physical activity, it is not available to areas involved in rumination (i.e., compulsively thinking about the distresses in one's life). For instance, endurance running has been found to result in hypofrontality—a below-baseline level of activity in the frontal lobes, which are critical for executive functions such as planning and worrying (Dietrich, 2002). Indeed, exercise has long been known to have a positive impact on affect (Morgan and O'Connor, 1988) and to be associated with stress reduction (Tomporowski, 2003).

When a person confronts a stressor, the body has a multifaceted response. The autonomic nervous system has two divisions, sympathetic and parasympathetic, and consists of neurons that control glandular activity and the functioning of the internal organs. Generally, the sympathetic division is activated by conditions that promote arousal, which include situations involving stressors. Activation of the sympathetic nervous system prepares the body for intense motor activity; the sort of activity that would be necessary for attack, defense, or escape—all of which have an obvious survival value. This is the well-known *fight-or-flight* system. It is characterized by the activation of the adrenomedullary system, so named because the center of the kidney (the adrenal medulla) is activated via the hypothalamic activity of the brain. Following activation, the adrenomedullary system secretes epinephrine (adrenaline) and norepinephrine. These affect the cardiovascular, digestive, and respiratory systems, allowing for speedy, life-saving behaviors. The digestive system is involved because the blood flow is diverted away from the digestive system in order to provide resources to the muscles. If you have ever felt a cold feeling in the pit of your stomach in a stressful situation, this is a result of the adrenomedullary response.

Exercise induces a slower neuroendocrine response via the hypothalamic–pituitary–adrenal (HPA) axis, so named because it follows a chain of activation from the hypothalamus to the pituitary gland to the adrenal cortex. The hypothalamus releases the corticotropin-releasing hormone (CRH) to the pituitary gland, which then releases the adrenocorticotropic hormone (ACTH). The ACTH acts on the adrenal cortex of the kidneys, which produces glucocorticoid hormones—mostly cortisol. Cortisol circulates in the bloodstream impacting a number of systems, resulting in a heightened level of blood sugar providing energy to cells. The peak levels of cortisol occur roughly 20–40 min following exposure to a stressor, after which there is a slow decline. This decline is initiated by the hippocampus. The hippocampus is sensitive to circulating cortisol, and when it detects sufficient cortisol in the bloodstream, it signals the hypothalamus to cease secreting the CRH, thus shutting the stress system down through a negative feedback loop.

The above description accounts for how the system functions in ideal circumstances. It is important to note that cortisol is toxic to the hippocampus. Too much cortisol results in hippocampal atrophy. In the presence of chronic stress, the stress response is continuously active, despite attempts by the hippocampus to shut it down. As a result, the hippocampus deteriorates, which makes it even harder to shut down the stress response, since shutdown is generally the function of the hippocampus. Thus, chronic stress can create a positive feedback loop of hippocampal destruction, such that the longer you experience stress, the less able your body is to halt the cycle.

The hippocampus is critical for learning and memory. Through stress relief, exercise preserves hippocampal function, providing a basis for enhanced cognitive functioning. In addition to facilitating the shutdown of toxic chronic stress systems, thereby preserving the hippocampus, exercise has been shown to result in an increased rate of neurogenesis (the forma-tion of new neurons) in the hippocampus (Brown et al., 2003; van Praag et al., 1999). Furthermore, recent research links exercise to increased gray matter (the dark tissue of the brain that consists of neuronal cell bodies and dendrites) in the hippocampus (Erickson et al., 2011; Pajonk et al., 2010). In addition to the hippocampus, brain imaging research has established a link between physical activity during middle age and gray matter volume in the frontal brain regions (which is thought to be important for executive func-tions) in later life (Rovio et al., 2010).

Recent research suggests that an additional boost may be realized when exercise is combined with cognitive training. Fabre et al. (2002) demon-strated that aerobic endurance training combined with cognitive training that is designed to enhance a variety of cognitive functions (e.g., memory, attention, spatial skills) was more effective than either exercise or cognitive training alone. These results make sense when the additional brain effects of exercise, namely, neuroplasticity, are considered. Neuroplastic enhance-ments that are related to physical activity include increases in dendritic spine density (Stranahan et al., 2007); enhanced long-term potentiation (increased signal strength between neurons) (van Praag et al., 1999); increased levels of the neurotransmitters serotonin, norepinephrine, and ACh (Lista and Sorrentino, 2010); increased dopamine receptor density (Fordyce and Farrar, 1991); and an augmented release of growth factors such as brain-derived neurotrophic factor (BDNF) (Knaepen et al., 2010) and insulin-link growth factor-1 (IGF-1) (Rojas Vega et al., 2010).

Neurotrophic factors are proteins that are responsible for the development and survival of nascent neurons, as well as the maintenance of mature neu-rons and the connections between neurons. Neurotrophic factors may also facilitate the regrowth of damaged neurons (Deister and Schmidt, 2006). Increased BDNF has been found following acute bouts of aerobic exercise (Gold et al., 2003), and the amount released seems contingent on the inten-sity of the exercise, with greater intensity eliciting a greater release (Ferris et al., 2007). Furthermore, the neurotrophic factor IGF-1 has been linked with resistance training (Cassilhas et al., 2012). Thus, the release of multiple neu-rotrophic factors may be achieved by combining exercise methods, perhaps explaining why combining regimes is particularly effective in producing cognitive benefits (Colcombe and Kramer, 2003). Thus, combined physical exercise may make the brain more pliable, facilitating the cognitive enhance-ment achieved via training by making the brain more capable of acquiring new information, resulting in gains that exceed those achieved by either intervention alone (Kempermann, 2008).

There is one additional observation to consider in the context of cognitive state—the so-called runner's high. This refers to a state of analgesia (inhibition of pain), sedation, and anxiolysis (inhibition of anxiety), and a general sense of well-being that is sometimes associated with prolonged physical activity. A prominent theory explaining this effect involves the release of endogenous opioid peptides or endorphins that function as neurotransmitters within the brain. However, the *endorphin hypothesis* has received little support (Tuson and Sinyor, 1993) and suffers from a number of serious problems (Kolata, 2002). A promising new line of research involves the release of endocannabinoids. Researchers have long been aware of the behavioral effects of tetrahydrocannabinol (THC), the major compound contained in marijuana. A cellular receptor for these compounds has been discovered within the brain (Devane et al., 1988). Following the identification of these receptors, termed *cannabinoid receptors*, brain areas were identified that exhibit significant cannabinoid receptor density. These areas include the cerebellum, hippocampus, globus pallidus, and substantia nigra. The identification of cannabinoid receptors raises the question, "Why does the human brain possess receptors for a compound present in a plant?" A few years following the discovery of cellular receptors for cannabinoids, researchers isolated substances in the brain with cannabinoid-like activity (Devane et al., 1992). These substances have become known as the *endocannabinoids*.

Endocannabinoids exert a variety of effects by acting on the cannabinoid receptors. For instance, in the hippocampus, endocannabinoids are produced by pyramidal neurons (the primary output neurons of this brain area), at which point they diffuse to the nearby terminals of interneurons that release the inhibitory neurotransmitter GABA. The endocannabinoids reduce the activity of GABAergic interneurons, lessening the inhibition of hippocampal pyramidal cells and permitting the pyramidal cells to fire more rapidly (Wilson and Nicoll, 2002). Given the effect that endocannabinoids are known to have on the brain (particularly the dialing up of activity in the hippocampal output neurons), the recent finding that exercise increases serum concentrations of endocannabinoids (Dietrich and McDaniel, 2004) presents a mechanism to explain the feeling of well-being that is associated with the aptly named *runner's high*.

Cognitive Enhancement through Meditation

While cognitive state manipulation is not necessarily the end goal of the interventions discussed in the previous sections, the objective of meditation is to achieve an altered cognitive state. While there are a number of meditation techniques, the method of mindfulness meditation has become a popular topic of research, and we will focus our discussion on this particular approach. There are two major varieties of mindfulness meditation: focused attention and open monitoring (Travis and Shear, 2010). Focused attention meditation entails fixating on an object or a process (e.g., a mantra, a visual stimulus, breathing); the meditator attempts to remove any distraction from this focus and if distracted, subsequently attempts to reengage his or her focus. Open monitoring involves the practice of becoming aware of the present moment. This includes focusing on sensory experiences as they arise, as well as cognitions and emotions; simply observing without judging or reacting.

Meditation can be incredibly difficult. It has been described as "the state of mind that occurs in the space between thoughts," but given the frequency of thoughts, there is a brief window at sporadic intervals to glimpse the cognitive state that one is attempting to achieve during meditation. Even though we experience a somewhat continuous stream of thoughts, this stream is prone to interruptions, which is not surprising given the multitude of distractions (both external and self-generated) that surround us. Achieving a relaxed, continuously focused state, or a state of observing without reacting, can be an incredibly foreign state of mind, so much so that it may take some time to recognize when this state has been achieved. It does not come naturally or easily; rather it requires practice, and like most things that require practice, the more you work at it, the easier it becomes. There is, of course, a payoff to becoming proficient at meditation.

Research has shown that mindfulness meditation can boost a variety of cognitive processes, including sustained attention (Kozasa et al., 2012), selective attention (Jha et al., 2007), and working memory (van Vugt and Jha, 2011), in addition to increased awareness, relaxation, insight, emotional well-being (Hölzel et al., 2011), resistance to impulses and negative affect (Witkiewitz et al., 2012), pain reduction (Zeidan et al., 2011), and improved self-control (Jenkins and Tapper, 2013). As with exercise, recent research has focused on elucidating meditation-induced changes that occur in the brain that help to explain these benefits.

In a recent study, it was demonstrated that individuals trained in focused attention mindfulness meditation were able to exert greater control over their brain alpha rhythms (associated with wakeful relaxation) (Kerr et al., 2011), which may relate to the ability to screen out distractions (Figure 7.3). This finding was supported by functional magnetic resonance imaging (fMRI) research indicating that the brain areas involved in voluntary control over attention (e.g., the rostral anterior cingulate cortex and the dorsal medial prefrontal cortex) tend to exhibit greater activity during mindfulness meditation (Hölzel et al., 2007). In addition to acute modulation of their brain activity, experienced meditators demonstrate greater cortical density in areas associated with attention, including the prefrontal cortex and the right anterior insula, which is positively associated with measures of cognitive performance (Lazar et al., 2005). The implications extend into the clinical realm, as alpha rhythm deregulation and deficits in attentional control are the hallmarks of individuals with attention-deficit hyperactivity disorder (ADHD) (Koehler et al., 2009), offering a potential intervention that is not based on pharmaceuticals. In fact, a 6-week mindfulness meditation training session was found to result in a significant reduction in symptoms in adolescents with ADHD (Harrison et al., 2004).

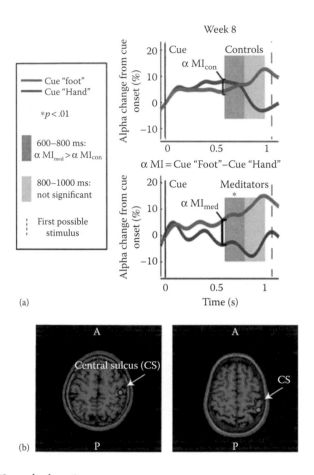

FIGURE 7.3 **(See color insert)**
(a,b) Peak alpha frequency for meditators and nonmeditators during sustained attention to body and breath-related sensations. (From Kerr, C.E., Sacchet, M.D., Lazar, S.W., Moore, C.I. and Jones, S.R., *Frontiers in Human Neuroscience*, 7, 1–15, 2013. With permission.)

A number of other benefits are strikingly similar to those achieved with exercise—notably, stress reduction and staving off the age-related decline in gray matter within the brain. One study recruited human resources managers and divided them into three groups (Levy et al., 2012). One group received mindfulness meditation training, one group received body relaxation training, and the third group did not receive training. The training lasted 8 weeks, and the participants were given a stressful multitasking test before and after their training. On the final test, the group that received mindfulness training stayed on task longer, made fewer task switches, reported less stress during the test, and showed improved memory for the task. The idea that meditation can reduce stress and improve task performance is supported by a study that enlisted participants to play a stressful computer game (Mohan et al., 2011). The participants received guided meditation before or after the task, and physiological measures of stress were recorded during task performance. Those who meditated prior to the task showed an attenuated stress response relative to the posttask meditators, and their memory capabilities increased. The brain basis of this stress reduction is thought to be a reduction in the connectivity strength between the areas of the brain that are involved in emotional response and the medial prefrontal cortex, which is involved in self-referential processing (Brewer et al., 2011). This means that when an unpleasant experience occurs, meditators are more effective in objectively assessing the situation without becoming distracted by bodily sensations or the idea that there is a threat. This is exactly what meditation trains individuals to do—observe without judging. Given the deleterious impact of chronic stress on cognitive functioning via a reduction in the hippocampal gray matter, this research indicates that meditation could provide a benefit for those individuals who often engage in stressful activities.

With regard to reductions in gray matter, as with exercise, long-term practitioners of meditation experience less brain shrinkage as they age (Luders et al., 2011). The idea that meditation allows the retention of gray matter is important since gray matter is associated with sensory perception, emotional stability, and intelligence (Haier et al., 2004). The same research team has noted that meditators also exhibit a greater degree of brain gyrification (Luders et al., 2012). Gryrification refers to the pattern and the degree of folding of the cerebral cortex. Greater gyrification is associated with faster brain processing and better memory formation (Luders et al., 2012). Notably, the researchers found that there was a positive correlation between the amount of gyrification and the number of years that the participant had practiced meditation. This raises the issue of time; how long must one practice meditation in order to glean benefits from it? The vast majority of the research concerning neurophysiological changes associated with mindfulness meditation has compared expert practitioners (often Buddhist monks with thousands of hours of experience) with nonmeditators (Davidson and Lutz, 2008). This has been done to maximize the likelihood of finding differences between meditators and nonmeditators on the basis of brain activity.

A number of researchers (e.g., Brewer et al., 2011; Hasenkamp et al., 2011; Jang et al., 2011) have found enhanced functional connectivity between regions of the default-mode network (DMN) and regions of the brain associated with self-monitoring, inhibition, and cognitive control—the posterior cingulate, anterior cingulate cortex, and dorsolateral prefrontal cortex. The DMN is implicated in mind wandering and rumination. Meditation increases focus and attention control by strengthening the ability of the frontal cortices to exert inhibitory control over activity associated with mind wandering. In at least one case, these changes occurred after only 8 weeks of meditation training and were associated with improved resistance to distraction, conflict monitoring, and working memory. Additional evidence suggesting that brief training may produce benefits comes from the aforementioned study by Kerr et al. (2011) in which meditators were able to exert an influence on their brain alpha waves. These participants started the study as novices and received a scant 3 months of training.

Behavioral research supports the idea that even a brief amount of meditation may be beneficial. One study found that mindfulness meditation can improve attention and self-regulation in as few as five 20-min sessions (Tang et al., 2007). Another demonstrated that in as few as 4 days of training, mindfulness meditation led to an improved ability to modulate the experience of pain (Zeidan et al., 2011). In the study mentioned earlier involving the effect of meditation on anticipatory stress occurring prior to a stressful task, participants had no prior meditation experience, yet still showed a benefit (Mohan et al., 2011). In fact, there are now a number of mindfulness training methods that are designed to improve cognitive functioning in as few as 8 weeks (Hölzel et al., 2011; Kerr et al., 2011).

Meditation, much like exercise, seems to offer both short- and long-term benefits that encompass a variety of cognitive functions. Mindfulness meditation involves several intervals in a cognitive cycle, starting with an attempt to focus. This is followed by mind wandering, awareness of mind wandering, shifting of attention back to the object or process that serves as the focal point, and finally, sustained attention (Hasenkamp et al., 2012). It is not surprising that practicing this type of focus and identifying distractions translate to an improved focus, even when one is not meditating. It is a practiced skill, and it may take thousands of hours to become an expert, much like most skills. However, even for those who do not invest the time to achieve expertise, a few sessions are sufficient to elicit a benefit. It is worth mentioning that there are a number of parallels between meditation and exercise, including the preservation of gray matter into advanced age, the reduction of stress, and the combination of acute and chronic benefits. This may be contrasted with caffeine use, which offers reliable benefits when used in moderation. This factor does not seem to be a concern with exercise or meditation and, indeed, there seems to be added benefit to the long-term practice of either exercise or meditation.

Concluding Thoughts and Future Directions

We have examined a number of interventions that alter the cognitive state as expressed through changes in the basic cognitive systems of attention, perception, memory, understanding, and learning, with particular emphasis on caffeine, nicotine, exercise, and meditation. These are only a few of the methods that are available. For instance, Ritalin is a psychostimulant drug that is often used in the treatment of ADHD and has found popularity in academic circles, where it is used by students to enhance their cognitive functioning (White et al., 2006). Likewise, a number of nutritional supplements are commonly used for the purposes of cognitive enhancement (e.g., ginkgo biloba extract), though their efficacy, adverse effects, and interactions are largely unknown (Cupp, 1999). The focus of this chapter has been on legal interventions that are relatively well understood and commonly used, for which practical advice may be offered. As such, a plethora of interventions fall beyond the scope of this chapter, though it is important to recognize that the world of cognitive enhancement is much larger.

One promising intervention is transcranial direct current stimulation (tDCS). This method of brain stimulation essentially consists of a 9 V battery connected to wet-sponge electrodes placed on the scalp. A very weak electrical current (1–2 mA) is passed through the sponges and is thought to alter the resting membrane potential of entire populations of neurons. This occurs in a polarity-specific fashion, such that anodal (positive electrode) stimulation results in increased excitability through the depolarization of the neurons, whereas cathodal (negative electrode) stimulation decreases excitability via hyperpolarization (Nitsche et al., 2002). Basically, the neurons in the region near the anode are able to fire more easily, while those beneath the cathode are suppressed.

The idea that electricity applied to the scalp can elicit benefits is actually a very old one. As early as AD 43, Scribonius Largus observed that the discharge of the black torpedo fish (an electric fish that is native to the Mediterranean Sea) delivered to a patient could be used to treat headaches, as well as gout and hemorrhoids, when applied to the appropriate areas (Kellaway, 1946). Pliny the Elder and the Greek physician Galen reported similar findings, with Galen realizing that the observed benefits were due to numbness and the narcotic effect that was induced by the electric fish (Kellaway, 1946). However, a systematic investigation of the therapeutic efficacy of electric current proved difficult without a reliable and convenient source. Because of technological limitations, the ancients were forced to rely on current-generating animals such as the torpedo fish or rubbing a nonconductor such as amber to produce static electricity.

While tDCS is being examined as a potential treatment for a variety of neurological and psychiatric disorders, including depression (Boggio et al., 2008), Alzheimer's disease (Boggio et al., 2009), multiple sclerosis (Mori et al., 2010), and rehabilitation after stroke (Ko et al., 2008), in recent years, there has been increasing interest in using electrical stimulation to enhance the cognitive abilities of healthy individuals. tDCS has been shown to positively impact a number of basic cognitive functions, including working memory (Fregni et al., 2005), language learning (Floel et al., 2008), motor learning (Antal et al., 2004), and simple somatosensory and visual motion perception learning (Antal and Paulus, 2008; Ragert et al., 2008). One recent study by Clark and colleagues demonstrated that anodal tDCS administered over the right inferior frontal cortex (RIFC) was effective in accelerating learning to detect concealed objects in a threat-detection task (Clark et al., 2012). A follow-up study suggests that at the root of this learning effect, tDCS is enhancing the basic cognitive process underlying attention (Coffman et al., 2012).

However, these findings need to be interpreted with caution as the effects of one stimulation session tend to be transient, and the effects of multiple sessions for the purposes of cognitive enhancement have yet to be systematically investigated. With chronic use, habituation becomes a concern. Consider how the chronic use of caffeine and nicotine impairs baseline functioning such that for habitual users, their consumption is necessary to alleviate withdrawal symptoms. There are currently no studies addressing habituation to tDCS, but given that the brain adapts and tends toward homeostasis, it is a potential cause for concern. Cautions, caveats, and concerns in mind, there are several distinct advantages to using tDCS.

One such advantage is affordability—the technology is relatively simple and, as a result, it is relatively cheap. In fact, several companies have developed tDCS units for personal as opposed to research use. For example, the foc.us headset is designed with video game players in mind (http://www.foc.us/) and currently costs approximately $250. A substantial do-it-yourself community has emerged around this technology, as evidenced by active forums devoted to tDCS on popular websites such as Reddit (http://www.reddit.com/r/tDCS). Another advantage is specificity. Our discussion of nicotine included mention of the wide distribution of nicotinic receptors, both in the brain and in the autonomic nervous system. This means that introducing nicotine into the bloodstream has a shotgun effect—you are forced to take the positive effects together with the negative effects. Relative to nicotine, tDCS may be considered more a scalpel—it directly targets specific brain regions rather than reaching the brain through an indirect delivery system that impacts other bodily systems.

Currently, many cognitive enhancement techniques (of which electrical stimulation is just one; others include gene alteration, hormone therapy, and nootropics) have not been evaluated with regard to their risks. Furthermore, it is currently difficult to obtain funding to research cognitive enhancement in healthy individuals, as opposed to using the same methods to correct a decrement in a clinical population. It could be argued that there is a fine line between the two. For instance, enhancing the memory of an individual with a naturally poor memory may result in someone with a memory that has improved relative to his or her own individual baseline, but is still poor. Thus, someone who has undergone cognitive enhancement may not necessarily possess above-average cognitive faculties—they have just improved relative to their baseline. The bottom line is that until more is known about the risks of long-term stimulation (and about the potential benefits as well), it is difficult to make an informed decision concerning repeated personal use for cognitive enhancement. However, current research suggests tDCS is a relatively low-risk intervention, and a future in which people wear some form of "smart cap" that stimulates particular areas during particular situations in order to provide a contextually relevant cognitive boost does not seem far-fetched.

Despite the potential benefits, there may be ethical concerns. Though addiction to such a method is not likely (the deep brain location of reward/craving centers makes them a difficult target when current is applied to the scalp, as in tDCS), issues of legitimacy are raised—not just for tDCS, but for cognitive enhancement methods in general. By this, it is meant that if certain cognitive abilities can be induced rather than "earned" in the traditional sense (i.e., through education or practice), does that cheapen the achievement?

The issue is muddled by the wide variety of enhancements that are already available, legal, and commonly used. When competing for scholarships or employment positions, the frequency of caffeine consumption, exercise, nicotine use, and so on, is a topic that is seldom if ever broached. In general, the interest is in the overall level of productivity that an individual is able to achieve rather than the means that the individual enlisted to achieve it. Cognitive enhancement is built into our society to such a degree that it is only noticed when people make use of methods in a fashion that is notable for its novelty, intensity, or legality. It remains to be seen how competitive societies handle issues raised by cognitive enhancement methods.

Acknowledgments

Sandia National Laboratories is a multiprogram laboratory managed and operated by Sandia Corporation, a wholly owned subsidiary of Lockheed Martin Corporation, for the US Department of Energy's National Nuclear Security Administration under contract DE-AC04-94AL85000. This work was supported in part by a Department of Energy Computational Science Graduate Fellowship, Grant No. DE-FG02-97ER25308.

References

Abbott, R.D., White, L.R., Ross, G.W., Masaki, K.H., Curb, J.D. and Petrovitch, H. (2004). Walking and dementia in physically capable elderly men. *The Journal of the American Medical Association, 292*(12), 1447–1453.

Albert, M.S., Jones, K., Savage, C.R., Berkman, L., Seeman, T., Blazer, D. and Rowe, J.W. (1995). Predictors of cognitive change in older persons: MacArthur studies of successful aging. *Psychology and Aging, 10*(4), 578–589.

Andel, R., Crowe, M., Pedersen, N.L., Fratiglioni, L., Johansson, B. and Gatz, M. (2008). Physical exercise at midlife and risk of dementia three decades later: A population-based study of Swedish twins. *The Journals of Gerontology, Series A, 63*(1), 62–66.

Angevaren, M., Aufdemkampe, G., Verhaar, H.J., Aleman, A. and Vanhees, L. (2008). Physical activity and enhanced fitness to improve cognitive function in older people without known cognitive impairment. *The Cochrane Database of Systematic Reviews, 16*(2), CD005381.

Antal, A., Nitsche, M.A., Kincses, T.Z., Kruse, W., Hoffmann, K.P. and Paulus, W. (2004). Facilitation of visuo-motor learning by transcranial direct current stimulation of the motor and extrastriate visual areas in humans. *European Journal of Neuroscience, 19*(10), 2888–2892.

Antal, A. and Paulus, W. (2008). Transcranial direct current stimulation and visual perception. *Perception, 37*(3), 367–374.

Attwood, A.S., Higgs, S. and Terry, P. (2007). Differential responsiveness to caffeine and perceived effects of caffeine in low and high regular caffeine consumers. *Psychopharmacology, 190*(4), 469–477.

Barenberg, J., Berse, T. and Dutke, S. (2011). Executive functions in learning processes: Do they benefit from physical activity? *Educational Psychology Review, 6*(3), 208–222.

Basheer, R., Porkka-Heiskanen, T., Strecker, R.E., Thakkar, M.M. and McCarley, R.W. (2000). Adenosine as a biological signal mediating sleepiness following prolonged wakefulness. *Biological Signals and Receptors, 9*(6), 319–327.

Benowitz, N.L., Jacob, P. 3rd, Jones, R.T. and Rosenberg, J. (1982). Interindividual variability in the metabolism and cardiovascular effects of nicotine in man. *Journal of Pharmacology and Experimental Therapeutics, 221*(2), 368–372.

Best, J.R. (2010). Effects of physical activity on children's executive function: Contributions of experimental research on aerobic exercise. *Developmental Review, 30*(4), 331–551.

Best, J.R. and Miller, P.H. (2010). A developmental perspective on executive function. *Child Development, 81*(6), 1641–1660.

Boggio, P.S., Khoury, L.P., Martins, D.C.S., Martins, O.E.M.S., De Macedo, E. and Fregni, F. (2009). Temporal cortex direct current stimulation enhances performance on a visual recognition memory task in Alzheimer disease. *Journal of Neurology, Neurosurgery and Psychiatry, 80*(4), 444.

Boggio, P.S., Rigonatti, S.P., Ribeiro, R.B., Myczkowski, M.L., Nitsche, M.A., Pascual-Leone, A. and Fregni, F. (2008). A randomized, double-blind clinical trial on the efficacy of cortical direct current stimulation for the treatment of major depression. *International Journal of Neuropsychopharmacology, 11*(2), 249–254.

Bostrom, N. and Sandberg, A. (2009). Cognitive enhancement: Methods, ethics, regulatory challenges. *Science and Engineering Ethics, 15*(3), 311–341.

Brewer, J.A., Worhunsky, P.D., Gray, J.R., Tang, Y., Weber, J. and Kober, H. (2011). Meditation experience is associated with differences in default mode network activity and connectivity. *Proceedings of the National Academy of Sciences of the United States of America, 108*(50), 20254–20259.

Brown, J., Cooper-Kuhn, C.M., Kempermann, G., Van Praag, H., Winkler, J., Gage, F.H. and Kuhn, H.G. (2003). Enriched environment and physical activity stimulate hippocampal but not olfactory bulb neurogenesis. *The European Journal of Neuroscience, 17*(10), 2042–2046.

Brownstein, M.J. (1993). A brief history of opiates, opioid peptides, and opioid receptors. *Proceedings of the National Academy of Sciences, USA, 90*, 5391–5393.

Brunyé, T.T., Mahoney, C.R., Liberman, H.R., Giles, G.E. and Taylor, H.A. (2010). Acute caffeine consumption enhances the executive control of visual attention. *Brain and Cognition, 74*(3), 186–192.

Bullitt, E., Rahman, F.N., Smith, J.K., Kim, E., Zeng, D., Katz, L.M. and Marks, B.L. (2009). The effect of exercise on the cerebral vasculature of healthy aged subjects as visualized by MR angiography. *American Journal of Neuroradiology, 30*(10), 1857–1863.

Cannon, W.B. (1927). The James-Lange theory of emotions: A critical examination and an alternative theory. *The American Journal of Psychology, 39*, 106–124.

Cassilhas, R.C., Lee, K.S., Fernandes, J., Oliveira, M.G., Tufik, S., Meeusen, R. and de Mello, M.T. (2012). Spatial memory is improved by aerobic and resistance exercise through divergent molecular mechanisms. *Neuroscience, 202*, 309–317.

Chaddock, L., Erickson, K.I., Prakash, R.S., Voss, M.W., VanPatter, M., Pontifex, M.B., Hillman, C.H. and Kramer, A.F. (2012). A functional MRI investigation of the association between childhood aerobic fitness and neurocognitive control. *Biological Psychology, 89*(1), 260–268.

Clark, V.P., Coffman, B.A., Mayer, A.R., Weisend, M.P., Lane, T.D., Calhoun, V.D., Raybourn, E.M., Garcia, C.M. and Wassermann, E.M. (2012). TDCS guided using fMRI significantly accelerates learning to identify concealed objects. *Neuroimage, 59*(1), 117–128.

Coffman, B.A., Trumbo, M.C. and Clark, V.P. (2012). Enhancement of object detection with transcranial direct current stimulation is associated with increased attention. *BMC Neuroscience, 13*(1), 108.

Colcombe, S. and Kramer, A.F. (2003). Fitness effects on the cognitive function of older adults: A meta-analytic study. *Psychological Science, 14*(2), 125–130.

Costill, D.L., Dalsky, G.P. and Fink, W.J. (1978). Effects of caffeine ingestion on metabolism and exercise performance. *Medicine and Science in Sports, 10*(3), 155–158.

Cupp, M.J. (1999). Herbal remedies: Adverse effects and drug interactions. *American Family Physician, 59*(5), 1239–1244.

Daly, J.W. and Fredholm, B.B. (1998). Caffeine—An atypical drug of dependence. *Drug and Alcohol Dependence, 51*(1–2), 199–206.

Davidson, R.J. and Lutz, A. (2008). Buddha's brain: Neuroplasticity and meditation. *IEEE Signal Processing Magazine, 25*(1), 176–174.

Davis, C.L., Tomporowski, P.D., McDowell, J.E., Austin, B.P., Miller, P.H., Yanasak, N.E., Allison, J.D. and Naglieri, J.A. (2011). Exercise improves executive function and achievement and alters brain activation in overweight children: A randomized, controlled trial. *Health Psychology, 30*(1), 91–98.

Deister, C. and Schmidt, C.E. (2006). Optimizing neurotrophic factor combinations for neurite outgrowth. *Journal of Neural Engineering, 3*(2), 172–179.

Devane, W.A., Dysarz, F.A. III, Johnson, M.R., Melvin, L.S. and Howlett, A.C. (1988). Determination and characterization of a cannabinoid receptor in rat brain. *Molecular Pharmacology, 34*(5), 605–613.

Devane, W.A., Hanus, L., Breuer, A., Pertwee, R.G., Stevenson, L.A., Griffin, G., Gibson, D., Mandelbaum, A., Etinger, A. and Mechoulam, R. (1992). Isolation and structure of a brain constituent that binds to the cannabinoid receptor. *Science, 258*(5090), 1946–1949.

Dietrich, A. (2002). Functional neuroanatomy of altered states of consciousness. *Consciousness and Cognition, 12*(2), 231–256.

Dietrich, A. and McDaniel, W.F. (2004). Endocannabinoids and exercise. *British Journal of Sports Medicine, 38*(5), 536–541.

Donnelly, J.E., Greene, J.L., Gibson, C.A., Smith, B.K., Washburn, R.A., Sullivan, D.K., DuBose, K., et al. (2009). Physical activity across the curriculum (PAAC): A randomized controlled trial to promote physical activity and diminish overweight and obesity in elementary school children. *Preventative Medicine, 49*(4), 336–341.

Erickson, K.I., Voss, M.W., Prakash, R.S., Basak, C., Szabo, A., Chaddock, L., Kim, J.S., et al. (2011). Exercise training increases size of hippocampus and improves memory. *Proceedings of the National Academy of Sciences of the United States of America, 108*(7), 3017–3022.

Etgen, T., Sander, D., Huntgeburth, U., Poppert, H., Forstl, H. and Bickel, H. (2010). Physical activity and incident cognitive impairment in elderly persons: The INVADE study. *Archives of Internal Medicine, 170*(2), 186–193.

Evans, S.M. and Griffiths, R.R. (1992). Caffeine tolerance and choice in humans. *Psychopharmacology, 108*(1–2), 51–59.

Fabre, C., Chamari, K., Mucci, P., Masse-Biron, J. and Prefaut, C. (2002). Improvement of cognitive function by mental and/or individualized aerobic training in healthy elderly subjects. *International Journal of Sports Medicine, 23*(6), 415–421.

Ferris, L.T., Williams, J.S. and Shen, C.-L. (2007). The effect of acute exercise on serum brain-derived neurotrophic factor levels and cognitive function. *Medicine and Science in Sports and Exercise, 39*(4), 728–734.

Floel, A., Rosser, N., Michka, O., Knecht, S. and Breitenstein, C. (2008). Noninvasive brain stimulation improves language learning. *Journal of Cognitive Neuroscience, 20*(8), 1415–1422.

Fordyce, D.E. and Farrar, R.P. (1991). Enhancement of spatial learning in F344 rats by physical activity and related learning-associated alterations in hippocampal and cortical cholinergic functioning. *Behavioural Brain Research, 46*(2), 123–133.

Foulds, J., Stapleton, J.A., Bell, N., Swettenham, J., Jarvis, M.J. and Russell, M.A.H. (1997). Mood and physiological effects of subcutaneous nicotine in smokers and never-smokers. *Drug and Alcohol Dependence, 44*(2–3), 105–115.

Foulds, J., Stapleton, J.A., Swettenham, J., Bell, N., McSorley, K. and Russell, M.A.H. (1996). Cognitive performance effects of subcutaneous nicotine in smokers and never-smokers. *Psychopharmacology, 127*(1), 31–38.

Fregni, F., Boggio, P.S., Nitsche, M., Bermpohl, F., Antal, A., Feredoes, E., Marcolin, M.A., et al. (2005). Anodal transcranial direct current stimulation of prefrontal cortex enhances working memory. *Experimental Brain Research, 166*(1), 23–30.

Gilbert, D.G. (1979). Paradoxical tranquilizing and emotion-reducing effects of nicotine. *Psychological Bulletin, 86*(4), 643–661.

Gilbert, R.M. (1984). Caffeine consumption. In G.A. Spiller (ed.), *The Methylxanthine Beverages and Foods. Chemistry, Consumption, and Health Effects*, pp. 185–213. New York: A.R. Liss Incorporation.

Glade, M.J. (2010). Caffeine: Not just a stimulant. *Nutrition, 26*(10), 932–938.

Gold, S.M., Schulz, K.H., Hartmann, S., Mladek, M., Lang, U.E., Hellweg, R., Reer, R., et al. (2003). Basal serum levels and reactivity of nerve growth factor and brain-derived neurotrophic factor to standardized acute exercise in multiple sclerosis and controls. *Journal of Neuroimmunology, 138*(1–2), 99–105.

Griesar, W.S., Zajdel, D.P. and Oken, B.S. (2002). Nicotine effects on alertness and spatial attention in non-smokers. *Nicotine and Tobacco Research, 4*(2), 185–194.

Griffiths, R.R., Evans, S.M., Heishman, S.J., Preston, K.L., Sannerud, C.A., Wolf, B. and Woodson, P.P. (1990). Low-dose caffeine physical dependence in humans. *The Journal of Pharmacology and Experimental Therapeutics, 255*(3), 1123–1132.

Haier, R.J., Jung, R.E., Yeo, R.A., Head, K. and Alkire, M.T. (2004). Structural brain variation and general intelligence. *Neuroimage*, 23(1), 425–433.

Hammami, M.M., Al-Gaai, E.A., Alvi, S. and Hammami, M.B. (2010). Interaction between drug and placebo effects: A cross-over balanced placebo design trial. *Trials*, 11(110), 1–10.

Harbaugh, W.T., Mayr, U. and Burghart, D.R. (2007). Neural responses to taxation and voluntary giving reveal motives for charitable donations. *Science*, 316(5831), 1622–1625.

Harrison, L., Manoch, R. and Rubia, K. (2004). Sahaja yoga meditation as a family treatment programme for children with attention deficit-hyperactivity disorder. *Clinical Child Psychology and Psychiatry*, 9(4), 479–497.

Hasenkamp, W., James, G.A., Boshoven, W. and Duncan, E. (2011). Altered engagement of attention and default networks during target detection in schizophrenia. *Schizophrenia Research*, 125(2–3), 169–173.

Hasenkamp, W., Wilson-Mendenhall, C.D., Duncan, E. and Barsalou, L.W. (2012). Mind wandering and attention during focused meditation: A fine-grained temporal analysis of fluctuating cognitive states. *Neuroimage*, 59(1), 750–760.

Hölzel, B.K., Lazar, S.W., Gard, T., Schuman-Olivier, Z., Vago, D.R. and Ott, U. (2011). How does mindfulness meditation work? Proposing mechanisms of action from a conceptual and neural perspective. *Perspectives on Psychological Science*, 6(6), 537–559.

Hölzel, B.K., Ott, U., Hempel, H., Hackl, A., Wolf, K., Stark, R. and Vaitl, D. (2007). Differential engagement of anterior cingulate and adjacent medial frontal cortex in adept meditators and non-meditators. *Neuroscience Letters*, 421(1), 16–21.

Hötting, K., Holzschneider, K. and Röder, B. (2012). A combined physical exercise and cognitive training modulate functional brain activations during spatial learning. In R. Riemann (ed.), *Kongress der Deutschen Gesellschaft für Psychologie*, vol. 48, pp. 46–47. Lengerich: Pabst Science Publishers.

Hötting, K. and Röder, B. (2013). Beneficial effects of physical exercise on neuroplasticity and cognition. *Neuroscience and Biobehavioral Reviews*, 37(9), 2243–2257.

Intlekofer, K.A. and Cotman, C.W. (2013). Exercise counteracts declining hippocampal function in aging and Alzheimer's disease. *Neurobiology of Disease*, 57, 47–55.

Jang, J.H., Jung, W.H., Kang, D.-H., Byun, M.S., Kwon, S.J., Choi, C.-H. and Kwon, J.S. (2011). Increased default mode network connectivity associated with meditation. *Neuroscience Letters*, 487(3), 358–362.

Jenkins, K.T. and Tapper, K. (2013). Resisting chocolate temptation using a brief mindfulness strategy. *British Journal of Health Psychology*. [Epub ahead of print.]

Jha, A.P., Krompinger, J. and Baime, M.J. (2007). Mindfulness training modifies subsystems of attention. *Cognitive, Affective, and Behavioral Neuroscience*, 7(2), 109–119.

Julien, R.M. (2001). *A Primer of Drug Action: A Concise Nontechnical Guide to the Actions, Uses and Side Effects of Psychoactive Drugs*. New York: Macmillan.

Kellaway, P. (1946). The part played by the electric fish in the early history of bioelectricity and electrotherapy. *Bulletin of the History of Medicine*, 20(2), 112–137.

Kempermann, G. (2008). The neurogenic reserve hypothesis: What is adult hippocampal neurogenesis good for? *Trends in Neurosciences*, 31(4), 163–169.

Kerr, C.E., Jones, S.R., Wan, Q., Pritchett, D.L., Wasserman, R.H., Wexler, A., Villanueva, J.J., et al. (2011). Effects of mindfulness meditation training on anticipatory alpha modulation in primary somatosensory cortex. *Brain Research Bulletin*, 85(3–4), 96–103.

Kerr, C.E., Sacchet, M.D., Lazar, S.W., Moore, C.I. and Jones, S.R. (2013). Mindfulness starts with the body: Somatosensory attention and top-down modulation of cortical alpha rhythms in mindfulness meditation. *Frontiers in Human Neuroscience*, 7(12), 1–15.

Knaepen, K., Goekint, M., Heyman, E.M. and Meeusen, R. (2010). Neuroplasticity—Exercise-induced response of peripheral brain-derived neurotrophic factor: A systematic review of experimental studies in human subjects. *Sports Medicine*, 40(9), 765–801.

Knott, V., Bosman, M., Mahoney, C., Ilivitsky, V. and Quirt, K. (1999). Transdermal nicotine: Single dose effects on mood, EEG, performance, and event-related potentials. *Pharmacology, Biochemistry, and Behavior*, 63(2), 253–261.

Ko, M.H., Han, S.H., Park, S.H., Seo, J.H. and Kim, Y.H. (2008). Improvement of visual scanning after DC brain polarization of parietal cortex in stroke patients with spatial neglect. *Neuroscience Letters*, 448(2), 171–174.

Koehler, S., Lauer, P., Schreppel, T., Jacob, C., Heine, M., Boreatti-Hummer, A., Fallgatter, A.J. and Herrmann, M.J. (2009). Increased EEG power density in alpha and theta bands in adult ADHD patients. *Journal of Neural Transmission*, 116(1), 97–104.

Kolata, G. (2002). Runner's high? Endorphins? Fiction say some scientists. *New York Times*, May 21, http://www.nytimes.com/2002/05/21/health/runner-s-high-endorphins-fiction-some-scientists-say.html?pagewanted=all&src=pm. Retrieved May 30, 2014.

Kozasa, E.H., Sato, J.R., Lacerda, S.S., Barreiros, M.A., Radvany, J., Russell, T.A., Sanches, L.G., Mello, L.E. and Amaro, E. (2012). Meditation training increases brain efficiency in an attention task. *Neuroimage*, 59(1), 745–749.

Lambourne, K. and Tomporowski, P. (2010). The effect of exercise-induced arousal on cognitive task performance: A meta-regression analysis. *Brain Research*, 1341, 12–24.

Lara, D.R. (2010). Caffeine, mental health, and psychiatric disorders. *Journal of Alzheimer's Disease*, 20(1), 239–248.

Laurin, D., Verreault, R., Lindsay, J., MacPherson, K. and Rockwood, K. (2001). Physical activity and risk of cognitive impairment and dementia in elderly persons. *Archives of Neurology*, 58(3), 498–504.

Lazar, S.W., Kerr, C.E., Wasserman, R.H., Gray, J.R., Greve, D.N., Treadway, M.T., McGarvey, M., et al. (2005). Meditation experience is associated with increased cortical thickness. *Neuroreport*, 16(17), 1893–1897.

Levy, D.M., Wobbrock, J.O., Kaszniak, A.W. and Ostergren, M. (2012). The effects of mindfulness meditation training on multitasking in a high-stress information environment. In *Proceedings of the 2012 Graphics Interface Conference*, pp. 45–52. Canadian Information Processing Society, Toronto, ON.

Lista, I. and Sorrentino, G. (2010). Biological mechanisms of physical activity in preventing cognitive decline. *Cellular and Molecular Neurobiology*, 30(4), 493–503.

Liu-Ambrose, T., Nagamatsu, L.S., Graf, P., Beattie, B.L., Ashe, M.C. and Handy, T.C. (2010). Resistance training and executive functions: A 12-month randomized controlled trial. *Archive of Internal Medicine*, 170(2), 170–178.

Luders, E., Clark, K., Narr, K.L. and Toga, A.W. (2011). Enhanced brain connectivity in long-term meditation practitioners. *Neuroimage*, 57(4), 1308–1316.

Luders, E., Kurth, F., Mayer, E.A., Toga, A.W., Narr, K.L. and Gaser, C. (2012). The unique brain anatomy of meditation practitioners: Alterations in cortical gyrification. *Frontiers in Human Neuroscience*, 6, 34.

Mohan, A., Sharma, R. and Bijlani, R. (2011). Effect of meditation on stress-induced changes in cognitive functions. *The Journal of Alternative and Complementary Medicine*, 17(3), 207–212.

Moody, P.M., Averitt, J.H. and Griffith, R.B. (1973). Current status of the core service smoking behavior studies. In *Proceedings of the University of Kentucky Tobacco and Health Research Institute Tobacco and Health Workshop Conference* (Conference Report 4, 18–30). University of Kentucky, Lexington, KY.

Morgan, W.P. and O'Connor, P.J. (1988). Exercise and mental health. In R.K. Dishman (ed.), *Exercise Adherence: Its Impact on Public Health*, pp. 91–121. Champaign, IL: Human Kinetics.

Mori, F., Codeca, C., Kusayanagi, H., Monteleone, F., Buttari, F., Fiore, S., Bernardi, G., Koch, G. and Centonze, D. (2010). Effects of anodal transcranial direct current stimulation on chronic neuropathic pain in patients with multiple sclerosis. *The Journal of Pain*, 11(5), 436–442.

Newhouse, M.T. (1999). Tennis anyone? The lungs as a new court for systemic therapy. *Canadian Medical Association Journal*, 161(10), 1287–1288.

Nijs, I.M., Muris, P., Euser, A.S. and Franken, I.H. (2010). Differences in attention to food and food intake between overweight/obese and normal-weight females under conditions of hunger and satiety. *Appetite*, 54(2), 243–254.

Nitsche, M.A., Liebetanz, D., Tergau, F. and Paulus, W. (2002). Modulation of cortical excitability by transcranial direct current stimulation. *Nervenarzt*, 73(4), 332–335.

Pajonk, F.G., Wobrock, T., Gruber, O., Scherk, H., Berner, D., Kaizl, I., Kierer, A., et al. (2010). Hippocampal plasticity in response to exercise in schizophrenia. *Archives of General Psychiatry*, 67(2), 133 143.

Parrott, A.C. (1999). Does cigarette smoking *cause* stress? *American Psychologist*, 54(10), 817–820.

Parrott, A.C. and Kaye, F.J. (1999). Daily uplifts, hassles, stresses and cognitive failures: In cigarette smokers, abstaining smokers, and non-smokers. *Behavioral Pharmacology*, 10(6–7), 639–646.

Posselt, W. and Reimann, L. (1828). Chemische untersuchungen des tabaks und darstellung des eigenthumlichen wirksamen princips dieser pflanze. *Geigers Magazin der Pharmazie*, 24, 138–161.

Ragert, P., Vandermeeren, Y., Camus, M. and Cohen, L.G. (2008). Improvement of spatial tactile acuity by transcranial direct current stimulation. *Clinical Neurophysiology*, 119(4), 805–811.

Richards, M., Hardy, R. and Wadsworth, M.E.J. (2003). Does active leisure protect cognition? Evidence from a national birth cohort. *Social Science and Medicine*, 56(4), 785–792.

Ritter, F.E. and Yeh, K-C.M. (2011). Modeling pharmacokinetics and pharmacodynamics on a mobile device to help caffeine users. In *Augmented Cognition International Conference 2011*, FAC 2011, HCII 2011, LNAI, vol. 6780, pp. 528–535. Berlin Heidelberg: Springer-Verlag.

Rodgers, P.J. and Dernoncourt, C. (1998). Regular caffeine consumption: A balance of adverse and beneficial effects for mood and psychomotor performance. *Pharmacology, Biochemistry, and Behavior*, 59(4), 1039–1045.

Rojas Vega, S., Knicker, A., Hollmann, W., Bloch, W. and Struder, H.K. (2010). Effect of resistance exercise on serum levels of growth factors in humans. *Hormone and Metabolic Research*, 42(13), 982–986.

Rovio, S., Kareholt, I., Helkala, E., Viitanen, M., Winblad, B., Tuomilehto, J., Soininen, H., Nissinen, A. and Kivipelto, M. (2005). Leisure-time physical activity at midlife and the risk of dementia and Alzheimer's disease. *The Lancet Neurology*, 4(11), 705–711.

Rovio, S., Spulber, G., Nieminen, L.J., Niskanen, E., Winblad, B., Tuomilehto, J., Nissinen, A., Soininen, H. and Kivipelto, M. (2010). The effect of midlife physical activity on structural brain changes in the elderly. *Neurobiology of Aging*, 31(11), 1927–1936.

Ruscheweyh, R., Willemer, C., Kruger, K., Duning, T., Warnecke, T., Sommer, J., Völker, K., et al. (2011). Physical activity and memory functions: An interventional study. *Neurobiology of Aging*, 32(7), 1304–1319.

Sherwood, N. (1993). Effects of nicotine on human psychomotor performance. *Human Psychopharmacology*, 8(3), 155–184.

Smith, A., Sturgess, W. and Gallagher, J. (1999). Effects of a low dose of caffeine given in different drinks on mood and performance. *Human Psychopharmacology: Clinical and Experimental*, 14(7), 473–482.

Smith, A.P., Kendrick, A.M. and Maben, A.L. (1992). Effects of breakfast and caffeine on performance and mood in late morning and after lunch. *Neuropsychobiology*, 26(4), 198–204.

Stice, E., Spoor, S., Bohon, C. and Small, D.M. (2008). Relationship between obesity and blunted striatal response to food is moderated by *TaqIA* A1 allele. *Science*, 322(5900), 449–452.

Stranahan, A.M., Khalil, D. and Gould, E. (2007). Running induces widespread structural alterations in the hippocampus and entorhinal cortex. *Hippocampus*, 17(11), 1017–1022.

Strickland, R.A. (1996). Ether drinking in Ireland. *Mayo Clinic Proceedings*, 71(10), 1015.

Tang, Y.-Y., Ma, Y., Wang, J., Fan, Y., Feng, S., Lu, Q., Yu, Q., et al. (2007). Short-term meditation training improves attention and self-regulation. *Proceedings of the National Academy of Sciences*, 104(43), 17152–17156.

Tomporowski, P.D. (2003). Effects of acute bouts of exercise on cognition. *Acta Psychologica (Amsterdam)*, 112(3), 297–324.

Travis, F. and Shear, J. (2010). Focused attention, open monitoring an automatic self-transcending: Categories to organize meditations from Vedic, Buddhist and Chinese traditions. *Consciousness and Cognition*, 19(4), 1110–1118.

Tuckman, B.W. and Hinkle, J.S. (1986). An experimental study of the physical and psychological effects of aerobic exercise on schoolchildren. *Health Psychology*, 5(3), 197–207.

Tuson, K.M. and Sinyor, D. (1993). On the affective benefits of acute aerobic exercise: Taking stock after twenty years of research. In P. Seraganian (ed.), *Exercise Psychology: The Influence of Physical Exercise on Psychological Processes*, pp. 80–121. New York: Wiley.

van Praag, H., Christie, B.R., Sejnowski, T.J. and Gage, F.H. (1999). Running enhances neurogenesis, learning, and long-term potentiation in mice. *Proceedings of the National Academy of Sciences of the United States of America*, 96(23), 13427–13431.

van Vugt, M.K. and Jha, A.P. (2011). Investigating the impact of mindfulness meditation training on working memory: A mathematical modeling approach. *Cognitive, Affective, and Behavioral Neuroscience*, 11(3), 344–353.

Volkow, N.D. and Wise, R.A. (2005). How can drug addiction help us understand obesity? *Nature Neuroscience, 8*(5), 555–560.

West, R. (1996). An application of prefrontal cortex function theory to cognitive aging. *Psychological Bulletin, 120*(2), 272–292.

White, B.P., Becker-Blease, K.A. and Grace-Bishop, K. (2006). Stimulant medication use, misuse and abuse in an undergraduate and graduate student sample. *Journal of American College Health, 54*(5), 261–268.

Wilson, R.I. and Nicoll, R.A. (2002). Endocannabinoid signaling in the brain. *Science, 296*(5568), 678–682.

Witkiewitz, K., Lustyk, M.K.B. and Bowen, S. (2012). Retraining the addicted brain: A review of hypothesized neurobiological mechanisms of mindfulness-based relapse prevention. *Psychology of Addictive Behaviors, 27*(2), 351–365.

Xu, X., Aron, A., Brown, L., Cao, G., Feng, T. and Weng, X. (2011). Reward and motivation systems: A brain mapping study of early-stage romantic love in Chinese participants. *Human Brain Mapping, 32*(2), 249–257.

Zeidan, F., Martucci, K.T., Draft, R.A., Gordon, N.S., McHaffie, J.G. and Coghill, R.C. (2011). Brain mechanisms supporting the modulation of pain by mindfulness meditation. *The Journal of Neuroscience, 31*(14), 5540–5548.

8

Expertise

Within any domain, a rough distinction may be drawn between experts, who are considered to have attained a notable level of proficiency, and novices, who are at various stages of development ranging from beginners to competent performers. Among those considered to be experts, a further distinction may be made with some of these individuals being elite, meaning that they are the best of the best, possessing skills or knowledge that are clearly superior to all others. The current chapter focuses on the basis for these distinctions from the perspective of behavioral differences and measurable differences in underlying neurophysiology.

Anders Ericsson and the Notion of Deliberative Practice

In 1993, Anders Ericsson and colleagues published a seminal paper advancing their contention that the attainment of elite status within any domain was a function of what they termed, "deliberative practice" (Ericsson et al., 1993). In this paper, Ericsson confronted long-popular conceptions that held that elite performance was attributable to hereditary factors, while laying out a theoretical framework to account for progression from novice to expert to elite performer. This contention has subsequently been popularized by the author Malcolm Gladwell (2008) through the often-quoted assertion that within any domain, there is a prerequisite of 10,000 h of practice to attain mastery.

In Ericsson and colleague's original paper, they first challenged the idea that practice alone was sufficient to attain elite status within a domain. While numerous examples ranging from chess to music to scientific writing may be cited to illustrate that approximately 10 years of practice is necessary to reach a level of eminence, extensive practice is not sufficient. It is a regular occurrence to see highly experienced individuals within a domain perform poorly, particularly where there is little motivation, or scrutiny of individual performance. It is argued that it is not mere practice, but instead deliberative practice that allows an individual to advance to the highest levels of skill.

Deliberative practice involves a concerted effort to assess one's weaknesses, undertake activities targeted to overcome these weaknesses, continuously monitor performance, and explore alternative strategies for performance improvement. Deliberative practice is unlike operational experience in that deliberative practice is focused on overcoming specific weaknesses, whereas operational experience may or may not expose those weaknesses. Likewise, it is emphasized that deliberative practice is not enjoyable in that it requires hard work, with one regularly failing, and experiencing the associated feelings of frustration. Furthermore, it is not a matter of merely accumulating hours of practice. Once practice has extended beyond a certain duration, there are diminishing returns such that few, if any, benefits are derived from continuing to practice beyond this point and one is better served to rest and recuperate. Thus, given that there is a limited duration in which one can productively benefit from practice, for performance improvement, it is essential to maximize practice time to achieve the greatest gains for the effort expended. The elite may work harder than others, but they do not necessarily work longer. This notion runs counter to popular belief that is rooted in our cultural embrace of a strong work ethic being the key to success. Many stories are told of athletes who attain their level of mastery through countless hours of practice, being the first to arrive in the gym every morning and the last to leave every evening. The reality is that mastery is accrued through regular, intense, focused practice that is geared to the improvement of specific skills, with its duration being relatively brief (e.g., a few hours each day) such that there is ample time to recuperate and consolidate the gains amassed through each practice session.

A goal of practice is often automation, which confers the benefit of liberating the cognitive resources necessary to complete a task. The increasing automaticity of a behavior, however, may be a double-edged sword, as once a behavior is automatic it becomes recalcitrant to change (Dovidio and Fazio, 1992). In order to adjust an automated procedure, it must be brought back into the realm of working memory and attention. One way to do this is via deliberate practice; in fact, Ericsson and colleagues specifically noted the utility of deliberate practice in altering otherwise automatic routines (Ericsson et al., 1993). The deliberate focus of attention during practice allows for the interruption of the automatic execution of a behavior, bringing it under conscious control and enabling its adjustment. When renowned golfer Tiger Woods decided that he must change the nature of his stroke to improve his golf game, he employed deliberate practice. During the transitory period of deliberate practice, his performance level suffered, but in the end, he was able to achieve a better swing (Quinton, 2009). Again, it is worthwhile considering the diminishing returns of practice. If one approaches mastery of a behavior, but that behavior is not optimal for the situation, it is better to adjust the behavior than to continue to master the inferior method.

Unlikely Elites

Few make the transition from being expert to becoming elite performers, which is understandable given the pain and costs incurred. I spent considerable time thinking of various individuals whose stories illustrated

the arduous process that one must endure and the personal characteristics that are essential to become an elite. However, I was dissatisfied
because most of the individuals were the typical examples with which
we are all familiar, such as athletes, entertainers, and business people.
Then, I stumbled on an unusual, yet compelling example of someone
who had done exactly what one must do to become an elite performer;
however, it is uncertain whether their elite status is often appreciated.

I am thinking of the journey that the four hobbits undertook in J.R.R.
Tolkien's *Lord of the Rings*. Elite status is not attained through mere practice and it requires more than an accumulation of hours exercising the
requisite skills. Instead, to become among the elite, one must subject oneself to a tortuous form of practice that repeatedly forces one to operate
beyond the limits of one's capabilities.

When the hobbits set out from the Shire, few of their kind had ever
ventured into the world beyond the borders of their home. Almost immediately, they were forced to evade the pursuit of the Ring Wraths, which
pitted them against as formidable an opponent as existed within middle-
earth. While their escape required cleverness and, eventually, substantial
assistance, they were forced to overcome their fears and resist helplessness, despite the seeming hopelessness of their situation. From the out-
set, the hobbits subjected themselves to challenges that exceeded their
capabilities and in doing so, exercised personal characteristics that had
never been tested so severely.

As the story unfolds, the hobbits face repeated challenges that
exceed their physical prowess, but they succeed through perseverance.
They are not destined to be great warriors or clever strategists, but
their status is rooted in their willingness to persist and find a way, no
matter how daunting the odds. Their talent lies in their determination. One typically does not think of such a characteristic as being a
talent in that this capability cannot be demonstrated or measured as
with musical skills or athletic performances. However, this capability
directly applies to everyday life and often distinguishes those who are
highly successful from those who are capable, yet achieve more modest accomplishments.

Perhaps, one might question if the hobbits were actually elite in any
respect. However, their story provides several lessons regarding expertise. First, sheer talent is not the basis for attaining elite status. Many
with innate talent never reach the potential attributed to them. In contrast, the hobbits attained the status of hero without having any noteworthy talents. Practice is not enough. The hobbits were surrounded
by legions of warriors that had likely practiced their skills extensively,
yet were supporting characters furnishing background to their story. If
the hobbits did possess a natural gift that destined them to greatness, it
was their willingness to persevere. However, they not only persevered,
but they also undertook challenges that were beyond their capabilities

and repeatedly pushed them beyond their limits. This is the hallmark of those who attain elite status. They combine determination with a penchant for challenging themselves to exceed their limitations. No matter how dire the situation, the hobbits never gave up, but embarked on each new challenge. Through these characteristics, they illustrate the most essential element in becoming an elite performer.

How Does Practice Change Brain Activity?

As practice is a critical component on the journey to mastering a skill, it is worth considering how practice impacts the brain in order to frame the discussion of what qualities characterize an expert. As discussed in previous chapters, the brain remains plastic even through adulthood, allowing for reorganization as a result of practice and experience (Kolb and Whishaw, 1998). This reorganization may occur at a number of levels, ranging from molecular and synaptic changes to sweeping changes in the cortical maps and large-scale neural networks (Buonomano and Merzenich, 1998). Given the complexity of the brain and the variety of ways in which it may change, a simple account in which greater expertise is reflected in greater brain activity is naïve. The corpus of neuroimaging literature research on the impact of practice on the brain reports three distinct findings: (1) an increase in activation in the brain areas involved in task performance; (2) a decrease in brain activation in other areas; and (3) a functional reorganization of brain activity (resulting in a mixed pattern of increased and decreased activation). These physiological changes are thought to result from one of two cognitive consequences of practice—increasing mastery over the previously utilized strategy or the development of a novel strategy (Jonides, 2004).

Decreasing brain activity as a result of practice is the most common finding, and is thought to be the result of increasing neural efficiency (Kelly and Garavan, 2005). The primary mechanism by which greater efficiency may occur, resulting in decreased neural activation, is that certain neurons within a network become dominant via a pattern of increased firing and concomitant inhibition of their neighbors. Only a small sample of neurons responds when performing a particular task, but they do so with a much greater signal-to-noise ratio than is present prior to practice (see figure 4 in Poldrack and Gabrieli, 2001). A decrease in activation brought about in this fashion may manifest as a contraction in cortical representations (i.e., less neurons fire) or as a simple reduction in neural activity (i.e., the same number of neurons fire, but they fire less) (Poldrack and Gabrieli, 2001). Conversely, an increase in activation may be the product of the expansion of cortical representations (i.e., more neurons fire) reflecting practice-induced recruitment of additional cortical units or increases in the strength of activation (i.e., the same number of neurons fire, but do so with greater frequency) (Poldrack and Gabrieli, 2001).

The reorganization of the functional brain anatomy (both increased and decreased activation) may be further divided into two categories: (1) redistribution and (2) true reorganization. Redistribution refers to quantitative increases and decreases in activation, such that the same brain areas remain active following practice, but to a greater or lesser extent. This situation has been explained using the framework of a scaffolding-storage process (Petersen et al., 1998). In this context, the brain areas that are active when performing a novel task through effortful performance provide scaffolding. With practice, performance becomes increasingly automatic. Consequently, there is a decrease in the activity of the brain areas related to generic processes such as attention and cognitive control (a falling away of the scaffolding). This is coupled with an increase in activation in the brain areas related to task-specific storage and processing. Thus, during initial, unskilled task performance, areas such as the prefrontal cortex and the anterior cingulate cortex (involved in cognitive control and attention) will exhibit relatively high levels of activity when compared with their activity following task mastery. Conversely, areas that are involved in task-specific performance even when the performance has become largely automated (e.g., primary and secondary sensory and motor cortices, parietal or temporal cortex) will exhibit relatively high levels of activation once mastery has been achieved.

The phenomenon of redistribution has been demonstrated in research conducted by Sakai et al. (1998). In their experiment, participants were tasked with learning the correct sequence of button presses in response to 10 pairs of targets. As the performance became automatic, the participants exhibited a decrease in activation in the left dorsolateral prefrontal cortex and the presupplementary motor area, coupled with an increase in activation in the precuneus and intraparietal sulcus. These changes were interpreted as a practice-induced transition from declarative processes that necessitate focus of attention and cognitive control to automatic procedural processes. Consistent with the scaffolding framework suggested by Petersen et al. (1998), this pattern of results is indicative of the gradual de-emphasis of the brain areas involved in generic attention and cognitive control, while activity in the brain areas related to task-specific performance increases. It is worth noting that for this button-press task, high-performing participants showed a more rapid decline in prefrontal activity relative to poor performers, indicating that poor performers required prolonged use of the attentional scaffolding in order to achieve task automaticity (see Figure 6 in Sakai et al., 1998).

True reorganization refers to a qualitative rather than a quantitative shift in the patterns of brain activity; that is, a change in the anatomical areas of activation (rather than levels) associated with a shift in the cognitive processes that are used to perform a task. Recall that with practice, one of two cognitive processes is likely to take place: (1) mastery over an initially utilized strategy; or (2) a shift in task strategy (Jonides, 2004). The redistribution of brain activity is associated with increasing mastery over a given strategy, whereas true reorganization is indicative of an explicit shift in task strategy (Bernstein et al., 2002; Glabus et al., 2003). Since a qualitative shift in brain activation is associated with a shifting task strategy, it may be said that with situations in which reorganization occurs, the task performed by a novice is both neurobiologically and cognitively different from the task performed by someone who has attained mastery.

Experimental evidence for reorganization comes from research performed by Poldrack et al. (1998) and Poldrack and Gabrieli (2001) in which participants performed a mirror reading task while functional magnetic resonance imaging (fMRI) data were collected. Brain imaging took place both before and after an extensive 2-week training period. The results indicated that practice was associated with a reorganization of the functional anatomy such that activation in the dorsal visual stream (the visual pathway concerned with visuospatial information and interaction with objects) decreased, while activation in the ventral visual stream (concerned with object identification and recognition) increased. Underlying this reorganization was a shift from a visuospatial strategy that involved the mental transformation of the mirror-oriented words to their usual format into a more automatic process centered on the recognition of mirror-reversed words (sight-reading). This is consistent with the idea that reorganization is associated with strategy shift rather than strategy mastery. Of course, the line blurs when it is considered that once there has been a strategy shift, practicing that strategy will generally lead to increasing mastery, such that reorganization may often be followed by redistribution.

A variety of additional factors, such as task domain and complexity, may also influence the way that the brain changes as a result of practice (Schiltz et al., 2001). In fact, different brain areas seem to respond to practice in different ways. For instance, Kolb and Gibb (2002) suggested that neurons in the prefrontal cortex may exhibit an increased density of their dendritic spines (a small protrusion on the dendrite of a neuron that acts as a receiver for the axon terminal of another neuron) as a result of practice, whereas the parietal and occipital cortices reflect experience via neurons altering the length of their dendrites. While there are a number of factors that may impact how the brain changes to reflect increasing task proficiency, it is not necessary for the brain to exhibit greater overall activation to generate practice-related improvement. Haier et al. (1992) observed a widespread decrease in the rate of glucose metabolism in the brain during the performance of a complex visuospatial/motor task following a period of training that lasted several weeks. This decrease in energy use was associated with an increase in performance, suggestive of an increase in the efficiency of the brain for task performance following practice. Likewise, Beauchamp et al. (2003) demonstrated that as participants exhibited greater proficiency on the Tower of London task (a problem-solving puzzle that requires significant planning), they manifested less prefrontal brain activity.

Thus, there seems to be a relationship between greater task proficiency and decreased brain activity, perhaps as a result of enhanced neural efficiency attained through practice, meaning that it is not necessarily true (perhaps even unlikely) that an expert devotes more brain power to a task than a novice does. However, behavior needs to be considered in conjunction with brain activity. It may be true that an expert uses less brain activity than a novice does in order to achieve equivalent levels of performance due to the expert's greater cognitive and neural efficiency. However, to achieve a level of performance that qualifies an individual as an expert, a level of brain activity beyond that of a novice may be required (Seidler et al., 2002). In other words, experts may receive greater bang for their cognitive and neural buck—a concept that should be kept in mind when discussing some of the other characteristics associated with experts.

What Makes an Expert Different?

Given Ericsson et al.'s (1993) assertions that the path to eminence within a domain requires many years of regular deliberative practice, one might ask what the factors are that distinguish the performance of an expert. Obviously, within domains where there are objective measures of performance (e.g., athletics), the expert demonstrates superior capabilities with respect to objective measures of performance. However, many domains do not lend themselves to objective measures of performance, yet some individuals are recognized to be superior, with this recognition acknowledging their capabilities and not merely their years of experience. Likewise, one might go a level deeper and ask, what is it that experts do that enables them to outperform their counterparts?

Patterns and the Subtle Reward Structure Inherent to an Activity

In a seminal series of publications, Gary Klein and colleagues (e.g., Klein et al., 1993) reported their observations of experts from various domains and the cognitive thought processes underlying their decision making. This research served to dispel common notions within the decision-making literature that characterized expert decision making as a process in which an individual would rationally appraise alternative courses of action, relying on logical thought processes to make the best choice. Unlike many of their predecessors who primarily studied decision making in laboratory settings, Klein and colleagues studied decision making within real-world settings where significant consequences could follow from a poor choice. Their findings revealed that expert decision making did not resemble a rational process of evaluating alternative courses of action or applying a series of complex rules. Instead, experts often did not evaluate any alternatives. The process, which has become known as *naturalistic decision making* or *recognition-primed decision making,* generally involved an appraisal of the situation and based on this appraisal, recognition of a pattern, with the appropriate course of action being implicit to the recognized pattern. When the pattern was not immediately apparent, the expert would often take steps to elicit additional information or cues, or in other cases, the expert might engage in activities described as mental simulation. Furthermore, when experts committed errors, these errors were generally the result of having confused the current situation with another similar situation from the past, implying a failure within the pattern recognition process (Norman et al., 1989).

This process is familiar to all of us. We have all had the experience of eating at different types of restaurants, where you go through somewhat different routines to get a table, and order and receive your food. In a full-service restaurant, you are met at the door and are escorted to your table, and someone comes to your table to take your order. In contrast, in fast-food restaurants, you generally order at the counter and select your own table, with your food brought to your table in some cases, but in other cases, there is a pickup counter where you retrieve your food. On walking in the door of a restaurant, most of us are able to quickly sense a few key cues and put these cues together to form a recognizable pattern that tells us the type of restaurant. Once we have recognized the pattern, the associated routines and expectations are immediately obvious. This familiar process is the same as that exhibited by experts when they enter into a new situation. They assess the cues and once a pattern has been recognized, they know what to do.

The recognition of meaningful patterns is a process that we all frequently engage in. For instance, read each row of letters below. After reading a row, look away for 5 s, and then see if you are able to recall the letters from the row in order.

j q m z
p l g r t v t
t w b x m j t g
g h j q w v z n p m

As you progressed down the rows, you likely found it more difficult to recall the entire set of letters as the number of letters increased. Try the same exercise with the following rows:

bubble clam bake
correct horse staple battery

It is unlikely that you had much difficulty recalling either of these rows, even though the first row consisted of 14 letters and the second row consisted of 25 letters. In contrast, the maximum number of letters contained in the first set of rows was 10. This example illustrates the process of *chunking,* or the mental grouping of connected elements. Words constitute a chunk, such that even though the word-based examples contain a relatively high number of letters, these rows consist of three and four chunked elements, respectively. Grouping the letter-only rows into chunks is difficult (note that these rows do not contain vowels, which makes it impossible to form words), so the number of elements contained in each row is equal to the number of letters, whereas the number of elements contained in the word-based examples is the number of words. Even though there are more letters, grouping the letters into a meaningful pattern means that the word-based examples actually contain fewer elements and thus, are easier to remember. Chunking is a common mechanism that people use to facilitate information processing—one that we all employ every time we read.

Previous research has demonstrated that experts within a domain exhibit a superior capacity to recognize patterns that are relevant to their domain of expertise. Within the field of chess, Chase and Simon (1973) presented a master player, an intermediate player, and a novice with 24–26 pieces aligned on a chessboard in positions taken from an actual chess game, for a period of 5 s. The participants were then asked to reconstruct the positions of the pieces. Although the master player was able to correctly place the most pieces, the critical finding was that when the board positions of the pieces were random rather than taken from the middle of an actual game, recall was equivalent regardless of experience. The conclusion drawn from this research is that experts are better at chunking meaningful information into larger units, which facilitates recall. Consequently, familiarity gained through practice provides a greater collection of meaningful configurations.

Within the domain of physics, one identified difference between novices and experts involves problem schemas—knowledge structures centered around understanding the type of problem that one is confronted with and how to solve it. This has been demonstrated by Chi et al. (1981), who presented physics novices and experts with various physics problems and asked them to categorize the problems based on the solution procedure. The results indicated that while the novices tended to group the problems by the physical objects listed within them (e.g., inclined planes or springs), the experts grouped the problems by the applicable laws of physics (e.g., conservation of momentum), which enabled the experts to readily access the equations relevant to the problem, allowing them to more readily solve the problems.

When considered as a whole, this body of research demonstrates that experts use extensive domain-specific knowledge in order to focus on relevant information and discard irrelevant information. The process of acquiring the background knowledge that is necessary to determine the relevance of information requires a great deal of experience and exposure to varied problems, which enable experts to recognize situations as instances of previously encountered problems and apply a solution that has worked well in the past. Research has demonstrated that teaching basic heuristics (i.e., general procedures) to novices is often ineffective, likely because without being taught how to implement the heuristics, novices lack knowledge that is essential to effectively apply the general rules (Schoenfeld, 1985).

To study the brain processes that underlie an expert's ability to effectively appraise situations to recognize meaningful patterns, Wan et al. (2011) studied expert Shogi players. Shogi is a Japanese board game that bears some resemblance to chess in that it requires players to make strategic decisions regarding moving their pieces, relative to an opponent. Decisions are made quickly on the basis of decision-making processes that often seem automated. When comparing amateurs with professional players, two brain regions exhibited greater levels of activation within the professionals. The first was the precuneus region of the parietal lobe, which was active during the appraisal of the layout of the pieces on the board, suggesting a functional role in perceptual pattern recognition. However, as has been demonstrated with grand master chess players, superior pattern recognition may require more than perceptual processes. In particular, with chess, it has been shown that during rapid play, the number of errors is no greater when blindfolded than when able to visually observe the chessboard (Chabris and Hearst, 2003). The second area for which the professional Shogi players showed greater activation was the caudate nucleus of the basal ganglia. This activation was associated with generating moves based on recognized patterns. Given that the activity of these two regions covaried in response to the demands of specific game situations, the authors proposed that these neural regions work in concert, enabling the perceptual recognition of patterns and the associated rapid response generation. Furthermore, it is through the experience accumulated by an expert that this circuit is exercised and elaborated to enable the highly refined, seemingly effortless performance of an expert.

It is worth mentioning that while expertise tends to be domain specific, improved performance on a trained task should bolster performance in additional domains and tasks to the extent that they rely on overlapping cognitive abilities or share neural systems (Dahlin et al., 2008). Interestingly, it has been suggested that the pattern recognition experience that leads to expertise within a given domain may produce a generalized superiority for pattern recognition (Abernethy et al., 2005). This was demonstrated in a study that considered the pattern recognition skills of subjects who were either experts or merely experienced players in netball games (e.g., basketball, field hockey). The subjects were shown defensive positions of players from sports other than the sport for which they were experienced. It was found that the experts showed a superior ability to recognize defensive patterns within sports for which they had little or no experience, as compared with the nonexperts. For example, basketball players were better on average at recognizing patterns associated with field hockey, despite being unfamiliar with the game. This suggests that training that gives rise to expertise within a given domain may serve to develop generalized cognitive skills that are transferable to other activities demanding the same cognitive skills.

Enhanced Perceptual Discrimination

Within many domains, expertise correlates with an ability to perceptually distinguish objects on the basis of minor details. Many skills involve a significant refinement of perceptual processes with regard to a specific sense and the patterns of sensory input associated with certain types of objects. For example, automobile experts not only develop a rich knowledge of the different makes and models of cars, but also an ability to accurately recognize the make and model, as well as the year, of a car after a relatively brief visual exposure. It has been demonstrated that enhanced capacities for perceptual discrimination that are found in many areas of expertise are accompanied by increased refinement of the brain areas associated with the categorization of perceptual objects (Gauthier et al., 2000) (Figures 8.1 and 8.2).

The fusiform gyrus is a region near the visual areas of the brain that has been associated with activities involving the perceptual categorization of objects, with much of this research focused on the recognition of faces. In a study by Gauthier et al. (2000), individuals with expertise in either cars or birds were asked to make categorical judgments regarding faces, familiar objects, cars, or birds. When viewing the cars or birds, the level of activation found in the fusiform gyrus correlated with a measure of each individual's relative expertise regarding these categories of objects. This finding suggests that with expertise, there is an elaboration of the neural circuits within the brain associated with making detailed distinctions between objects on the basis of perceptual details. This research was extended through a study in which participants were trained over a period of time to discriminate figures that combined different geometrical shapes and could be categorized based on the presence and configuration of these geometrical shapes. As the subjects became increasingly adept at making these discriminations, there was increased activation of the fusiform gyrus, which correlated with the participants' ability to make discriminations on the basis of the holistic properties of the objects (Gauthier and Tarr, 2002).

Self-Regulation

Elite performers exhibit an enhanced capacity for regulating their emotional and cognitive state. Within high-stress environments, the accompanying physiological arousal can have a debilitating effect on one's ability to process complex information and make effective decisions. Furthermore, extended periods of arousal can be fatiguing, draining one's mental and physiological resources. In a series of studies, Simmons et al. (2012) assessed the emotional responsiveness and the associated self-regulation of emotions in US Navy SEALs. This is a group of military special operations forces that are recognized for their elite status within the domain of combat operations. In these studies, off-duty Navy SEALs were compared with healthy, age-matched volunteer subjects with regard to their response to images that were selected

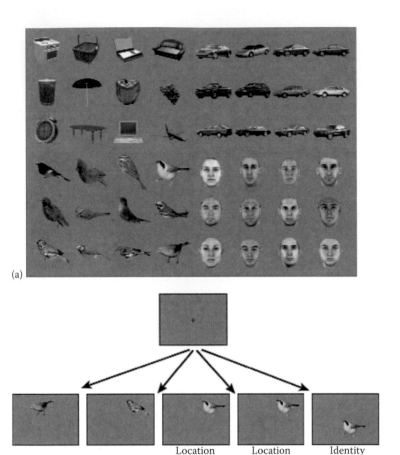

FIGURE 8.1

(a,b) Stimuli used by Gauthier et al. to assess the brain representation of categorical expertise. Subjects were presented with stimuli and were required to recall either the identity or location of the stimulus on the previous trial. (From Gauthier, I., Skudlarski, P., Gore, J.C., and Anderson, A.W., *Nature Neuroscience*, 3, 191–197, 2000. With permission.)

to elicit an emotional response. Different-colored geometric shapes were used to prime subjects to expect either a positive or a negative image. The positive images reflected pleasant scenes in which individuals displayed expressions of happiness. The negative images depicted combat scenes. The subjects' task was to respond as quickly as possible to the geometric shapes by pressing a button on the left when they saw a circle and a button on the right when they saw a square. Ordinarily, in this type of study, there is an effect of the emotional imagery, with subjects responding more slowly to the shapes. The prime serves to prepare the subject for the upcoming emotional image and, generally, when primed, there is a reduced effect on the

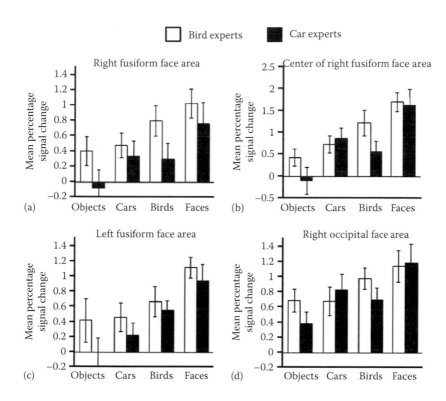

FIGURE 8.2
(a–d) Changes in the signal intensity of the fusiform face area for bird experts and car experts while performing recall tasks involving either the identity or the location for either car, bird, or face stimuli. (From Gauthier, I., Skudlarski, P., Gore, J.C., and Anderson, A.W., *Nature Neuroscience*, 3, 191–197, 2000. With permission.)

response time resulting from the negative images. In the current study, the prime generally coincided with the image, with positive primes preceding positive images and negative primes preceding negative images. However, there were trials in which the prime and the image did not coincide. Having established through previous studies that the Navy SEALs exhibit a differential adaptive response to emotional images based on whether or not they represent a potential threat (Paulus et al., 2010), the researchers were interested to see if the Navy SEALs would be more adaptive when presented with trials in which the emotions elicited by the images differed from what was expected on the basis of the primes. The results confirmed this expectation. There was significantly less slowing in response to the shapes in the trials in which the prime and image did not match for the Navy SEALs, as compared with the control group (see Figure 8.3). Furthermore, the Navy SEALs had greater activation of the brain regions associated with emotional self-regulation (i.e., middle insula and bilateral frontal lobes). This highlights the ability of these elite performers to better manage their physiological response

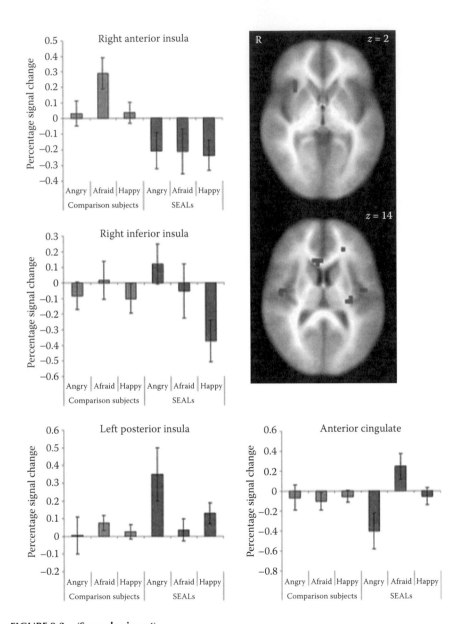

FIGURE 8.3 **(See color insert)**
US Navy SEALs showed greater activation of the right insula in response to angry faces than control subjects did, suggesting greater sensitivity and awareness of potential threats. (From Paulus, M.P., Simmons, A.N., Fitzpatrick, S.N., Potterat, E.G., Van Orden, K.F., Bauman, J., and Swain, J.L., *PLoS ONE*, 5, e10096, 2010.)

to emotional situations. Thus, this points to a capacity that may extend to elite performers across different domains to better regulate their mental and physical resources, allowing them to better cope with the demands of high-stress situations.

Michael Zotov and colleagues at Saint Petersburg State University have developed measures to assess an individual's capacity for self-regulation and examined the use of these measures as a basis for evaluating expertise within a domain (Zotov et al., 2009). Their research has focused on the use of heart-rate variability as an indicator of self-regulatory capacity. Normally, an individual exhibits moment-to-moment variability in key components of the heart rate. However, when stressed, there is a reduction in this variability. The reduction in heart-rate variability has been attributed to a failure of mechanisms that normally allow the body to adapt to ongoing demands. Zotov and colleagues compared novice and experienced train drivers as they completed scenarios on a locomotive simulator that is used for training. Their results showed that during nonstressful periods, there was a slight difference, with the experienced train drivers exhibiting greater heart-rate variability than the novices. However, this difference was substantial when the subjects were presented with a critical incident, which dramatically increased the task demands. Both the novices and the experts displayed reduced heart-rate variability, but the reduction was much greater in the novices, with this reduction correlated with behavioral measures of the errors committed and slowed response times. These findings suggest that the experts possessed a greater capacity for self-regulation and, as a result, they better adapted to the stressful conditions, maintaining some degree of moment-to-moment responsiveness to the environmental demands.

In a subsequent study, Zotov and colleagues examined these findings more closely using a laboratory paradigm known as the *multiattribute test battery* (MAT-B; Zotov et al., 2011). The MAT-B presents subjects with four simultaneous tasks that they must perform and it allows the experimenter to selectively adjust the demands associated with each task. The subjects underwent extensive training, which resulted in significant improvements in their ability to cope with the simultaneous demands of the MAT-B tasks. However, there was a range in the level of skill attained by the subjects. When the researchers considered those subjects who exhibited the highest levels of skill, it was found that as these subjects performed the task under demanding conditions, they did not exhibit the reductions in heart-rate variability that were observed with the less-skilled performers. The ability for self-regulation, evidenced in the variability present within the heart rate, correlated with the level of skill attained by the individual subjects. Subsequently, Zotov et al. (2011) measured heart-rate variability in air traffic controllers as they performed under stressful conditions. As with the previous studies, experts exhibited greater variability. However, when the researchers looked at points within the scenarios that involved a critical incident, with heightened task demands and associated stress, the reduction in heart-rate variability that occurred with novice air traffic controllers was of significantly longer durations than that with the experts. This finding suggests that when presented with a stressful situation, both experts and novices show reductions in heart-rate variability. However, the experts quickly recover, while the impact on the novices persists for an extended period of time. Thus, experts not only show greater self-regulatory capacities, but they are also capable of recovering more quickly following periods of extreme demands.

Based on the findings reported by the research group at Saint Petersburg State University, the capacity for self-regulation offers a basis for measuring the resilience of training to stressful conditions. Within a training scenario, it can be expected that there will be periods during which demands are high and elevated levels of physiological arousal would be expected. During these periods, students should show elevated arousal evidenced by a reduction in heart-rate variability. The absence of an arousal response would be a reason for concern in that it suggests that a student may not appreciate the significance of the situation. In contrast, the scenario should also contain periods during which demands are low and there should be a relatively low level of physiological arousal. During these intervals, a high level of arousal would indicate that a student is struggling. This is important because the student may very well perform at an acceptable level based solely on behavioral measures of performance. However, the fact that the student is mustering all of his or her resources to attain this level of performance suggests that the student's training may be relatively fragile and is likely to break down under the stresses of the operational environment.

High levels of arousal during periods of low demand indicate that the student may have a weak understanding of the overall task environment. Experts understand when conditions warrant heightened levels of attention and know to get themselves up for these situations. Likewise, experts understand when demands are low and that there is an opportunity to relax and recover. In contrast, a novice may lack this basic understanding of the task environment and continuously operate at a high level of arousal, even when the circumstances of the task do not demand his or her full attention. The result is that the novice will more quickly expend his or her resources and become fatigued, with associated reductions in performance. Thus, while the initial performance of the novice may be adequate, a precipitous letdown may follow as he or she becomes fatigued and can no longer sustain the requisite levels of attention to the task environment.

The use of biofeedback offers the potential to improve students' capacity for self-regulation. For example, with expert marksmen, it has been demonstrated that a key component of their success involves the cognitive state that they achieve prior to taking a shot (Hatfield et al., 1984). Specifically, expert marksmen exhibit a capacity to quiet the brain in regions that are normally associated with the ongoing internal dialogue that we associate with our moment-to-moment thoughts. This is evidenced through greater synchronization of activity in the 8–13 Hz, or alpha bandwidth, over temporal regions of the brain. Given this finding, it has been shown that subjects trained to reproduce the patterns of brain activation observed in expert marksmen using electroencephalogram (EEG) biofeedback exhibited greater performance improvements than comparable students who merely practiced their marksmanship skills (Behneman et al., 2012). This suggests that in many cases, enhanced performance may be attained through approaches that focus on training the self-regulatory skills that characterize expertise within a given domain.

Given the above observations concerning expert marksmen, it is worth noting that the experience of choking, or failing to produce expected or normal levels of performance in stressful situations, has been linked to excessive internal dialogue. It is believed that this internal dialogue (e.g., worrying about how one will be perceived if one fails) competes for key cognitive resources such as working memory, placing the performer at a disadvantage (Beilock, 2010). Again, this points to the importance of self-regulation, or in this case, the ability to regulate one's internal thought processes.

Recovery from Errors

One might conclude that a marker of expertise is that these individuals do not make mistakes, or at least, they make substantially fewer mistakes than those who are less adept. This would be an erroneous conclusion. Experts do make mistakes, with their expertise making them more prone to certain types of errors (Dror, 2011). However, experts exhibit a capacity to recover from errors more quickly and effectively.

In an earlier chapter, there was discussion of the brain's intrinsic response to the realization that an error has been committed. This has been referred to as *error-related negativity*, based on the electrophysiological response that is observed. When an individual realizes that he or she has committed an error, a wave of activity that originates in the cingulate region of the brain extends over a broad area. The size of the response varies in relation to the magnitude of the error and there is a response whether feedback concerning the error occurs immediately or is delayed for some duration. Using a perceptual categorization task that called on skills similar to those exhibited by experts in many domains (e.g., evaluating collectibles), it was shown that as one gains proficiency, the magnitude of the error response increases (Krigolson et al., 2009). This suggests that with greater levels of proficiency, there is an increased sensitivity to feedback indicative of having committed an error. Furthermore, this sensitivity extends to situations where one observes someone else committing an error. In a study involving nonmusicians, amateur musicians, and expert musicians, the participants listened to pieces of music that had been constructed to include certain tonal irregularities (Oeschslim et al., 2012). These tonal irregularities created a violation of expectations and produced the expected neurophysiological response observable within fMRI brain images. The results showed that the magnitude of the response to the irregularities correlated with the participants' level of expertise. The subjects with the greatest expertise exhibited a more pronounced response to violations of expectations in the pieces to which they were asked to listen.

Much of the research concerning the neurophysiological basis of expertise has involved musicians. With expert musicians, it has been shown that they are not only sensitive to having committed an error, but within their brains, the response to having committed an error may precede the actual error. For example, as shown in Figure 8.4, when expert pianists were asked to play different scales and patterns, it was observed that there was a detectable electrophysiological response 100 ms prior to the pianist playing an erroneous note (Maidhof et al., 2009). Similarly, in a study in which expert pianists were asked to recall memorized music pieces at a rapid tempo, there was brain activity indicative of an error 70 ms prior to having committed the error (Ruiz et al., 2009). Furthermore, the presence or absence of feedback concerning errors did not affect the response prior to committing the error, yet it did have the expected effect on the subsequent neural response that accompanied the realization that an error had occurred.

In practice, when one observes experts, they often appear to perform flawlessly. They effectively carry out their objectives, responding to moment-to-moment demands. Some things may not go as planned, but they seem to confidently adapt and make appropriate adjustments. However, it is often surprising when, during debrief, an expert readily confesses to having made any number of errors. If it is a group of experts, they may chide one another for their individual miscues. To the casual onlooker, there was nothing

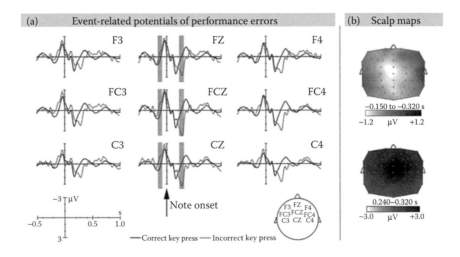

FIGURE 8.4

(a,b) The EEG-evoked response as an expert pianist played incorrect notes. The error signifies the point at which the incorrect note was played, with the electrophysiological response commencing approximately 100 ms prior to the erroneous performance. (From Maidhof, C., Rieger, N., Prinz, W., and Koelsch, S., *PLoS ONE*, 4, e5032, 2009.)

amiss; however, the expert is generally keenly aware of every misstep. Yet, the expert had the knowledge and skill to recover, leaving an impression of a perfect performance.

Mental Toughness, Motivation, and Self-Confidence

It has long been recognized that elite performers exhibit certain psychological traits that distinguish them from other equally capable performers. These traits have often been lumped under the more general trait referred to as *mental toughness* (Crust, 2007). Mental toughness has been described in various ways, but generally refers to the observation that elite performers display a capacity to persevere and continually push themselves despite adversity arising from fatigue, misfortune, or disappointing outcomes. Furthermore, those possessing mental toughness are thought to have an unusually strong conviction and commitment to achieving their goals, accompanied by self-confidence and an unshakable faith that they control their own destiny (Clough et al., 2002). It has been asserted that in certain competitive athletic settings, as much as 50% of successful outcomes may be attributed to mental toughness (Loehr, 1986). Athletes possessing mental toughness are said to be disciplined thinkers who respond to pressure by remaining calm, relaxed, and energized. This has been demonstrated in a study of participants in competitive Wushu (a performance-oriented style of Chinese martial arts) in which it was shown that the most successful performers were those who displayed a capacity to remain focused on their task, while controlling the negative emotions associated with the competition (Kuan and Roy, 2007). Furthermore, evidence suggests that there may be a genetic component with the traits giving rise to mental toughness being somewhat heritable and linked to heritable personality characteristics (Horsburgh et al., 2009). With regard to specific personality attributes, based on the traits identified in the five-factor model of personality (Costa and McCrae, 1992), mental toughness was positively correlated with extraversion, open-mindedness, agreeableness, and conscientiousness, while being negatively correlated with neuroticism.

This is not to say that experts are immune to the effects of pressure. The phenomenon of *choking*, in which an individual performs below expectations with regard to a well-learned skill while under pressure, is likely one that we have all witnessed in the realm of athletics. Pressure may come in the form of monetary performance–based incentives, peer pressure, or social evaluation. Beilock and Carr (2001) examined the differential impact of these types of pressure in a series of experiments using a golf-based scenario. In the first experiment, there were three groups of participants: experienced golfers, experienced athletes who were new to golf, and nonathletes who were new to golf. These groups completed three rounds of putting, with the first two rounds followed by a questionnaire asking the participants to detail the steps involved in making a putt in general, and the final questionnaire asking the participants to describe the steps involved in making a specific putt—the last one taken by the participants. The results indicated that while the expert golfers were able to provide more detailed accounts of the generic process involved in putting than the other groups, the inexperienced golfers provided greater detail concerning the particular instance of a putt. This supports the idea that during performance, expert golfers have largely automated the task of putting to the point where they do not attend to the process as thoroughly as a novice, and thus are unable to recall as many of the specifics.

The second experiment repeated the procedure used in the first, but this time some of the participants were given a deformed putter, which required expert golfers to change their routine for putting. Under the "funny putter" condition, it was found that experienced golfers were still able to give more detailed generic descriptions of putting, but instead of exhibiting a detriment in recalling specific instances, the experts were able to provide a more detailed account than the less-experienced golfers. The explanation for this result was that the oddly shaped putter forced the experts to attend closely to their putting, and their golfing experience combined with this increased attention led to their recall of a specific putting episode that exceeded all other groups.

In the third and fourth experiments, either early on or following training, participants were told that they would receive a monetary award for successfully completing the task and that their performance would be videotaped for the purposes of training other participants. The results indicated that with instructions given early in training, pressure may facilitate skill acquisition by providing motivation to focus on the fundamentals of the task. However, once a skill has been mastered, it becomes susceptible to the detrimental effects of pressure, leading to interruption of an otherwise automated, fluidly performed skill.

This result was explained via the explicit monitoring theory, which states that under pressure, an expert may pay too much attention to processes that would otherwise be performed with fluidity, leading to an outcome that is less than optimal. Think back to our discussion of how brain activity changes with practice. Often, less neural activation is associated with the superior performance of experts, reflecting a decreased need for attention and cognitive control of mastered abilities, such that "overthinking" or consciously exerting cognitive control over an otherwise automated behavior results in a performance decrement. This series of experiments suggests that pressure may facilitate the performance of novices by motivating them to focus their cognitive resources on a task, thereby increasing their chances of competently performing the task fundamentals; whereas, for an expert who has already mastered and automated the fundamentals, pressure may have a detrimental impact. This goes back to the idea of deliberate practice, which entails focusing attention on a task in order to exert cognitive control over it for purposes of improvement. As mentioned during our discussion at the beginning of the chapter, the process of deliberate practice resulted in a temporary performance decrease for Tiger Woods, though once he was able to adjust his routine and reautomate the process via extensive practice, the end result was a better swing.

Although you have probably witnessed choking under pressure play out in the realm of athletics, additional work by Beilock et al. (2004) suggests that choking under pressure may occur for cognitive tasks as well, such as when solving mathematical problems. It is worth mentioning that while explicit monitoring seems to account for choking under pressure when a task is sensorimotor in nature, choking under pressure on a cognitive task is more likely to be the result of divided attention, such that pressure serves to split an individual's attention between the task at hand and worry concerning the outcome of the task (Beilock et al., 2004). On the bright side, recent research indicates that individuals who possess high expectations regarding their ability to perform under pressure may actually perform better in high-pressure, as opposed to low-pressure scenarios—even if their expectancies have been artificially inflated (e.g., false survey results) rather than forged through past experience (McKay et al., 2012). This underscores the importance of self-confidence when considering expert performance in high-pressure situations.

To date, there has been little research addressing the neurophysiological factors that underlie the motivational components of expert and elite performance. One may speculate that similar motivational processes occur in laboratory paradigms involving sustained effort to achieve an objective. For instance, in rats, a depleted level of dopamine within the reward system, and particularly, the nucleus accumbens, has been linked to the capacity of animals to work harder to obtain food rewards (Salamone et al., 2010). Similarly, it has been shown that drugs that counteract the effects of adenosine (e.g., block the adenosine receptors, which are colocated with dopamine receptors within the nucleus accumbens reward system) increase the willingness of animals to work to achieve a reward (Nunes et al., 2010). Interestingly, as noted in an earlier chapter, it is believed that a primary mechanism by which caffeine operates is through blocking the adenosine receptors. The brain regions identified in these studies correspond to the regions within the human brain that have been identified as common motivational nodes that modulate the level of effort exerted for both physical and mental tasks (Schmidt et al., 2012).

Some insight may be gained regarding the factors that underlie extreme levels of motivation from a consideration of the mechanisms that are linked to deficits in motivation. In a study using positron emission tomography to obtain detailed images of the brain, Volkow et al. (2011) found that the prevalence of the dopamine receptors and molecules involved in dopamine transport was negatively correlated with measures of intrinsic motivation. Other research has shown that the modulation of activity in the nucleus accumbens reward circuits that normally occurs in response to the relative magnitude of rewards is less evident in adolescents who are relatively unresponsive to incentives (Bjork et al., 2004). Given that deficits in motivation seem attribut-able to a reduced responsiveness of the dopamine-mediated reward circuits of the brain, it may be suggested that the intense levels of motivation seen in elite performers could be the product of their unusually sensitive reward systems. Such an assertion is consistent with observations that elite perform-ers often exhibit a greater drive to be successful, while being able to sustain this drive despite unfavorable outcomes. Furthermore, an explanation cen-tering on an unusually responsive reward system would also correspond to observations that elite performers often seem to experience a greater level of pleasure from their activities and related achievements (Loehr, 1986), sug-gesting that these individuals simply enjoy themselves more and as a result, feel more compelled to persist and exert themselves.

However, an alternative explanation, or perhaps an additional factor, involves the impact of success on basic neurophysiological processes, with it suggested that these effects may translate into heightened levels of self-confidence. Fuxjager et al. (2010) conducted studies using a species of mouse (i.e., the California mouse) that is territorial and aggressive in defending its territory. With this species of mouse, the researchers were able to engineer situations where they could control which mouse won and loss individual disputes. In other words, the researchers were able to create winners and losers, as well as to make a winner a loser or make a loser a winner. The researchers found that the experience of winning disputes increased the expression of androgen hormonal receptors in the reward circuits of the ani-mals' brains. Thus, the experience of winning changed the brain in a way that would have promoted a willingness to engage in subsequent disputes. In subsequent research, it was shown that the maximum effect on later behavior resulted from a combination of winning disputes and high base-line levels of testosterone (Fuxjager et al., 2011). Either factor alone produced only a moderate effect on behavior. With respect to humans, a summary of research studies assessing the hormonal levels of participants in competitive sporting events found that while there are various factors that modulate hor-mone levels (e.g., personal assessments of performance), winning produces elevated levels of testosterone (Brondino et al., 2013). Interestingly, the mag-nitude of this effect was equivalent for both contact and noncontact sports.

There may be many who, due to intrinsic factors, exhibit a level of drive and perseverance that ensures some degree of success. These intrinsic factors may then be amplified through the neurohormonal effects that follow the experi-ence of having succeeded. This creates conditions for a feedback loop where intrinsic factors lay the groundwork for rewarding experiences that then intensify the intrinsic motivational drive. However, one should be cautious in concluding that we are relegated to a world where only a lucky few have any chance of attaining elite status or routinely enjoying success. The bright spot lies in the winner's effect and the fact that the experience of winning can produce changes in basic neurophysiology. Consequently, whether or not one is intrinsically endowed, the experience of winning can be transformative.

Within organizations, competition can be both motivating for the would-be winners and demoralizing for the losers. Likewise, it must be appreciated that the benefits of competition are often diminished when institutional processes reward everyone equally. This can be observed in organizations that employ merit-based annual pay increases, yet the difference in rewards between the highest and lowest achievers is marginal. In these situations, it is difficult for the high-achievers to avoid cynicism regarding the process and there is little incentive for the low-performers to find ways to improve their contributions. It seems that many organizations are stuck at either end of the continuum. Either their institutional processes reward a few, leaving most demoralized by the competitive process, or they reward everyone equally, with there being little incentive for anyone to do better. However, organizations do have the opportunity to create a variety of opportunities for individuals to compete and have the experience of winning. Models can be found in events that judge competitors and give awards for a range of different categories, as well as in competitive sports where there are many different conferences or divisions with champions at every level. Thus, while some prizes may carry more prestige and a greater reward, there may be many different areas or levels in which individuals and teams may compete, and winning in any area or level has the potential to produce a winner's effect and the subsequent motivational results and sense of well-being among the winners.

Faster Reactions

There are definite benefits to being able to react faster than one's competitors in activities that emphasize rapid perceptual-motor responses, but faster reactions are also often beneficial in activities that rely more on judgment and decision making. With respect to perceptual-motor performance, experts exhibit a capacity to respond more quickly to perceptual cues. Placed in a situation in which a response is imminent, yet it is uncertain exactly when the cue eliciting the response will appear, activity may be observed within the circuits of the brain that will produce the eventual response. This is not enough activity to evoke a response, but it serves to ready the brain by providing a higher level of baseline activity within the essential neural circuits. As a result, once the cue appears, a response may be generated more quickly. This preparatory activity is referred to as a *readiness potential*. In research conducted with elite table tennis players, subjects were presented with a task in which they had to quickly respond with either their left or right hand (Hung et al., 2004). Initially, a cue was presented that indicated the direction of the forthcoming response, although in a small proportion of the trials, this cue was invalid and signaled the wrong response direction. Following the preparatory cue, a second cue served to prompt the response, including the actual direction of the response. While all the subjects in the study reacted faster to validly than invalidly cued responses, overall the elite table tennis players exhibited faster reactions across conditions. This corresponded to these subjects exhibiting more pronounced readiness potentials, indicating a higher level of preparatory activation of neural circuits in response to the directional cues. However, it was also noted that the elite table tennis players exhibited a more pronounced neural response on trials involving invalid cues. Based on these results, it was suggested that the mechanism by which the elite table tennis players achieved their superior reactions oriented around their preparing for the expected response, yet simultaneously directing attention to the unexpected response. Consequently, on validly cued trials, they were prepared to respond faster, but on invalidly cued trials, they more quickly recognized and responded to the discrepancy between the expected and the actual response.

In addition to evidence indicating that elite performers more effectively execute the perceptual-motor processes producing a response, it has been suggested that expertise within a given domain results in increased efficiency within the corresponding neural circuits. Efficiency implies that neural circuits have been more deeply engrained, such that lower levels of energy are required to produce a response. This translates into faster, less ambiguous responses, accompanied by lower levels of neural activation. Babiloni et al. (2010) compared expert karate athletes with novices as they judged videos in which various karate techniques were demonstrated. It was believed that the experts had a deep understanding of and familiarity with the techniques and would be able to quickly distinguish well-executed techniques from poorly executed techniques. Within the brain, when performing a task for which there is a low level of demand, there is an increased synchronization of neural circuits oscillating in the 8–13 Hz bandwidth. As tasks become increasingly more demanding, there is diminished synchronization indicating a broader recruitment of neural processes. Babiloni et al. (2010) found less desynchronization in the expert karate athletes as they judged the performances. This suggested that their familiarity with the activities allowed them to more readily interpret and assess the performances, and as a result, the engagement of neural processes was less extensive, suggesting a more efficient neural response.

The ability of elite and expert performers to react to situations more quickly appears to also have a perceptual component. Studies have been conducted for various sports using either temporal or spatial occlusion techniques to determine the points at which experts begin to sense the information that will be critical to their subsequent response. In temporal occlusion, a scene is shown (e.g., a tennis player serving the ball), and at various points in time the video is stopped and subjects are asked to predict the subsequent event (e.g., the direction of the ball following the serve). The subjects are then compared based on the accuracy of their responses. These studies show that experts are able to accurately predict events at an earlier point in the sequence of activities than novices. This has been demonstrated for sports such as tennis (Jones and Miles, 1978), cricket (Renshaw and Fairweather, 2000), and squash (Abernethy, 1990). Thus, expert performers have the capacity to anticipate future events and initiate processes that allow them to respond more quickly, giving them the ability to routinely be a few milliseconds faster than less-experienced performers.

In addition to reacting more quickly to perceptual cues, expert and elite athletes also appear to have a capacity to focus on the most critical perceptual features. An experimental technique known as spatial occlusion has been used to investigate the use of specific perceptual information by athletes. In spatial occlusion, a portion of a scene is occluded from view and the subject is asked to predict what will happen. For example, with soccer, expertise is associated with the ability to recognize and effectively react to offensive and defensive sequences of movement on the field. Expert players not only recognize the corresponding patterns using actual video, but they do so when the players are replaced by point sources of light and the action is depicted as patterns of moving lights (Williams et al., 2006). However, when either the images of players within a video or lights depicting players are occluded, the expert no longer has an advantage in anticipating future events. Similarly, with cricket, the position of the hand and arm of a bowler prior to pitching the ball has been shown to be critical to a batsman's ability to anticipate the trajectory of the pitch (Müller et al., 2006). Furthermore, with tennis, it has been shown that training that is focused on learning to attend to the perceptual cues utilized by experts led to measurable increases in performance for novice athletes, compared with their counterparts who merely practiced returning serves (Williams et al., 2002).

The Myth of Talent

A counterpoint to the importance of acquiring a vast body of domain-specific knowledge is the idea that some individuals possess an innate predisposition that enables high performance in a general domain (e.g., art, athletics, math), such as in the theory of multiple intelligences posited by Gardner (1983). We refer to this inborn ability as a *talent*, and while a truly exceptional performance within a domain is thought to result from a combination of acquired knowledge and talent (Winner, 2000), a body of work conducted by Ericsson (2002) suggests that the view of talent as a critical component for exceptional achievement may be wrong. Rather, as discussed previously, the level of proficiency in a discipline, whether intellectual or artistic, seems to be a direct function of the total amount of deliberate practice—a form of methodical practice that emphasizes perfection through repetition. For instance, violinists in a music academy who were thought to be the best of their class were found to have spent an averaged total of 7410 h practicing by age 18, as opposed to the 5301 h spent on average by those considered merely "good" (Ericsson, 2002). This work suggests that talent is essentially a myth in as much as there is no evidence for it and any results demonstrating exceptional performance may be explained in terms of the total amount of deliberate practice.

It was thought that individuals with savant syndrome provided a counterpoint to the idea that expertise must be earned via deliberate practice. While restricted in most mental activities, savants are characterized by extraordinary competence in one particular domain; this is why such individuals were, until recently, referred to as *idiot savants*—as a reference to the gulf between their incredible aptitude within one domain and their limited functioning in all others. Smith and Tsimpli (1995) described one such person, who was severely brain damaged since infancy. As a result, he was unable to care for himself, was considered severely mentally retarded, and required institutionalization. However, his sister would occasionally bring technical papers home from work that involved foreign languages, and as a teenager, he quickly acquired these languages, leading to linguistic ability in Danish, Dutch, Finnish, French, German, Greek, Hindi, Italian, Norwegian, Polish, Portuguese, Russian, Spanish, Swedish, Turkish, and Welsh, ranging from a rudimentary understanding to fluency.

This feat is even more impressive given that the boy never received formal training in linguistics and in fact found it difficult to play games such as checkers due to an inability to comprehend the rules of the game. The rules of language, however, did not seem to be as insurmountable as a grasp of checkers. On the surface, this case suggests that there may be a way to alter the brain such that language acquisition becomes trifling. However, the reality is that the boy spent a great deal of time studying languages. This may be because despite extensive brain damage, the areas of the brain that are responsible for language acquisition continued to function quite well, and due to either external reinforcement or self-satisfaction, he invested substantial time and energy practicing the one skill that he was able to exercise normally. This may explain why those with savant syndrome often demonstrate unusual aptitude in a unique area, such as being able to recall the weather when provided with a calendar date. An individual who possesses normal brain function is capable of this same mastery. However, it is unlikely that someone capable of engaging in a panoply of activities would find the process of memorizing weather patterns and calendar dates sufficiently rewarding to persevere to the same extent as a savant (Thioux et al., 2006). In the absence of pathology, most people are able to find mental outlets that are more rewarding and entertaining than the activities for which various savants have been reported to have mastered.

Related to the concept of a savant is that of a prodigy—an individual who achieves expertise at a young age, such as Bobby Fisher in the field of chess or Mozart in the realm of musical composition. At first blush, these individuals seem to contradict the idea that a great deal of practice is necessary, given that their achievements occurred at an age at which most individuals would not have had the opportunity to sufficiently practice a skill to achieve expert status. However, a careful study of such individuals reveals that the same processes that generally lead to expertise (external encouragement, access to effective coaching, deliberative practice) are at play with these individuals as well. Mozart typifies this finding, as contrary to claims that he seemed to write music in bursts without the need for editing, evidence shows that he did in fact spend a great deal of time editing his work in a fashion similar to that of other composers of his stature (Ross, 2006).

The discussion of savants and prodigies fits in with what we know about those individuals considered elite in their field. While high performers are often recognized as "talented," this designation trivializes the years of effortful practice that these individuals have put in. Bloom and Sosniak (1985) studied a group of 120 Americans considered the top performers across six professions, and concluded that just about any person could accomplish the same feats given the right conditions, emphasizing the importance of deliberative practice and discarding the notion of native ability. This notion is consistent with findings by Ericsson (2002) and repeated by Gladwell (2008) in asserting that elite performers typically invest 10,000 h or more of intense study. Keep in mind that it is more than simply time on task that results in this performance—the hours spent practicing must be spent in deliberative, focused practice, and there are a number of other factors that contribute to an individual's willingness to engage in and persevere in this type of practice (e.g., mental toughness, reinforcement). Perhaps, talent is better thought of in terms of those factors that incite individuals to engage in the arduous process of deliberate practice. Motivation to excel is what ties talent and time on task together; individuals persevere because they are good at something and believe themselves capable of mastering it (Winner, 2000).

It is important to recognize that talent is not the driving explanation for mastery of a skill. Often, people assume that proficiency is the critical factor—you are either good at something or you are not, and there is little you can do to change it. This applies not just to the realms of art or athletics, but to highly cognitive domains as well. Likely, we all know someone who is "just not good at math" and as a result, spends little effort attempting to get better. Actually, what people mean when they say they are not good at math (or art or reading or science) is that they have spent little time engaged in deliberative practice within these domains, perhaps because they lack the motivation to do so or do not find the process rewarding. Without a belief that improvement is possible, people are unlikely to devote time to a task.

Starting down the road to expertise is often the most difficult part, as skill acquisition without background domain knowledge may prove difficult. The more expertise that is developed in a particular domain, the easier it becomes to acquire new knowledge in that domain—a situation known as the *Mathew Effect*. Also referred to as *accumulated advantage*, this is a concept taken from the field of sociology, coined by Robert Merton (1968), which may be summarized as, "the rich get richer and poor get poorer." The name comes from a line in the biblical Gospel according to Matthew that reads "For unto every one that hath shall be given, and he shall have abundance: but from him that hath not shall be taken even that which he hath" (Mt 25: 29, King James Version). Initial success or reinforcement is met with a cascade of consequences including additional practice, greater skill acquisition, and better access to resources that facilitate expertise (mentorship, funding, gym facilities, etc.), all of which continue a feedback loop that, if unbroken, leads to expertise. Conversely, initial failure or lack of reinforcement may lead to the idea that someone is just "not good" at a particular activity, and as a result, there is no additional practice, access to resources, or reinforcement, and he or she ceases the activity—the poor get poorer. This idea—that deliberative practice with access to resources is key to expertise—does not mean that anyone can be president. It means that anyone with the proper motivation, time commitment, and access to resources may achieve proficiency in a given domain. Experts are forged in the crucible of intense practice, not simply born, although it does not hurt to be born amid the resources that are necessary for fostering skill development.

Acknowledgments

Sandia National Laboratories is a multiprogram laboratory managed and operated by Sandia Corporation, a wholly owned subsidiary of Lockheed Martin Corporation, for the US Department of Energy's National Nuclear Security Administration under contract DE-AC04-94AL85000.

References

Abernethy, B. (1990). Anticipation in squash: Differences in advance cue utilization between expert and novice players. *Journal of Sports Sciences, 8*(1), 17–34.

Abernethy, B., Baker, J. and Cote, J. (2005). Transfer of pattern recall skills may contribute to the development of sport expertise. *Applied Cognitive Psychology, 19*(6), 705–718.

Babiloni, C., Marzano, N., Infarinato, F., Iacoboni, M., Rizza, G., Aschieri, P., Cibelli, G., Soricelli, A., Eusebi, F. and Del Percio, C. (2010). "Neural efficiency" of experts' brain during judgment of actions: A high-resolution EEG study in elite and amateur karate athletes. *Behavioural Brain Research, 207*(2), 466–475.

Beauchamp, M.H., Dagher, A., Aston, J.A. and Doyon, J. (2003). Dynamic functional changes associated with cognitive skill learning of an adapted version of the Tower of London task. *Neuroimage, 20*(3), 1649–1660.

Behneman, A., Berka, C., Stevens, R., Vila, B., Tan, V., Galloway, T., Johnson, R.R. and Raphael, G. (2012). Neurotechnology to accelerate learning: During marksmanship training. *IEEE Pulse, 3*(1), 60–63.

Beilock, S. (2010). *Choke: What the Secrets of the Brain Reveal About Getting It Right When You Have To*. New York: Free Press.

Beilock, S.L. and Carr, T.H. (2001). On the fragility of skilled performance: What governs choking under pressure? *Journal of Experimental Psychology: General, 130*(4), 701–725.

Beilock, S.L., Kulp, C.A., Holt, L.E. and Carr, T.H. (2004). More on the fragility of performance: Choking under pressure in mathematical problem solving. *Journal of Experimental Psychology: General, 133*(4), 584–600.

Bernstein, L.J., Beig, S., Siegenthaler, A.L. and Grady, C.L. (2002). The effect of encoding strategy on the neural correlates of memory for faces. *Neuropsychologia, 40*(1), 86–98.

Bjork, J.M., Knutson, B., Fong, G.W., Caggiano, D.M., Bennett, S.M. and Hommer, D.W. (2004). Incentive-elicited brain activation in adolescents: Similarities and differences from young adults. *Journal of Neuroscience, 24*(8), 1793–1802.

Bloom, B. and Sosniak, L. (1985). *Developing Talent in Young People.* New York: Ballantine Books.

Brondino, N., Lanati, N., Giudici, S., Arpesella, M., Roncarolo, F. and Vandoni, M. (2013). Testosterone level and its relationship with outcome of sporting activity. *Journal of Men's Health, 10*(2), 40–47.

Buonomano, D.V. and Merzenich, M.M. (1998). Cortical plasticity: From synapses to maps. *Annual Review of Neuroscience, 21*, 149–186.

Chabris, C.F. and Hearst, E.S. (2003). Visualization, pattern recognition and forward search: Effects of playing speed and sight of the position on grand master chess errors. *Cognitive Science, 27*(4), 637–648.

Chase, W.G. and Simon, H.A. (1973). The mind's eye in chess. In W.G. Chase (ed.), *Visual Information Processing*, pp. 215–278. New York: Academic Press.

Chi, M.T.H., Feltovich, P.J. and Glaser, R. (1981). Categorization and representation of physics problems by experts and novices. *Cognitive Science, 5*(2), 121–152.

Clough, P., Earle, K. and Sewell, D. (2002). Mental toughness: The concept and its measurement. In I. Cockerill (ed.), *Solutions in Sport Psychology*, pp. 32–45. London: Thomson.

Costa, P.T. and McCrae, R.R. (1992). *The Revised NEO Personality Inventory (NEO–PI–R) and the NEO Five-Factor Inventory (NEO-FFI) Professional Manual.* Odessa, FL: Psychological Assessment Resources.

Crust, L. (2007). Mental toughness in sport: A review. *International Journal of Sport and Exercise Psychology, 5*(3), 270–290.

Dahlin, E., Neely, A.S., Larsson, A., Backman, L. and Nyberg, L. (2008). Transfer of learning after updating training mediated by the striatum. *Science, 320*, 1510–1512.

Dovidio, J.F. and Fazio, R.H. (1992). New technologies for the direct and indirect assessment of attitudes. In J. Tanur (ed.), *Questions About Questions: Inquiries into the Cognitive Bases of Surveys*, pp. 204–237. New York: Russell Sage Foundation.

Dror, I.E. (2011). The paradox of human expertise: Why experts get it wrong. In N. Kapur, A. Pascualeone and V. Ramachandran (eds), *The Paradoxical Brain*, pp. 177–188. Cambridge: Cambridge Press.

Ericsson, K.A. (2002). Attaining excellence through deliberate practice: Insights from the study of expert performance. In M. Ferrari (ed.), *The Pursuit of Excellence Through Education. The Educational Psychology Series*, pp. 21–55. Hillsdale, NJ: Erlbaum.

Ericsson, K.A., Krampe, R.T. and Tesch-Romer, C. (1993). The role of deliberative practice in the acquisition of expert performance. *Psychological Review, 100*(3), 363–406.

Fuxjager, M.J., Forbes-Lorman, R.M., Coss, D.J., Auger, C.J., Auger, A.P. and Marler, C.A. (2010). Winning territorial disputes selectively enhances androgen sensitivity in neural pathways related to motivation and social aggression. *Proceedings of the National Academy of Science of the United States of America*, 107(27), 12393–12398.

Fuxjager, M.J., Oyegbile, T.O. and Marler, C.A. (2011). Independent and additive contributions of postvictory testosterone and social experience to the development of the winner effect. *Endocrinology*, 152(9), 3422–3429.

Gardner, H. (1983). *Frames of Mind: The Theory of Multiple Intelligences*. New York: Basic Books.

Gauthier, I., Skudlarski, P., Gore, J.C. and Anderson, A.W. (2000). Expertise for cars and birds recruits brain areas involved in face recognition. *Nature Neuroscience*, 3, 191–197.

Gauthier, I. and Tarr, M.J. (2002). Unraveling mechanisms for expert object recognition: Bridging brain activity and behavior. *Journal of Experimental Psychology: Human Perception and Performance*, 28(2), 431–446.

Glabus, M.F., Horwitz, B., Holt, J.L., Kohn, P.D., Gerton, B.K., Callicott, J.H., Meyer-Lindenberg, A. and Berman, K.F. (2003). Interindividual differences in functional interactions among prefrontal, parietal and parahippocampal regions during working memory. *Cerebral Cortex*, 13(12), 1352–1361.

Gladwell, M. (2008). *Outliers: The Story of Success*. New York: Little, Brown and Company.

Haier, R.J., Siegel, B.V. Jr., MacLachlan, A., Soderling, E., Lottenberg, S. and Buchsbaum, M.S. (1992). Regional glucose metabolic changes after learning a complex visuospatial/motor task: A positron emission tomographic study. *Brain Research*, 570(1–2), 134–143.

Hatfield, B.D., Landers, D.M. and Ray, W.J. (1984). Cognitive processes during self-paced motor performance: An electroencephalographic profile of skilled marksmen. *Journal of Sport Psychology*, 6, 42–59.

Horsburgh, V.A., Schermer, J.A., Veselka, L. and Vernon, P.A. (2009). A behavioural genetic study of mental toughness and personality. *Personality and Individual Differences*, 46(2), 100–105.

Hung, T.M., Spalding, T.W., Santa Maria, D.L. and Hatfield, B.D. (2004). Assessment of reactive motor performance with event-related brain potentials: Attention processes in elite table tennis players. *Journal of Sport and Exercise Psychology*, 26(2), 317–337.

Jones, C.M. and Miles, T.R. (1978). Use of advance cues in predicting the flight of a lawn tennis ball. *Journal of Human Movement Studies*, 4, 231–235.

Jonides, J. (2004). How does practice makes perfect? *Nature Neuroscience*, 7, 10–11.

Kelly, A.M.C. and Garavan, H. (2005). Human functional neuroimaging of brain changes associated with practice. *Cerebral Cortex*, 15(8), 1089–1102.

Klein, G.A., Orasanu, J., Calderwood, R. and Zsambok, C.E. (1993). *Decision Making in Action: Models and Methods*. Norwood, CT: Ablex.

Kolb, B. and Gibb, R. (2002). Frontal lobe plasticity and behavior. In D.T. Stuss and R.T. Knight (eds), *Principles of Frontal Lobe Function*, pp. 541–556. London: Oxford University Press.

Kolb, B. and Whishaw, I.Q. (1998). Brain plasticity and behavior. *Annual Review of Psychology*, 49, 43–64.

Krigolson, O.E., Pierce, L.J., Holroyd, C.B. and Tanaka, J.B. (2009). Learning to become an expert: Reinforcement learning and the acquisition of perceptual expertise. *Journal of Cognitive Neuroscience, 21*(9), 1833–1840.

Kuan, G. and Roy, J. (2007). Goal profiles, mental toughness and its influence on performance outcomes among Wushu athletes. *Journal of Sports Science and Medicine, 6*(CSSI-2), 28–33.

Loehr, J.E. (1986). *Mental Toughness Training for Sports: Achieving Athletic Excellence.* Lexington, MA: Stephen Greene Press.

Maidhof, C., Rieger, N., Prinz, W. and Koelsch, S. (2009). Nobody is perfect: ERP effects prior to performance errors in musicians indicate fast monitoring processes. *PLoS ONE, 4*(4), e5032. http://www.plosone.org/article/info%3Adoi%2F10.1371%2Fjournal.pone.0005032.

McKay, B., Lewthwaite, R. and Wulf, G. (2012). Enhanced expectancies improve performance under pressure. *Frontiers in Psychology, 3*, 8.

Merton, R. (1968). The Matthew Effect in science. *Science, 159*(3810), 56–63.

Müller, S., Abernethy, B. and Farrow, D. (2006). How do world-class cricket batsmen anticipate a bowler's intention? *The Quarterly Journal of Experimental Psychology, 59*(12), 2162–2186.

Norman, G.R., Rosenthal, D., Brooks, L.R., Allen, S.W. and Muzzin, L.J. (1989). The development of expertise in dermatology. *JAMA Dermatology, 125*(8), 1063–1068.

Nunes, E.J., Randall, P.A., Santerre, J.L., Given, A.B., Sager, T.N., Correa, M. and Salamone, J.D. (2010). Differential effects of selective adenosine antagonists on the effort-related impairments induced by dopamine D1 and D2 antagonism. *Neuroscience, 170*(1), 268–280.

Oeschslim, M.S., van de Ville, D., Lazeyras, F., Hauert, C.A. and James, C.E. (2012). Degree of musical expertise modulates higher order brain functioning. *Cerebral Cortex, 23*(9), 2213–2224. http://cercor.oxfordjournals.org/content/early/2012/07/23/cercor.bhs206.short.

Paulus, M.P., Simmons, A.N., Fitzpatrick, S.N., Potterat, E.G., Van Orden, K.F., Bauman, J. and Swain, J.L. (2010). Differential brain activation to angry faces by elite warfighters: Neural processing evidence for enhanced threat detection. *PLoS ONE, 5*(4), e10096. http://www.plosone.org/article/info%3Adoi%2F10.1371%2Fjournal.pone.0010096.

Petersen, S.E., van Mier, H., Fiez, J.A. and Raichle, M.E. (1998). The effects of practice on the functional anatomy of task performance. *Proceedings of the National Academy of Science of the United States of America, 95*(3), 853–860.

Poldrack, R.A., Desmond, J.E., Glover, G.H. and Gabrieli, J.D. (1998). The neural basis of visual skill learning: An fMRI study of mirror reading. *Cerebral Cortex, 8*(1), 1–10.

Poldrack, R.A. and Gabrieli, J.D. (2001). Characterizing the neural mechanisms of skill learning and repetition priming: Evidence from mirror reading. *Brain: A Journal of Neurology, 124*(1), 67–82.

Quinton, C. (2009). An understanding of Tiger Woods' new golf swing. Retrieved from http://www.oneplanegolfswing.com/golf-instruction/Tour_Pros/Tiger-Woods/index.php.

Renshaw, I. and Fairweather, M.M. (2000). Cricket bowling deliveries and the discrimination ability of professional and amateur batters. *Journal of Sports Sciences, 18*(12), 951–957.

Ross, P.E. (2006). The expert mind. *Scientific American*, 295(2), 64–71.

Ruiz, M.H., Jabusch, H.C. and Altenmuller, E. (2009). Detecting wrong notes in advance: Neuronal correlates of error monitoring in pianists. *Cerebral Cortex*, 19(11), 2625–2639.

Sakai, K., Hikosaka, O., Miyauchi, S., Takino, R., Sasaki, Y. and Putz, B. (1998). Transition of brain activation from frontal to parietal areas in visuomotor sequence learning. *The Journal of Neuroscience: The Official Journal of the Society for Neuroscience*, 18(5), 1827–1840.

Salamone, J.D., Correa, M., Farrar, A.M., Nunes, E.J. and Collins, L.E. (2010). Role of dopamine-adenosine interactions in the brain circuitry regulating effort-related decision making: Insights into pathological aspects of motivation. *Future Neurology*, 5(3), 377–392.

Schiltz, C., Bodart, J.M. and Crommelinek, M. (2001). A pet study of human skill learning: Changes in brain activity related to learning an orientation discrimination task. *Cortex*, 37(2), 243–265.

Schmidt, L., Lebreton, M., Cléry-Melin, M.L., Daunizeau, J. and Pessiglione, M. (2012). Neural mechanisms underlying motivation of mental versus physical effort. *PLoS Biology*, 10(2), e1001266.

Schoenfeld, A.H. (1985). *Mathematical Problem Solving*. Orlando, FL: Academic Press.

Seidler, R.D., Purushotham, A., Kim, S.G., Ugurbil, K., Willingham, D. and Ashe, J. (2002). Cerebellum activation associated with performance change but not motor learning. *Science*, 296(5575), 2043–2046.

Simmons, A.N., Fitzpatrick, S.N., Strigo, I.A., Potterat, E.G., Johnson, D.C., Matthews, S.C., Orden, K.F., Swain, J.L. and Paulus, M.P. (2012). Altered insula activation in anticipation of changing emotional states: Neural mechanisms underlying cognitive flexibility in special operations forces personnel. *NeuroReport*, 23(4), 234–239.

Smith, N. and Tsimpli, I.M. (1995). *The Mind of a Savant: Language Learning and Modularity*. Oxford: Basil Blackwell Ltd.

Thioux, M., Stark, D.E., Klaiman, C. and Schultz, R.T. (2006). The day of the week when you were born in 700 ms: Calendar computation in an autistic savant. *Journal of Experimental Psychology: Human Perception and Performance*, 32(5), 1155–1168.

Volkow, N.D., Wang, G.J., Newcorn, J.H., Kollins, S.H., Wigal, T.L., Telang, F., Fowler, J.S., et al. (2011). Motivation deficit in ADHD is associated with dysfunction of the dopamine reward pathway. *Molecular Psychiatry*, 16(11), 1147–1154.

Wan, X., Nakatani, H., Ueno, K., Asamizuya, T., Cheng, K. and Tanaka, K. (2011). The neural basis for intuitive best next-move generation in board game experts. *Science*, 331(6015), 341–346.

Williams, A.M., Hodges, N.J., North, J.S. and Barton, G. (2006). Perceiving patterns of play in dynamic sport tasks: Investigating the essential information underlying skilled performance. *Perception*, 35(3), 317.

Williams, A.M., Ward, P., Knowles, J.M. and Smeeton, N.J. (2002). Anticipation skill in a real-world task: Measurement, training, and transfer in tennis. *Journal of Experimental Psychology: Applied*, 8(4), 259.

Winner, E. (2000). Giftedness: Current theory and research. *Current Directions in Psychological Science*, 9(5), 153–156.

Zotov, M., Forsythe, C., Petrukovich, V. and Akhmedova, I. (2009). Physiological-based assessment of the resilience of training to stressful conditions. *Foundations of Augmented Cognition. Neuroergonomics and Operational Neuroscience Lecture Notes in Computer Science, 5638*, 563–571.

Zotov, M., Forsythe, C., Voyt, A., Akhmedova, I. and Petrukovich, V. (2011). A dynamic approach to the physiological-based assessment of the resilience to stressful conditions. *Foundations in Augmented Cognition. Directing the Future of Adaptive Systems Lecture Notes in Computer Science, 6780*, 657–666.

9

Teams and Groups

"Man is by nature a social animal"

(Aristotle)

Philosophers as far back as Aristotle have realized that individuals who do not partake of society or belong to groups are simply not human. Indeed, groups are a fact of human life. Each of us is born into a family within a social and cultural setting. At school, we study as part of a class. At work, we form work groups. We voluntarily join groups of one sort or another, such as sports teams, social clubs, unions, and political parties, based on shared occupations, beliefs, and interests. Groups impact our lives in both obvious and subtle ways by influencing how we behave, how we think of ourselves, and how others think of us, while connecting us to larger social aggregates. Several decades ago, Mills (1967) estimated that an average individual belonged to five or six groups at any given time. With the opportunities provided by Internet technology to join and leave virtual communities, the number is surely much larger now.

Groups have their origins in human evolution (Van Vugt and Schaller, 2007). As an adaptive strategy, living in groups enabled our ancestors to develop and benefit from the ability to work together. In pursuit of shared goals in hunting, foraging, migrating, and child rearing, group behavior afforded our ancestors a much greater capacity to survive, reproduce, and colonize. As Charles Darwin stated, "with those animals which were benefited by living in close association, the individuals which took the greatest pleasure in society would best escape various dangers, while those that cared least for their comrades, and lived solitary, would perish in greater numbers" (*The Descent of Man*). The evolution of human social behavior and the associated psychological mechanisms and neural processes that support a predisposition toward group living are a product of millions of years of group living. Human social behavior was initially shaped by our ancestors' capacity to adapt to their environment through social cooperation. This has since evolved into more sophisticated needs, including the need to develop intimate relations with others (i.e., psychological needs), to exchange information (i.e., informational needs), and to have a positive social identity (i.e., self-esteem needs) (Levine, 2012).

The industrial revolution brought on the institutionalization of work and the associated division of work into tasks allocated across a workforce. Since then, we have become increasingly reliant on teamwork for performing

253

complex tasks in various work environments, such as cockpits, hospitals, and nuclear power plants. Group behavior is critical to our ability to cope with many of the demands of modern life. This has prompted a growing appreciation that human cognition is social in nature. The mind operates within the context of groups, with social factors serving as determinants of perceptual and cognitive processes; with thoughts, beliefs, and memories shared among those inhabiting a common social environment (Hogg and Tindale, 2008).

Defining Groups

It is instructive to specify the characteristics that make a collection of individuals a group. In general, a group has the following characteristics (Levi, 2001; Shaw, 1971).

- *Individual motivation.* A group satisfies its members' physical and psychological needs, so that individuals are motivated to continue to participate. Groups that fail to satisfy members' needs usually disintegrate.
- *Group goals.* People join groups in order to achieve common goals.
- *Membership perception.* Group members have a collective perception of unity and are aware of their relationships to others.
- *Interdependence.* Group members recognize that they collectively share a common fate.
- *Interaction.* Group members communicate and interact with one another. This is the essential feature that distinguishes a group from a simple aggregate.
- *Group structure.* Group members' behavior is regulated by group structural elements, such as roles, norms, and statuses.
- *Mutual influence.* Group members influence each other, and the desire to remain in the group increases the potential for mutual influence.

A distinction may be drawn between groups and teams. The most critical difference between teams and groups is the differentiation of roles or task-relevant knowledge and the degree of interdependence between members (Orasanu and Salas, 1993). Group members tend to be homogeneous with interchangeable functions. They work independently, produce individual work products, and thus focus on individual goals. In contrast, a team consists of members with complementary skills and different functions, who work interdependently toward a defined common goal for which everyone in the team is held mutually accountable. To accomplish the common goal, team members rely on coordinated interaction and active cooperation. Therefore, teams may be considered a special subset of groups, whereas *groups* is a more inclusive term and can be applied to a larger number of social and organizational forms. Another dimension to distinguish teams from groups is the number of members. Groups range in size from two to thousands, while the size of teams tends to be smaller.

Social Psychology and Neuroscience

With distinct historical origins, perspectives, and theoretical frameworks, the fields of social psychology and neuroscience have tended to offer incompatible explanations for human behavior. Traditional neuroscience has treated individuals as the fundamental unit of analysis with a focus on cellular processes and the neural substrates of behavior. The influence of social environments on biological events and processes has received little attention. As Llinás (1989) stated, "to the extent that social factors were suspected of being relevant, their consideration was thought to so complicate the study of brain and behavior that they were not a priority." Social psychologists have tended to treat individuals as being immune to biological influences and have focused on social forces instead (Cacioppo et al., 2010, 2011). It is now recognized that social behavior has a biological basis, and our brain and biological functioning have a social origin and context. Consequently, an integrative analysis of both biological and social factors is needed to provide a comprehensive theory of human behavior. Thus, social neuroscience has emerged as an interdisciplinary field of research that investigates the interplay between biological and social phenomena, synthesizing the complementary perspectives, techniques, and knowledge from social psychology, neuroscience, and other related areas (Cacioppo et al., 2010, 2011). More specifically, social neuroscience capitalizes on biological concepts and methods to inform and refine theories of social behavior, and it uses social and behavioral constructs and data to advance theories of neural organization and function (Cacioppo et al., 2010, 2011).

Cooperation and Altruism

Cooperation and teamwork have evolved in a small number of species. From an evolutionary point of view, cooperation increases the fitness of the cooperators, when the cooperators can collect more resources than the sum of resources collected by each individual. Compared with other social species (e.g., ants, bees, and termites), the complexity of human cooperation is unparalleled. Increased interdependence and sophisticated forms of social interaction due to societal division of labor are believed to have promoted our ancestors' brain growth, which served to enable sophisticated forms of cooperation. Cooperation is the core behavioral principal of human social life and it has served as the foundation of human civilization.

Kin selection is an evolutionary strategy that favors the reproductive success of an organism's relatives, even at a cost to the organism's own survival and reproduction. Charles Darwin was the first to discuss this concept in his 1859 book, *The Origin of Species*. Reciprocal altruism is a behavior whereby an organism acts in a manner that temporarily reduces its fitness while increasing another organism's fitness, with the expectation that the other organism will act in a similar manner at a later time. That is, reciprocal altruism refers to cooperative behavior that is favored due to the likelihood of future, mutually beneficial interactions.

According to the theory of reciprocal altruism, there are two forms of reciprocal exchange: direct reciprocity and indirect reciprocity. Direct reciprocity is established on the principle of "help someone who may later help me." That is, there is an expectation that altruistic acts will be reciprocated by the recipient. However, people often dispense favors without expectation of a return. Therefore, indirect reciprocity was proposed to explain such altruistic acts. Indirect reciprocity is based on the principle of "I won't scratch your back if you won't scratch their backs." This implies a moral system, in which the reputation and status, or "image score," of an individual reflect whether the individual has helped others. Accordingly, a hypothetical image score is continuously assessed and reassessed by others and impacts the likelihood that an individual will be helped by others in future social interactions.

Rilling et al. (2002) used functional magnetic resonance imaging (fMRI) to examine the neural activity of 36 women as they played the prisoner's dilemma game with either another woman or a computer. In the game, players independently chose to either cooperate with each other or defect, and the awards that they received after each round were determined by their choices. The blood oxygen level–dependent (BOLD) responses of the subjects to the game outcome and their BOLD responses while deciding whether to cooperate or defect were analyzed. Overall, the study offered evidence of reward-related neural activity reinforcing cooperative behavior. For example, when looking at the subjects' reaction to mutual cooperation, Rilling et al. (2002) detected consistent activation of the brain regions associated with processing rewards (i.e., ventromedial frontal and orbitofrontal cortexes, and anteroventral striatum). This suggest that there is a rewarding effect of participating in a mutually cooperative social interaction. In contrast, when cooperation was met with defection, the anteroventral striatum was often deactivated, an observation that has been linked to the omission of expected rewards. Furthermore, it was found that the most significant activation associated with a cooperative outcome was in the somatosensory association cortex of the medial posterior parietal lobe, which is implicated in emotional experiences. Combined, these findings suggest that cooperative acts may be reinforced by feelings and social emotions, such as trust and comradery that occur as a result of the activation of the orbitofrontal cortex and anteroventral striatum during mutual cooperation.

Additionally, Rilling et al. (2002) found that the decision to cooperate was associated with activation in the ventromedial frontal cortex, which has been associated with sensitivity to distant rewards and punishments, and the rostral anterior cingulate cortex, which has been linked to processing conflict-related emotions. This is understandable given the conflict that may arise within the prisoner's dilemma game—immediate gratification with the prospect of future punishments for defection versus delayed but greater gains through cooperation. The activation of the ventromedial frontal cortex and the rostral anterior cingulate cortex may correspond to the inhibition of the desire for short-term gain in favor of long-term and higher rewards. Another finding from the study is that activation of the ventromedial frontal and orbitofrontal cortexes, but not the rostral anterior cingulate cortex or the anteroventral striatum, occurred when the second player was a computer. This suggests that the rostral anterior cingulate cortex and striatal activations may relate specifically to cooperative social interactions with human partners.

Group Intelligence

In the investigation of individual versus group performance, cognitive ability at the group level has been operationally defined as either the maximum, average, minimum, or standard deviation of the intelligence of group members. In a meta-analysis, Devine and Philips (2001) examined the correlations between four group cognitive ability indices and group performance. It was found that the standard deviation of member cognitive ability was not related to group performance, although the other three indices were positively correlated with group performance in most cases, with average intelligence being somewhat more predictive than the maximum or minimum intelligence of group members. This suggests that although groups do capitalize on the available cognitive resources of group members, the three indices are weakly predictive of group-level intelligence. In addition, the predictive efficacy of the three indices appears dependent on other factors, including task complexity, degree of physical activity, and task familiarity. For example, the indices may be marginally predictive of performance for simple and familiar tasks that involve repetitive physical activities, whereas they may be good predictors for tasks involving intellectual activities.

Unlike other researchers who tried to explain group-level intelligence in terms of individual-level intelligence, Woolley et al. (2010) examined whether a group's general ability to perform different activities was a stable property of the group itself, or just of its members. By assessing how well a single group performed a wide range of tasks, they demonstrated that groups, like individuals, do have characteristic levels of intelligence, which can be measured and used to predict group performance. That is, group intelligence does exist and it functions in the same way for groups as general intelligence does for individuals. In their study, they first assessed the intelligence of individual subjects using the Wechsler Adult Intelligence Scale. Afterward, the subjects were assigned to groups consisting of either two, three, four, or five members. The groups were then given various tasks to complete that required some degree of coordination of the group members. Examples of tasks assigned to the groups included solving visual puzzles, brainstorming, making collective moral judgments, and negotiating limited resources. When the performance across tasks was considered, the researchers found that a group who did well on one task tended to do well on other tasks. Furthermore, a factor analysis revealed a single factor that not only accounted for a large portion of the variance in group performance, but also had a statistically significant effect on group performance; hence, researchers referred to the factor as "collective intelligence."

One stunning finding from Woolley et al.'s (2010) study is that group performance does not appear to be related to individual intelligence, as no significant correlations were found between group performance and the maximum or average group member intelligence. This, combined with Devine and Philips' (2001) findings regarding the weak relationship between individual intelligence and group performance, suggests that group intelligence involves something more than the average intelligence of the group members. The implications are profound for efforts to assemble effective teams, especially given that many organizations seek to fill positions based on secondary measures of individual intelligence (e.g., grade point average) with the expectation that these individuals will effectively work within the context of a team.

Woolley et al. (2010) also examined a number of individual and group factors to discover the determinants of collective intelligence. Group cohesion, motivation, and satisfaction were not significant predictors of collective intelligence. A moderate correlation between collective intelligence and the maximum or average group member intelligence suggested that collective intelligence does depend on the composition of a group; however, the dependence is moderated by two other important factors that determine the internal dynamics of a group. The first concerned the level of turn taking within conversations. Groups that exhibited relatively equal distributions with regard to the time that each group member spoke or the number of occasions that each group member spoke performed better than groups that had less equal distributions. Thus, within superior groups, each group member is allowed an opportunity to express his or her perspective and participate in the decision-making processes of the group. Second, groups that on average scored high with regard to their social sensitivity to one another performed better. Social sensitivity was measured using a test known as the *Reading the Mind in the Eyes* test. In this test, a subject views a series of faces that show only the eyes and the surrounding areas of the face and is asked to indicate the associated emotional expression. This finding suggests that groups that perform well have a stronger capacity to sense the ongoing emotional and cognitive state of group members and adapt their interactions accordingly. Perhaps most significantly, the authors noted that these are traits that can be trained. This is important because it suggests that largely independent of intelligence, individuals may be taught skills that will enable them to effectively function within the context of a group, enabling levels of performance to be attained by the group that may exceed the performance one might expect given the makeup of the individual group members.

Individuals differ in their patterns of brain activity, the relative amount of neural activation, and the efficacy of interactions among different brain areas. These individual differences may affect group performance (Woolley et al., 2007). Woolley et al. (2007) studied the effect of the complementarity of group members' task-specific cognitive abilities on group effectiveness. They focused on two independent visual systems: the ventral visual system, which plays a central role in processing object properties such as shapes, color, and texture; and the dorsal visual system, which plays a central role in processing spatial relations. The two systems are located in different parts of the brain and evidence suggests that individuals with a strong object-processing ability tend not to have a strong spatial-processing ability, and vice versa. In the study, individuals were teamed to form two-person teams. Their task required the two members to work together with one member performing a spatial subtask and the other an object-properties subtask. The task involved navigating through a three-dimensional virtual world and remembering the locations where different objects were observed. The members' role assignments to the subtasks were either congruent or incongruent with their individual abilities. For congruent teams, an individual who was adept at object processing performed the object-processing task and an individual who was adept at spatial processing performed the spatial processing task. For incongruent teams, the roles were reversed and for semicongruent teams, one individual performed the task for which he or she possessed an aptitude and the other did not.

Teams for which roles were congruent with their abilities performed better than incongruent teams and semicongruent teams. In addition, the researchers found that when individuals were assigned roles that were congruent with their abilities, the level of communication between team members was unrelated to team performance. In contrast, in incongruent teams, communication was correlated with their performance and it appeared to be helpful in compensating for the misplacement of abilities. Interestingly, the performance of the semicongruent teams was negatively correlated with their communication. Woolley et al.'s study underscores the importance of considering individual cognitive proficiencies in composing effective teams. That is, a team should have the right abilities and the individuals need to be assigned to appropriate roles or tasks.

Good Team, Bad Team

For several years, I have worked with programs focused on engaging youth in science, technology, engineering, and math (STEM) through various activities. Much of this time has involved leading teams that have competed in the robotics tournaments that are coordinated through the US First program. This program emphasizes team competition, and teamwork is one of the criteria on which the teams are scored during the tournaments. Consequently, in preparing teams to compete in these tournaments, a considerable amount of time is devoted to teaching and practicing good teamwork skills.

One of the exercises that I have done with the children that has always been a lot of fun and that I believe is very informative with respect to team processes and team performance is a game I have called, "good team, bad team." In conducting this exercise, I always start by giving the children a task such as to build a model of some object using Lego bricks and to do it as a good team. This part of the exercise is not very informative because the children are always on their best behavior and they do all the things that you might expect them to do. They take turns, they complement each other, they try and help each other, and they do not talk over each other. It is much more interesting when I next ask them to do the same task as a bad team. This is their chance to let out their negative impulses and usually by the time they are finished, it has become so outrageous that no one can stop laughing.

In the behavior of the bad team, one sees many of the characteristics that distinguish effective from ineffective teams. There is no turn taking. Everyone speaks at once and no one listens to what anyone else has to say. Similarly, with the activity, everyone tries to do it at the same time, interfering with one another, with it generally devolving to the point that everyone is essentially working alone and independently doing what he or she wants to do. There is no sensitivity to one another. They say what they are thinking regardless of how it might affect the other members of the team. This includes various personally disparaging remarks and blunt criticisms. The other noteworthy observation is the self-centeredness that arises. Each member of the team becomes the focal point with the assumption that what he or she is doing is all that matters and everyone else should be working in service to this team member.

While the children provide an exaggerated version of the behaviors that underlie ineffective team processes, these same behaviors emerge within professional settings, yet more subtly. In meetings, one often sees one or more dominant individuals who drive the conversation, saying more and speaking longer than anyone else. Likewise, you see competition for limited resources, with many continuing to pursue resources well beyond the point at which they have secured more resources than they can actually consume. In professional settings, there are rarely outward expressions of negativity toward one another. These expressions occur in a veiled manner through an unwillingness to be helpful and competition fueled by jealously and animosity. The self-centeredness arises in an individual's infatuation with his or her own ideas and the insistence with which they are expressed, accompanied by a dismissal of other ideas, and an elevation of the "not invented here" syndrome to one better described as "not invented by me."

I have come to the conclusion that in most professional settings, highly effective teams are often the exception. Individuals become highly skilled in concealing, masking, and rationalizing their self-centered behavior. However, the behavior is present and undermines the effectiveness of team activities. Granted, this is often a product of the culture in which people are asked to work, particularly where the culture hinges on competition over limited resources. However, it is often the exception to see one sacrifice one's own potential gains for the betterment of the group, or to put aside one's own ambitions, so that everyone in the group can share in a larger bounty. In youth, I have seen a clear understanding of this distinction and a willingness to put aside personal gains for the benefit of the overall team. Likewise, in adults, I have seen near universal acknowledgement of the principles that underlie effective teamwork, but countless illustrations of behavior that may seem reasonable on the surface, but one layer deep, is contrary to these same principles.

Social Cognition, Metacognition, and Mentalization

Social cognition refers to the cognitive processes by which we make sense of ourselves, the people around us, and ourselves in relation to others within the social environment or culture in which we live. It provides human beings with a significant advantage over other creatures—the ability to work together in groups. Indeed, the fact that brain regions (e.g., medial prefrontal cortex [mPFC], superior temporal sulcus [STS], and lateral parietal cortex) that are associated with social-cognitive tasks have a higher baseline activity (i.e., higher resting metabolic rates) than average suggests that social cognition forms part of a default state of human cognition (Gusnard et al., 2001; Gusnard and Raichle, 2001; Raichle et al., 2001). That is, the human brain spontaneously engages in social-cognitive processing.

Our brains and minds are in continuous interaction with other people within a group environment, detecting and influencing what others are doing. It is not only the physical presence, but also the mental image of another person that can affect the state of one's brain, behavior, and attitude. Humans do not simply act together; rather, they work together by adopting a group-oriented perspective on activities. Each group member's behavior is guided by his or her understanding of other group members' behavior and intention. For instance, the first step of a joint action—the decision to collaborate with another person—is determined by judging the willingness of a prospective partner to collaborate based on an interpretation of his or her goals and intentions.

The ability to understand the behavior and intentions of other people relies heavily on two other abilities. First, individuals must recognize one another as intentional agents who are driven by internal mental states rather than external mechanistic forces. That is, human behavior is not driven by the actual state of the external world, but instead by an internal representation of the possible states of the external world. Second, individuals must possess cognitive skills essential to ascribe meaning to other people's actions by making inferences concerning their internal mental states. Social cognition allows us to develop a shared representation of the mental states of the self and others, and the relationship between these mental states, by taking account of our own and other people's knowledge, beliefs, goals, feelings, and enduring dispositions. Shared mental states provide a fundamental basis for social interactions, enabling us to predict how our own behavior will impact the mental states of others. As mentioned in the previous section, groups that can more efficiently perceive and share their members' emotions (i.e., greater social sensitivity) are more collectively intelligent.

Metacognition and mentalization are two important aspects of social cognition. Metacognition concerns the higher-order processes by which we monitor and control our own cognitive processes. It is often defined as *cognition about cognition* or *knowing about knowing*. Mentalization refers to our ability to impute the mental states underlying the overt behavior of other people. It is sometimes referred to as *perspective taking* or *theory of mind* (ToM). Mentalization can also be thought of as a special case of metacognition where metacognition is applied to others, rather than one's self.

Brain localization studies suggest a dissociation of social cognition from nonsocial cognition. It has been found that social reasoning tasks (e.g., consideration of a person's mental state and prediction of a person's behavior) trigger greater neural activity than nonsocial-cognitive tasks (e.g., consideration of a person's physical characteristics and prediction of an inanimate object's behavior) in a set of brain regions, including the mPFC, STS, and lateral parietal cortex. As shown in Figure 9.1, differential engagement of these regions can be induced by manipulating subjects' beliefs (Gallagher et al., 2002; McCabe et al., 2001). For example, in an interactive game (e.g., the game of "rock, paper, scissors") that requires second-guessing one's

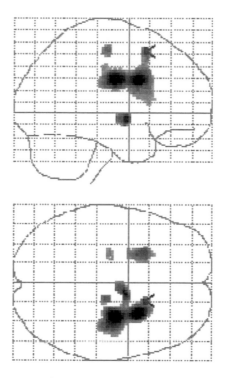

Fitted response and peristimulus time histogram

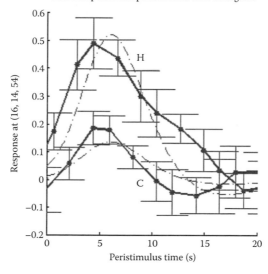

FIGURE 9.1

Brain regions showing greater activation when subjects believed that they were playing against a human partner as opposed to a computer partner. (From McCabe, K., Houser, D., Ryan, L., Smith, V., and Trouard, T., *Proceedings of the National Academy of Science of the United States of America*, 98, 11832–11835, 2001. With permission.)

opponent, enhanced activation of the mPFC, STS, and lateral parietal cortex is observed when subjects who are playing against a computer believe that they are playing against another human. This suggests that the neural activity in the mPFC, STS, and lateral parietal cortex is associated with inferences concerning the mental states of others. Interestingly, the mentalization impairments that are observed in autistic children are independent of other general cognitive abilities (Leslie and Thaiss, 1992). These findings suggest that social cognition draws on a specialized set of cognitive processes that are distinct from those subserving nonsocial aspects of thought. However, this does not mean that social-cognitive abilities are completely independent of nonsocial-cognitive abilities, as both rely on various basic cognitive processes (Mitchell, 2006).

It has been proposed that the specialized set of social-cognitive abilities found in humans is innate and represents an evolutionary result of our ancestors adapting to social challenges arising from their interactions with conspecifics within a social group environment (Mason and Macrae, 2008). Although infants and young children are generally assumed to be unaware that people have different mental perspectives, they exhibit precursors of the capacity to intuit other people's intentions and desires. For example, young infants are more attracted to and show enhanced neural processing in response to cues that signal intentionality, such as human faces, compared with other objects. Within the first few months of life, infants begin to follow the direction of an adult caregiver's line of sight. By the age of one, they start to engage in spontaneous role-taking and pretend play, showing an increased capacity to reason nonegocentrically. It appears that social cognition evolves with the development of other cognitive abilities and is subject to environmental and cultural influences (Mason and Macrae, 2008).

Research has demonstrated the dissociations between different aspects of social cognition as well as the overlap between social cognition and other forms of cognitive processing, suggesting that the cognitive processes that are deployed for social cognition vary as a function of the content of mentalization. For instance, the STS appears to play a critical role in integrating cues indicative of intentional movement and ascribing meaning to them (Mason and Macrae, 2008). The junction of the temporal and parietal cortices (TPJ) subserves inferences about others' beliefs (Saxe and Kanwisher, 2003; Saxe and Wexler, 2005). In addition, construing the behavior of similar versus dissimilar others has been associated with different mPFC regions. Specifically, the ventral mPFC is engaged in mentalization about similar others and a more dorsal region of the mPFC is engaged in mentalization about dissimilar others (Jenkins et al., 2008). Given that the ventral mPFC is also involved in tasks that require self-referential thought, there seems to be a link between introspection about self and mentalization about similar others. This points to a "simulationist" view of social cognition, which contends that we spontaneously reference our own mental states to infer those of other individuals to the extent that we believe that the other individuals have comparable mental experiences (Jenkins et al., 2008).

The discussion above suggests that social cognition is highly contingent on the interpretation of others' behavior from our own perspective. One implication is that social cognition is susceptible to error and bias—the price for easy access to the inner workings of another's mind (Mason and Macrae, 2008). For example, we often exhibit a discrepancy between how we understand and justify our own and other people's actions. Specifically, we tend to attribute our own actions to situational constraints but attribute other people's actions to trait characteristics. Furthermore, there is evidence that we are less accurate in recognizing the causes of our own actions than inferring the causes of other people's actions (Pronin et al., 2007). Therefore, our understanding of our own actions can benefit from others' comments. Additionally, when using self-reflection to guide inferences, an individual may be incorrectly misjudged as an in-group or an out-group member. Even if we correctly identified an individual as an in-group member, we may fail to account for differences between ourselves and that individual with respect to mentalization. Finally, mentalization error and bias are likely to increase when out-group members behave ambiguously or information contradicts stereotypes. We are also less willing to acknowledge that out-group members have the same mental experiences as in-group members. These considerations highlight the complexities and ambiguities that plague everyday social interactions.

Neural Synchronization and Correlation During Group Processes

As discussed in a previous chapter, our brains possess what has been referred to as mirror neurons that selectively respond to the actions of another person (Rizzalotti and Craighero, 2004). For example, as one observes an actor performing a familiar routine (e.g., putting on socks and shoes), the mirror neuron system becomes active with the activation somewhat mirroring that which would occur if one was performing the activity oneself. In a series of studies reported by Stephens et al. (2010), the researchers asked if similar processes might be evident during everyday verbal communications. Initially, brain-imaging data were collected from subjects as they verbally told a story of a real-life experience from their past. Then, a different set of subjects listened to these stories while brain-imaging data were collected. The researchers compared the patterns and timing of the brain activity in the storytellers and listeners. The results revealed a correlation such that the patterns of activity in the listeners tended to mirror that of the storytellers. Generally, there was a slight lag with the corresponding activation in the story listener following that of the storyteller by 1–3 s. The areas for which a coupling was observed included areas normally associated with speech comprehension (e.g., Wernicke's area), as well as regions associated with processing semantic and social cues (e.g., precuneus, dorsolateral prefrontal cortex, orbitofrontal cortex, striatum, and mPFC). To demonstrate that the effect was attributable to the communication between the teller and the listener, the procedure was repeated with the storyteller speaking in Russian for story listeners who were non-Russian speakers. In this condition, the neural coupling was not observed, suggesting that it was the communicative properties of the story that produced the synchronization of neural processes between the storytellers and the listeners.

Stephens and colleagues next considered if the neural coupling between storytellers and story listeners was related to the degree to which the listener comprehended the storyteller. Listeners were assessed with respect to the extent to which they understood the story told by the storyteller. When listeners were ranked with respect to those showing the strongest to the weakest coupling between their brain activity and that of the storyteller, this ranking correlated with story understanding. Those subjects who exhibited the greatest degree of neural synchrony also had the greatest comprehension of the story. Furthermore, when the researchers considered the different time delays between the neural activation of the storyteller and the story listener, it was observed that often the corresponding activation of the listener would precede that of the teller, suggesting that the listener was anticipating the storyteller. Further analysis revealed that the extent to which story listeners exhibited this anticipatory coupling was also predictive of their comprehension of the story. Thus, those listeners who not only mirrored the neural activation of the storyteller, but also got ahead of the storyteller, anticipating what would come next, were the story listeners who most thoroughly understood the story and connected with the storyteller. This suggests that during everyday social interactions, to the extent that there is a coupling or synchronization of the neural activity of individuals interacting with one another, there will be a more effective and meaningful exchange of information. Consequently, one might reasonably ask what mechanisms, beyond mere familiarity, may be introduced that would serve to promote neural synchronization. Stephens et al. (2010) noted that there were significant differences in the extent to which their subjects exhibited neural coupling, with some subjects showing substantially stronger coupling than others. One hypothesis is that processes that involve highly structured routines will be more conducive to neural synchrony than more open-ended activities.

Within military and other similar domains, operational activities, including communications, are often highly structured. This involves choreographed sequences of activity in which each individual has a specific responsibility, with associated tasks, and the activities of the group are interleaved with the actions of the individuals who make up the group. Lindenberger et al. (2009) recorded the electroencephalogram (EEG) of eight pairs of guitarists as they played a short melody together. They observed synchronized brain activity between the guitarists during two periods. First, there was a preparatory period prior to playing the melody during which the guitarists set their tempo with the use of a metronome. Second, synchronization accompanied the start of play, and persisted throughout play, although at a reduced level. Then, once the melody was complete, the synchronization vanished. Interestingly, synchronization primarily occurred for lower-frequency brain activity, specifically delta (1–3 Hz) and theta (4–7 Hz). This may be attributable to the metronome being set at a similar frequency, yet it was noted that theta has been linked to the initiation of motor activities. These findings suggest that much like the storytellers and listeners, when individuals perform joint actions, their brains exhibit some degree of coordinated activation.

Whereas the studies discussed above involved somewhat isolated activities, groups operating in the real world must often cope with varying activities that impose different demands on group members for coordinated and individual task performance. Dodel et al. (2011) studied the neural synchronization of groups as they performed a simulated combat mission. The groups consisted of either expert operators with extensive operational experience in airborne battlespace management, or novice operators with sufficient experience to successfully complete the scenarios used in the experiment, but no operational experience. The tasks required that the groups use radar displays to monitor an ongoing battlespace, while working together to coordinate the activities of various entities within the battlespace, as well as to provide their command with an overall situation awareness. The researchers employed an approach that combined the activity from EEG recordings of the group members across frequency bands and used statistical techniques to construct a model of this activity. In this approach, the neural synchronization between group members corresponded to a simpler model with fewer dimensions. It was observed that the expert groups exhibited a lower dimensionality in their models, as compared with the novices, suggesting greater synchronization of their brain activity.

Similarly, Stevens et al. (2009) demonstrated the neural synchronization of groups engaged in a coordinated problem-solving task using EEG indicators of mental workload and engagement. The results have been extended to illustrate the presence of neural synchronies based on the same measurement techniques within the more free-flowing activities of submarine piloting and navigation teams (Stevens et al., 2012). It is suggested that real-time measurement of this nature could provide a basis for assessing ongoing operations, with the understanding that often when coping with challenging situations, there is a breakdown in group coordination. Such an idea would provide value in a training context as an indicator of group proficiency and as a diagnostic tool for intervening to improve group processes, but it might also be employed operationally as a high-level status indicator regarding the group work component of situation awareness.

Neuroeconomics

Economics underlie human social behavior, whether in the context of work, commerce, or recreation. For instance, various approaches may be employed to incentivize certain behaviors or to motivate performance. Decisions are constantly being made based on the subjective value that is assigned to objects and experiences. Trade permeates almost every human activity, whether oriented around goods, services, information, or opportunities. The responses to these situations are somewhat universal, such as the sense that someone has taken advantage of us, or the expression of status through the objects that we possess or activities in which we engage. Likewise, events in which human behavior results in unintended consequences routinely involve an overlooked economic element. A prime example has come to be known as the "Cobra Effect." The ruling government in the Indian city of Delhi became concerned about the large number of venomous snakes and offered a reward for anyone who killed a cobra and turned in the dead body. While a seemingly rational solution to the problem, the program actually made the problem worse. Entrepreneurial individuals began to breed cobras to kill and turn in for the bounty, causing the government to suspend the rewards. With there no longer being an incentive for keeping the snakes, the cobra breeders released them. As a result, having not thoroughly considered the economics that shapes human behavior, the program incentivized activities, snake breeding, which resulted in there being more dangerous snakes within the city.

Within economics, research has sought to elucidate tenets of human behavior that can be broadly generalized across different situations. Within the past decade, various groups have sought to link these behavioral tendencies to underlying neurophysiological processes. This work has given rise to a field of multidisciplinary science known as "neuroeconomics." While neuroeconomics covers a broad range of topics, the following sections provide a summary of a few pertinent topics with direct bearing on the design and engineering of systems, and associated human behavior within these systems.

Differential Response to Losses and Gains

One must frequently weigh alternative decisions with regard to potential losses and gains. Given the opportunity to change jobs, one might consider the gains associated with an increased salary and opportunities to expand one's skills and experience, but weigh these gains against losses such as losing generous health benefits and the need to frequently be away from family due to the travel required by the prospective job. When weighing alternatives of this nature, people tend to be loss averse, meaning that they assign much greater weight to potential losses than potential gains (Tversky and

Kahneman, 1992). In the laboratory, loss aversion has been studied using gambling paradigms in which given the odds of winning and the potential gains and losses, subjects must decide if they are willing to take a risk. Presented with a 50/50 chance of winning or losing, the gains must be almost double the losses before the subjects exhibit a willingness to accept the risk. Thus, given 50/50 odds, if the penalty for losing is $50, the gains for winning must be nearly $100 to induce a majority of the subjects to accept the gamble. Similarly, in studies where subjects are given an object and are allowed to use the object as their wager, the return on winning must be substantially greater than the amount the subjects would have actually paid for the object before they are willing to accept the risk of potentially parting with the object (Kahneman et al., 1990).

When subjects are posed with a decision involving potential risks, there is a differential response across a broad region of the brain that varies in proportion to the risk (Tom et al., 2007). Subjects were presented with hypothetical decisions in which there was a 50/50 chance of winning and the ratio of gains resulting from a win to losses resulting from a loss was varied. As the ratio of potential gains to losses increased, there was increasing activation of a collection of brain sites associated with the anticipation of rewards, which included the striatum, the prefrontal cortex, and the anterior cingulate cortex. In contrast, as the ratio of potential losses to gains increased, there was deactivation of this same circuit. The results did not suggest that separate circuits processed gains and losses, but that both were assessed by the same circuit, with the relative level of activation either increasing or decreasing, respectively. It was also shown that losses produced a more profound effect on the activation of this circuit than gains, with the level of decreased activation resulting from a potential loss being substantially greater than the level of increased activation resulting from an equivalent gain. Furthermore, the subjects varied in their individual sensitivity to potential gains and losses, with some being much more sensitive than others. Specifically, the subjects differed in their level of aversion to losses, with those showing the least aversion also showing the least reduction in neural activation associated with potential losses. These findings suggest that there is an innate tendency to weigh potential losses more heavily than potential gains, with this behavior based on the differential sensitivity of the brain reward systems. This trait may be manifested in a propensity to avoid risky decisions and perhaps an undue willingness to sacrifice potential gains in favor of avoiding potential losses.

Brain Basis for Subjective Value

Many decisions are not made on the basis of gains versus losses, but instead on the basis of one option being preferred over another. This type of decision is particularly prevalent in consumer purchases. Perusing the flavors offered in an ice-cream shop, I may find acceptable, even like, every option.

However, I may also select rocky road 9 times out of 10 because it is my favorite of all the flavors.

In a study by Lebreton et al. (2009), subjects were first shown images of faces, houses, or paintings and were asked to rate each with respect to its pleasantness. One month later, the subjects were shown pairs and were asked to choose which they preferred from each pair. The intent was to isolate the neural circuits that differentially responded to the subjective response to different stimuli from brain regions involved in choosing between two stimuli. This is an important distinction because our subjective assessment of various experiences, whether in the workplace or at home, during recreational or leisure activities, and so on, is based on incidental subjective responses to the environment, people, objects, and events. The results indicated that the same striatal reward circuit described previously with respect to our response to potential wins and losses, mediates our subjective responses to various stimuli.

It was noted that each category of stimuli—faces, houses, and paintings—produced activation within brain regions that are normally associated with processing stimuli corresponding to the category. For example, regions associated with processing facial stimuli were active when viewing facial stimuli. Furthermore, there was activation of the hippocampus, which may reflect the retrieval of memories associated with different stimuli. Yet, input from each of these areas fed into the reward circuits, which then produced the subjective assessment. In related research, Levy and Glimcher (2011) compared subjects' response to food, water, and monetary rewards in conditions where the subjects were exposed to varying degrees of food and water deprivation. Following deprivation, the subjects exhibited a more pronounced neural response to food or water within the reward circuits, which was accompanied by activation within distinct circuits associated with processing food, water, and monetary stimuli. Thus, it appears that there is a common brain system associated with making valuative judgments, independent of the category of items or experiences being evaluated.

In the study by Lebreton et al. (2009) where subjects indicated their preferences regarding faces, houses, and paintings, it was noted that the subjects varied in their preferences for different stimuli and that these preferences correlated with the level of activation associated with specific stimuli. A subject who generally preferred one type of house over another would consistently show greater activation for the former, whereas a subject who preferred the latter would show greater activation for the latter. Thus, the differential response represented individual subjective assessments, as opposed to a generalizable response to the universal characteristics of the stimuli. It is not that certain objects are better than others and everyone agrees, with the neural response merely reflecting recognition of superior aesthetic qualities. Instead, the response is a subjective, individual assessment, perhaps based on the sum of past experiences with similar items from each category.

From the perspective of design, these findings suggest that individuals are constantly making subjective assessments of their surroundings, including people, objects, and experiences, and that these assessments involve differential activation of circuits within the brain that are associated with the anticipation of rewards. It would be easy if certain characteristics were universally considered to be more rewarding. However, individuals differ with respect to their subjective assessments. For example, one person may view a feature within an online service favorably because it is similar to another service that has been the source of many rewarding experiences. At the same time, another individual may view the same feature negatively because he or she has had a frustrating experience elsewhere with a similar feature. One mechanism to accommodate these individual differences is to understand cultural factors and the extent to which common cultural experiences may predispose groups to view elements of design similarly. Yet, ideally, where experiences can be tailored to specific individuals, there is an opportunity to maximize the overall subjective response by tapping into the differential propensity of individuals to react positively to certain characteristics of their experiences.

Subjective Value, Now or Later

People favor immediate rewards, and will often sacrifice their overall return in favor of an immediate return. Through various experimental paradigms, it has been shown that given a choice involving either receiving an immediate reward (e.g., $5 gift card) or waiting for some duration (e.g., a week) and receiving a larger reward (e.g., $10 gift card), people will often take the immediate reward, despite it being substantially less than the delayed reward. The immediacy of a reward factors into its value with more immediate rewards perceived to be of greater value than delayed rewards. This finding has been referred to as "temporal discounting" (Frederick et al., 2002).

In research by Kable and Glimcher (2007), subjects were presented with a series of choices in which they could choose between an immediate reward of $20 or a delayed reward, which varied from trial to trial. The value of the delayed reward ranged from $20.25 to as much as $110, and the time delay varied from 6 h to 180 days. This technique allowed the researchers to calculate a discounting function for each individual, which reflected his or her willingness to sacrifice an immediate gain for a larger, yet delayed gain. The extent to which the subjects exhibited discounting, or the tendency to take an immediate reward and forgo a greater delayed gain, was correlated with the level of neural activity in three regions of the brain (ventral striatum, mPFC, and posterior cingulate cortex). These regions include the reward circuits discussed previously with respect to subjective value and suggest that the immediate reward is often perceived to be of greater value, with this associated with a more pronounced response within the reward circuits of the brain than the larger delayed reward. Similarly, differential levels of neural activation have also been shown to correlate with the extent to which discounting occurs in regard to the probability of receiving a reward (Peters and Buchel, 2009). In this case, subjects exhibit a differential tendency to accept a smaller high likelihood reward in favor of a larger, yet low likelihood reward (i.e., probability discounting). While the brain regions associated with probability discounting only partially overlap with those involved in temporal discounting, the reward circuits of the ventral striatum remain a key component. The propensity to accept a smaller reward in favor of a larger, yet riskier, reward was proportional to the level of activation of the ventral striatum reward circuits. These findings indicate that individual differences in discounting behavior are manifested in individual neural responses to subjective value.

From a systems engineering perspective, the research findings concerning discounting highlight the need to recognize individual differences in the tendency to respond to various incentives. An incentive program that is highly effective with some individuals may be modestly effective or perhaps ineffective with other individuals. Some individuals may be highly motivated by small, yet immediate rewards, but unresponsive to programs that promise substantial rewards if they are willing to wait. This applies not only to motivational incentives, but also to consumer choices. Thus, some individuals will be willing to sacrifice the quality and longevity of products in favor of lower costs. In contrast, other individuals will be content to delay a reward in favor of maximizing their gains over a longer time span. For instance, these individuals would be willing to work for lower wages given the assurance of greater long-term benefits through pension plans and health-care programs. Likewise, these individuals would be more inclined to delay purchases in favor of more expensive, higher-quality goods for which they can expect a longer service life. Within any given system, it must be recognized that participants will vary with respect to their propensity for discounting and this will affect their response to various forms of incentives, while impacting other decisions as well (e.g., purchasing, investment, etc.).

Unfairness

An ultimatum is when one person offers another a choice between two or more options and insists that he or she must pick between these options. This scenario has been incorporated into a game known as the *ultimatum game*, which offers insight into how people respond in situations perceived to be unfair. In the ultimatum game, there are two players and some item of value (e.g., money) that must be split between the two players. When the game is played with money, one player makes an offer of how to split the money. The second player may then accept or reject the offer. If the second player accepts the offer, then both players keep the money. If the second player rejects the offer, then neither player receives any of the money. From a rational perspective, the offerers should propose a split in which they retain the maximal sum and the responders should accept the offer on the basis that they have the opportunity to get something that they do not have without having to do anything for it. However, within Western cultures, players generally split the money roughly evenly and when offered a low sum (approximately 20% of the total), responders generally reject the offer (Thaler, 1988).

Research has identified the brain regions involved when players are engaged in the ultimatum game and particularly when posed with the decision to accept or reject an unfair offer (Sanfey et al., 2003). In this study, participants played the game with either a human partner or a computer, knowing that their partner was either human or a computer. It was noted that when playing against the human partner, the subjects were more willing to reject unfair offers (e.g., an $8 to $2 split or a $9 to $1 split) than when playing against a computer. When presented with an unfair offer, there was activation of the anterior insula, dorsolateral prefrontal cortex, and anterior cingulate cortex, with the activation of these regions more pronounced when playing against a human than when playing against a computer partner. Furthermore, activation of the anterior insula correlated with the relative unfairness of the offer, responding more prominently to the more disparate offers. This is interesting because research has linked the anterior insula with the experience of negative emotions and, particularly, the experience of anger and disgust. Given that much of the research concerning the anterior insula has involved the reaction to unpleasant odors and tastes, the researchers suggested that the reaction that a person experiences when presented with an unfair offer may involve the same circuits that give rise to a disgust reaction when exposed to unpleasant odors or smells. Subsequent research using skin conductance as an alternative measure of emotional reactions has confirmed this assertion (van't Wout et al., 2006). This study showed that there was indeed an emotional response when participants received an unfair offer and, similarly, this response was more pronounced when the partner was a human player, as opposed to a computer player.

In a related study involving the ultimatum game that measured the testosterone levels of players, men with higher levels of testosterone were quicker to reject low offers (Burnham, 2007). It was suggested that the low offers were perceived as challenges, triggering an emotional response comparable with that provoked when faced with a potential confrontation. The acceptance of an offer that is perceived to be unfair, yet is motivated by monetary gain, presents a conflict. One must suppress one's negative emotional reaction. In these circumstances, increased activation in the regions of the brain associated with emotional regulation (i.e., ventrolateral prefrontal cortex) has been observed (Tabibnia et al., 2008). Interestingly, given equivalent monetary gains, responses vary with regard to the perceived fairness of an offer (Tabibnia et al., 2008). In conditions in which a certain monetary gain is perceived to be unfair, but the subject accepts it, there is activation of the brain circuits associated with the suppression of negative emotions. In contrast, the exact same monetary gain accepted in conditions that are perceived to be fair produces broad activation of the reward circuits within the brain, as well as a self-reported sense of happiness with the transaction.

Within organizational systems, there is a tendency to assume that individuals and groups will react to policies in a rational manner. Furthermore, there is often surprise when seemingly benevolent offers are rejected on grounds that seem largely irrational and are based on unjustified emotions. However, it is important to remember that fairness is in the eyes of the beholder and what may seem generous to one party in a transaction may seem unfair to the other party. These outcomes are not based on simple economics, but reflect perceptions regarding the overall distribution of goods, wealth, or power and involve deeply rooted emotional processes that generally serve to protect an individual. It may be conjectured that the emotional reaction that one expresses when presented with an unfair offer may also serve to communicate a valuable lesson to the offerer. In particular, the rejection and the associated emotional reaction convey to the offerer that one will not readily allow the other to take advantage of them, and that one is not a "chump."

Unfairness toward Others

In the course of everyday activities, one may be a bystander, merely witnessing the unfair treatment of another person or group. As discussed in the previous section, there are distinct brain responses when an individual believes that he or she is being treated unfairly. Other research has considered how people respond when the subject of unfair treatment is someone else. In these studies, subjects played a variation of the prisoner's dilemma game that had been modified so that it involved economic decisions (Singer et al., 2006). In this game, there are two players who do not know about one another's actions and are not allowed to communicate. The players are asked to make a decision with the outcome of the decision based on their willingness to cooperate with one another. If neither player cooperates, they both lose. If both players cooperate, there is a modest gain. However, if one player cooperates and the other does not cooperate, the player who does not cooperate gains at the expense of the player who chose to cooperate.

The subjects in the studies by Singer et al. (2006) did not actually play the game, but merely watched as two other individuals whom they did not know played several rounds of the game. During the game, it was apparent that one of the players assumed a cooperative strategy, whereas the other player repeatedly sought to take advantage of him or her. In a subsequent analysis, the subjects revealed that they perceived the former player to be "fair" and "more likable," whereas they perceived the latter player to be "unfair" and "less likable." Afterward, the subjects and each of the players were exposed to a mildly painful stimulus (electric shock applied to the hand). The results showed that when the subjects witnessed the likable subject receiving the painful stimulus, there was activation of the same brain regions that were active when they themselves received the electric shock (i.e., anterior insula, fronto-insular cortex, and anterior cingulate cortex). This suggests that the experience of witnessing a likable individual in pain elicits an empathetic response. One has a subjective experience that is similar to the experience that one has when experiencing pain.

In contrast, when observing the unfair player experiencing pain, there was less activity in the brain circuits associated with the experience of pain than when observing the fair player in the same condition. This suggests that people tend to experience less empathy toward others who are perceived to be unfair. It was also found that with men, there was increased activation of the reward circuits of the brain (ventral striatum and nucleus accumbens) when observing the unfair player experiencing pain. This finding corresponded to a subsequent analysis that revealed an increased desire for revenge toward the unfair player in men, as compared with women. Thus, for men at least, there is a sense of satisfaction and perhaps even pleasure, associated with seeing those who are perceived to have behaved unfairly, punished for their behavior.

From a systems perspective, these findings point to the importance of there being a broad sense of fairness. It is not enough to single out individuals and take measures to ensure that they perceive themselves to be treated fairly. These experiences are not isolated to the individual. Instead, unfairness is experienced by all, and especially, when the unfairness is exhibited toward individuals or groups that are generally liked. Furthermore, when there is perceived unfairness, at least among men, there is a desire to see the unfairness punished, with this desire accompanied by a sense of satisfaction in knowing that the punishment has been administered.

Charitable Giving versus Taxation

It is common that provided sufficient resources, people exhibit a willingness to sacrifice some of those resources for the greater good. While there are tremendous individual differences in philanthropy, its existence raises questions about the internal processes that sustain the willingness to give away one's own resources. Charitable contributions may be considered in comparison to taxation whereby one is mandated to give up some portion of one's own resources for the overall civic good. In both cases, one sacrifices resources with little or no promise that one will personally benefit. However, with charity, the sacrifice is made voluntarily, and with taxation, the sacrifice is mandatory.

To study the neural processes associated with charitable giving, as opposed to taxation, researchers asked subjects to play the dictator game (Harbaugh et al., 2007). In this game, each subject received $100. The subjects were then presented with the opportunity to voluntarily contribute funds to a local food bank. At the same time, they witnessed funds being withdrawn from their account (i.e., taxation), which were also directed to the food bank. As expected, as the amount going to the charity increased and the cost to the giver decreased, there was an increasing willingness to donate funds to the charity. When the subjects received a payout to themselves, there was activation of the ventral striatal reward circuits. Similarly, there was activation of these same reward circuits when the subjects voluntarily gave away their resources. Thus, the brain experiences the same positive sensation when giving away one's resources as when receiving resources from someone else. Interestingly, the same response occurred when there was a mandatory transfer of the subjects' funds to the charity. Whether the transfer occurred through voluntary or mandatory mechanisms, there was a positive emotional experience associated with giving their resources to the charity. However, the satisfaction ratings associated with voluntary transfers were greater than those for mandatory transfers, and the voluntary transfers produced broader, more pronounced activation of the reward circuits. Subsequent research has shown that these processes are mediated by social considerations and, in particular, the magnitude of activation in the reward circuits associated with giving is greater when there are observers present than when comparable decisions are made in solitude (Izuma et al., 2010).

Harbaugh et al. (2007) next grouped subjects with respect to those who exhibited the largest activation of the reward circuits in response to receiving funds (i.e., "egoists") and those who exhibited the largest activation in response to giving funds to the charity (i.e., "altruists"). Those subjects categorized as altruists chose to contribute money to the charity twice as often as those categorized as egoists. This suggests that there exist individual differences such that those who most value receiving resources (i.e., exhibit the most pronounced response in the reward circuits of the brain) are the least inclined to give away those same resources. Likewise, those who exhibit the most activation of their reward circuits in response to sacrificing their personal resources show the greatest propensity toward charitable giving. However, the rewarding experience that is generated through charitable giving is modulated by individual social contexts. When subjects were presented with the choice to either contribute or not contribute to different charitable organizations that varied in their objectives, activation of the reward circuits was accompanied by activation of the brain regions associated with social attachment (Moll et al., 2006). When choosing to contribute to charitable organizations that shared a subject's moral perspectives, there was activation of the subgenual area of the cingulate cortex, which is a region linked to social attachment and is active when viewing photographs of one's close personal relationships (i.e., children, romantic partners). In contrast, choices involving organizations that did not share the subject's moral perspectives produced activation of the lateral orbitofrontal areas, which is a region that is responsive to social aversions. Related work has shown activation in the ventromedial prefrontal cortex in association with decisions regarding charitable contributions (Hare et al., 2010). It is suggested that this activation reflects processes associated with an appraisal of the relative value of secondary rewards, integrating input from brain regions responsive to positive and negative social influences, as a basis for making a decision.

The research described here regarding the relationship between behaviors associated with generosity, attainment of resources and charitable giving, and activation of the brain's reward circuits has important implications for behavior within organizational settings. Frequently, decisions must be made concerning the allocation of funds within an organization. Those making the decisions may act in their own self-interest, directing funds in a manner that benefits them and their close associates. This is in contrast to decisions that serve to benefit the organization as a whole, yet may offer no direct benefit to the individual decision maker. As noted, there are individual differences, with some exhibiting a greater propensity toward generosity and an accompanying willingness to sacrifice resources for the greater social good. In contrast, there are others who show a pronounced response in situations in which they are the recipient of rewards. These individuals are more likely to make decisions that promote their own self-interest, perhaps accompanied by a belief that what is in their best interest is in the best interest of the overall organization. It is noteworthy that social influences modulate the activity of the brain's reward circuits within these contexts. Consequently, by linking requests with the strongly held beliefs of decision makers, there is an opportunity to diminish the potential influence of self-interest. Furthermore, self-interest should have a diminished impact where decisions must be made in the presence of observers who have the capacity to make consequential social judgments regarding individual decision makers.

While economic decisions that occur within the workplace have a measurable impact, the same factors may similarly affect other behaviors. For instance, people regularly make decisions to either extend help to others or refrain from doing so, whether in the form of physical activities, championing other's ideas and achievements, or serving as mentors or advisors. While somewhat intangible, this help generally comes at a cost in that the helpers are sacrificing their time and energy, and sometimes putting their reputation at stake. The same neurobehavioral processes that mediate economic decision making may be extended to these situations. For example, it may be expected that individuals inclined toward altruism with respect to monetary resources would similarly be inclined toward altruism with respect to contributing their time, energy, knowledge, and social and political influence.

Trust and Cheating

No matter the currency (money, time and energy, information or knowledge, or influence and support), trust is a core element in economic transactions. Many institutional processes have evolved as a mechanism to facilitate commerce through the assurance of trust (e.g., legal contracts, commercial law, regulation of finances and business). Furthermore, trust conveys a dividend with extra costs for transactions where there is no assumed basis for trust.

In general, the human ability to trust is a mechanism to reduce the overhead associated with everyday transactions with it being more effortful to undertake transactions in which the other party cannot be trusted as compared with transactions where there is mutual trust.

To study the neurobehavioral basis for trust, researchers have employed a game called the *trust game*. In this game, experimental test subjects are assigned to pairs. Each member of the pair is informed that for showing up and agreeing to participate in the experiment, he or she will receive a payment of $10. However, the subjects must play a game in which one member of the team, the "giver," must make a decision to either keep the $10 or give some to the second member of the pair, the "reciprocator." There is a key stipulation that however much the giver agrees to transfer to the reciprocator, that amount will be quadrupled. Consequently, if the giver transfers all $10 to the reciprocator, he or she could earn as much as $40 for participating in the experiment. Once the giver has made a decision regarding transferring his or her funds to the reciprocator, the reciprocator must then make a decision to either give back some of the money or to keep it all. When subjects play this game, generally, at least three-quarters of the givers will send money to the reciprocators and an even larger portion of the reciprocators will send money back to the givers (Zak et al., 2005). On average, the givers finish the transaction with $14, whereas the reciprocators finish with $17. While there remains a disparity, these findings suggest that presented with an open expression of trust, there is a general tendency to reciprocate through sharing the bounties of that trust.

Zak et al. (2005) asked subjects to play the trust game following the conditions described above. After the transactions, blood samples were obtained from the participants. They found significantly higher levels of the neurohormone oxytocin in reciprocators following transactions in which a giver had expressed trust by transferring some of his or her money to them. This was in comparison to a condition in which the choice was made randomly by a computer and there was no intentionality on the part of the giver. Furthermore, the level of oxytocin correlated with the willingness of the reciprocators to then transfer money back to the giver. Thus, the experience of trust corresponded to an elevation in the levels of oxytocin, which was then associated with a greater tendency to reward that trust. The causal relationship between oxytocin and trusting behavior was demonstrated in a later study where subjects were administered either oxytocin or a placebo prior to playing the trust game (Kosfeld et al., 2005). The subjects who were administered oxytocin were significantly more likely to transfer funds to the giver than those receiving the placebo. This suggests that oxytocin release makes one more receptive to friendly overtures and more willing to reciprocate.

Subsequent research involving a variation of the trust game has utilized brain imaging to identify the brain regions associated with the willingness to transfer funds on the basis of trust that the recipient will reciprocate (Krueger et al., 2007). The willingness of the giver to trust the second member of their pair to reciprocate was correlated with activity in the paracingulate cortex. Interestingly, this is a region of the brain associated with Theory of Mind (ToM), or the capacity to infer the mental state, thoughts, and intentions of other individuals. Thus, situations involving trust recruit brain processes involved in imagining and assessing the mental state of another person.

In experiments involving the trust game, subjects are generally not allowed to actually see one another as they are making their decisions. In face-to-face encounters, oxytocin may have an even greater effect. Hurlemann et al. (2010) conducted a study in which subjects were required to learn category relationships through a series of decisions in which they were presented with three-digit numbers and asked to indicate if the numbers belonged to one of two categories. On each trial, feedback was presented in the form of either colored circles, with green indicating a correct response and red indicating an incorrect response, or faces, with a happy face indicating a correct response and an angry face indicating an incorrect response. In general, the subjects exhibited better learning performance for the category associations when presented with the facial feedback cues than the colored circles. However, the subjects who were administered oxytocin showed even greater learning with the facial feedback cues. This suggests that oxytocin enhances one's sensitivity to emotional cues, with facial expressions being a primary mechanism for communicating emotional states. In a related study, this was demonstrated in tests showing that those who were administered oxytocin showed higher levels of emotional empathy.

De Dreu et al. (2010, 2011) studied the effects of oxytocin on behavior within the context of team performance. In their study, subjects played a version of the prisoner's dilemma game. The subjects were given money that they could either keep for themselves or place in a pool that would be shared by all the members of their team. The subjects who were administered oxytocin were more willing to contribute to the pool, suggesting a greater willingness to trust the members of their team to similarly make contributions to the pool. In contrast, when there was another team and the subjects were told that if the other team did not contribute to the pool, they might not get as much money, the subjects who were given oxytocin were less likely to make contributions. Thus, it would appear that the trust-promoting effects of oxytocin may only operate in the context of one's own social group. Oxytocin may have the opposite effect in a context where there is a competing group, making one less likely to trust others and eliciting defensive behavior to protect one's personal assets. Furthermore, oxytocin has been shown to strengthen one's favoritism toward members of an in-group as measured by the willingness to ascribe favorable traits and exhibit emotional empathy toward individuals. At the same time, oxytocin increases the willingness to degrade members of an out-group, lessening the emotional empathy shown toward these individuals. Thus, the neurochemical properties that promote closeness and trusting relationships among people perceived to be in one's in-group, serve to fuel animosity, degradation, and dehumanization toward individuals perceived to be members of an opposing or competing group.

Related research suggests that testosterone may play an additional role in mediating our relationships with others and our willingness to exhibit trust and reciprocity (Bos et al., 2012). Subjects were presented with faces and were asked to rate the faces with regard to their being trustworthy as opposed to untrustworthy. A region of the brain known as the amygdala has been associated with a range of human emotions and, particularly, negative emotional reactions such as fear. Ordinarily, the frontal cortex and, specifically, the orbitofrontal cortex, function to regulate the response of the amygdala, allowing us to effectively cope with uncertain situations where we do not know whether there exists a basis for concern. When the subjects were administered testosterone, there was a reduction in the modulation of the amygdala responses to faces judged to be untrustworthy. This suggests that testosterone operates to diminish the capacity to squelch emotional reactions. Consequently, this may be manifested in a reduced willingness to exhibit trust. In practical contexts, testosterone may function to promote apprehensiveness in uncertain situations, as well as a tendency to impose demands for assurances to counteract mistrust of other groups and individuals.

Acknowledgments

Sandia National Laboratories is a multiprogram laboratory managed and operated by Sandia Corporation, a wholly owned subsidiary of Lockheed Martin Corporation, for the US Department of Energy's National Nuclear Security Administration under contract DE-AC04-94AL85000.

References

Bos, P.A., Hermans, E.J., Ramsey, N.F. and van Honk, J. (2012). The neural mechanisms by which testosterone acts on interpersonal trust. *NeuroImage, 61*(3), 730–737.

Burnham, T.C. (2007). High-testosterone men reject low ultimatum game offers. *Proceedings of the Royal Society B: Biological Sciences, 274*(1623), 2327–2330.

Cacioppo, J.T., Berntson, G.G. and Decety, J. (2010). Social neuroscience and its relation to social psychology. *Social Cognition, 28*, 675–684.

Cacioppo, J.T., Berntson, G.G. and Decety, J. (2011). A history of social neuroscience. In A.W. Kruglanski and W. Stroebe (eds), *Handbook of the History of Social Psychology*, pp. 123–136. New York: Psychology Press.

De Dreu, C.K., Greer, L.L., Handgraaf, M.J., Shalvi, S., Van Kleef, G.A., Baas, M. and Feith, S.W. (2010). The neuropeptide oxytocin regulates parochial altruism in intergroup conflict among humans. *Science*, *328*(5984), 1408–1411.

De Dreu, C.K., Greer, L.L., Van Kleef, G.A., Shalvi, S. and Handgraaf, M.J. (2011). Oxytocin promotes human ethnocentrism. *Proceedings of the National Academy of Science of the United States of America*, *108*(4), 1262–1266.

Devine, D.J. and Philips, J.L. (2001). Do smarter teams do better: A meta-analysis of cognitive ability and team performance? *Small Group Research*, *32*(5), 507–532.

Dodel, S., Cohn, J., Mersmann, J., Luu, P., Forsythe, C. and Jirsa, V. (2011). Brain signatures of team performance. In D.D. Schmorrow and C.M. Fidopiastis (eds), *Foundations of Augmented Cognition. Directing the Future of Adaptive Systems (Lecture Notes in Computer Science)*, Vol. 6780, pp. 288–297. Berlin and Heidelberg: Springer-Verlag.

Frederick, S., Loewenstein, G. and O'Donoghue, T. (2002). Time discounting and time preference: A critical review. *Journal of Economic Literature*, *40*, 351–401.

Gallagher, H.L., Jack, A.I., Roepstorff, A. and Frith, C.D. (2002). Imaging the intentional stance in a competitive game. *Neuroimage*, *16*(3), 814–821.

Gusnard, D.A., Akbudak, E., Shulman, G.L. and Raichle, M.E. (2001). Medial prefrontal cortex and self-referential mental activity: Relation to a default mode of brain function. *Proceedings of the National Academy of Science of the United States of America*, *98*, 4259–4264.

Gusnard, D.A. and Raichle, M.E. (2001). Searching for a baseline: Functional imaging and the resting human brain. *Nature Reviews Neuroscience*, *2*, 685–694.

Harbaugh, W.T., Mayr, U. and Burghart, D.R. (2007). Neural responses to taxation and voluntary giving reveal motives for charitable donations. *Science*, *316*(5831), 1622–1625.

Hare, T.A., Camerer, C.F., Knoepfle, D.T., O'Doherty, J.P. and Rangel, A. (2010). Value computations in ventral medial prefrontal cortex during charitable decision making incorporate input from regions involved in social cognition. *Journal of Neuroscience*, *30*(2), 583–590.

Hogg, M.A. and Tindale, R.S. (2008). Preface. *Blackwell Handbook of Social Psychology: Group Processes*. Oxford: Blackwell.

Hurlemann, R., Patin, A., Onur, O.A., Cohen, M.X., Baumgartner, T., Metzler, S. and Kendrick, K.M. (2010). Oxytocin enhances amygdala-dependent, socially reinforced learning and emotional empathy in humans. *Journal of Neuroscience*, *30*(14), 4999–5007.

Izuma, K., Saito, D.N. and Sadato, N. (2010). Processing of the incentive for social approval in the ventral striatum during charitable donation. *Journal of Cognitive Neuroscience*, *22*(4), 621–631.

Jenkins, A.C., Macrae, C.N. and Mitchell, J.P. (2008). Repetition suppression of ventromedial prefrontal activity during judgments of self and others. *Proceedings of the National Academy of Science of the United States of America*, *105*(11), 4507–4512.

Kable, J.W. and Glimcher, P.W. (2007). The neural correlates of subjective value during intertemporal choice. *Nature Neuroscience*, *10*(12), 1625–1633.

Kahneman, D., Knetsch, J.L. and Thaler, R.H. (1990). Experimental tests of the endowment effect and the Coase theorem. *Journal of Political Economy*, *98*(6), 1325–1348.

Kosfeld, M., Heinrichs, M., Zak, P.J., Fischbacher, U. and Fehr, E. (2005). Oxytocin increases trust in humans. *Nature*, *435*(7042), 673–676.

Krueger, F., McCabe, K., Moll, J., Kriegeskorte, N., Zahn, R., Strenziok, M. and Grafman, J. (2007). Neural correlates of trust. *Proceedings of the National Academy of Science of the United States of America, 104*(50), 20084–20089.

Lebreton, M., Jorge, S., Michel, V., Thirion, B. and Pessiglione, M. (2009). An automatic valuation system in the human brain: Evidence from functional neuroimaging. *Neuron, 64*(3), 431–439.

Leslie, A.M. and Thaiss, L. (1992). Domain specificity in conceptual development: Neuropsychological evidence from autism. *Cognition, 43*, 225–251.

Levi, D. (2001). *Group Dynamics for Teams*. Thousand Oaks, CA: Sage Publications.

Levine, J.M. (2012). *Group Processes*. Hoboken, NJ: Taylor and Francis.

Levy, D.J. and Glimcher, P.W. (2011). Comparing apples and oranges: Using reward-specific and reward-general subjective value representation in the brain. *Journal of Neuroscience, 31*(41), 14693–14707.

Lindenberger, U., Li, S.C., Gruber, W. and Muller, V. (2009). Brains swinging in concert: Cortical phase synchronization while playing guitar. *BMC Neuroscience, 10*, 22, http://www.biomedcentral.com/1471-2202/10/22.

Llinás, R.R. (1989). *The Biology of the Brain: From Neurons to Networks*. New York: W.H. Freeman.

Mason, M.F. and Macrae, C.N. (2008). Perspective-taking from a social neuroscience standpoint. *Group Processes and Intergroup Relations, 11*(2), 215–232.

McCabe, K., Houser, D., Ryan, L., Smith, V. and Trouard, T. (2001). A functional imaging study of cooperation in two-person reciprocal exchange. *Proceedings of the National Academy of Science of the United States of America, 98*, 11832–11835.

Mills, T.M. (1967). *The Sociology of Small Groups*. Englewood Cliffs, NJ: Prentice-Hall.

Mitchell, J.P. (2006). Mentalizing and Marr: An information processing approach to the study of social cognition. *Brain Research, 1079*(1), 66–75.

Moll, J., Krueger, F., Zahn, R., Pardini, M., de Oliveira-Souza, R. and Grafman, J. (2006). Human fronto-mesolimbic networks guide decisions about charitable donation. *Proceedings of the National Academy of Science of the United States of America, 103*(42), 15623–15628.

Orasanu, J. and Salas, E. (1993). Team decision making in complex environments. In G.A. Klein, J. Orasanu, R. Calderwood and C.E. Zsambok (eds), *Decision Making in Action: Models and Methods*, pp. 327–345. Norwood, NJ: Ablex.

Peters, J. and Buchel, C. (2009). Overlapping and distinct neural systems code for subjective value during intertemporal and risky decision making. *Journal of Neuroscience, 29*(50), 15727–15734.

Pronin, E., Berger, J. and Molouki, S. (2007). Alone in a crowd of sheep: Asymmetric perceptions of conformity and their roots in an introspection illusion. *Journal of Personality and Social Psychology, 92*(4), 585–595.

Raichle, M.E., MacLeod, A.M., Snyder, A.Z., Powers, W.J., Gusnard, D.A. and Shulman, G.L. (2001). A default mode of brain function. *Proceedings of the National Academy of Science of the United States of America, 98*, 676–682.

Rilling, J.K., Gutman, D.A., Zeh, T.R., Pagnoni, G., Berns, G.S. and Kilts, C.D. (2002). A neural basis for social cooperation. *Neuron, 35*(2), 395–405.

Rizzalotti, G. and Craighero, L. (2004). The mirror-neuron system. *Annual Review of Neuroscience, 27*, 169–192.

Sanfey, A.G., Rilling, J.K., Aronson, J.A., Nystrom, L.E. and Cohen, J.D. (2003). The neural basis of economic decision-making in the Ultimatum Game. *Science, 300*(5626), 1755–1758.

Saxe, R. and Kanwisher, N. (2003). People thinking about thinking people: The role of the temporo-parietal junction in "theory of mind". *Neuroimage, 19*(4), 1835–1842.

Saxe, R. and Wexler, A. (2005). Making sense of another mind: The role of the right temporo-parietal junction. *Neuropsychologia, 43*(10), 1391–1399.

Shaw, M.E. (1971). *Group Dynamics: The Psychology of Small Group Behavior*. New York: McGraw-Hill Book Company.

Singer, T., Seymour, B., O'Doherty, J.P., Stephan, K.E., Dolan, R.J. and Frith, C.D. (2006). Empathic neural responses are modulated by the perceived fairness of others. *Nature, 439*(7075), 466–469.

Stephens, G.J., Silbert, L.J. and Hassan, U. (2010). Speaker-listener neural coupling underlies successful communication. *Proceedings of the National Academy of Science of the United States of America, 107*(32), 14425–14430.

Stevens, R.H., Galloway, T., Berka, C. and Sprang, M. (2009). Can Neurophysiological synchronies provide a platform for adapting team performance? *Foundations of Augmented Cognition. Neuroergonomics and Operational Neuroscience (Lecture Notes in Computer Science)*, vol. 5638, pp. 658–667. Berlin: Springer.

Stevens, R.H., Galloway, T., Wang, P. and Berka, C. (2012). Cognitive neurophysiologic synchronies: What can they contribute to the study of teamwork? *Human Factors, 54*(4), 489–502.

Tabibnia, G., Satpute, A.B. and Lieberman, M.D. (2008). The sunny side of fairness: Preference for fairness activates reward circuitry (and disregarding unfairness activates self-control circuitry). *Psychological Science, 19*(4), 339–347.

Thaler, R.H. (1988). Anomalies: The ultimatum game. *Journal of Economic Perspectives, 2*(4), 195–206.

Tom, S.M., Fox, C.R., Trepel, C. and Poldrack, R.A. (2007). The neural basis of loss aversion in decision-making under risk. *Science, 315*(5811), 515–518.

Tversky, A. and Kahneman, D. (1992). Advances in prospect theory: Cumulative representation of uncertainty. *Journal of Risk and Uncertainty, 5*(4), 297–323.

Van't Wout, M., Kahn, R.S., Sanfey, A.G. and Aleman, A. (2006). Affective state and decision-making in the ultimatum game. *Experimental Brain Research, 169*(4), 564–568.

Van Vugt, M. and Schaller, M. (2007). Evolutionary approaches to group dynamics: An introduction. *Group Dynamics: Theory, Research, and Practice, 12*(1), 1–6.

Woolley, A.W., Chabris, C.F., Pentland, A., Hashmi, N. and Malone, T.W. (2010). Evidence for a collective intelligence factor in the performance of human groups. *Science, 330*, 686–688.

Woolley, A.W., Hackman, J.R., Jerde, T.E., Chabris, C.F., Bennett, S.L. and Kosslyn, S.M. (2007). Using brain-based measures to compose teams: How individual capabilities and team collaboration strategies jointly shape performance. *Social Neuroscience, 2*(2), 96–105.

Zak, P.J., Kurzban, R. and Matzner, W.T. (2005). Oxytocin is associated with human trustworthiness. *Hormones and Behavior, 48*(5), 522–527.

10

Neurotechnology

A 2007 study conducted by the Potomac Institute for Policy Studies projected that neurotechnology would be the basis for the next revolution in technology (McBride, 2007). The study recognized that the potential ramifications of neurotechnology could be on a scale comparable with those that resulted from the earlier agricultural, manufacturing, and digital revolutions. The study also envisioned a range of capabilities given the precise measurement of brain processes and effective interventions to enhance and in deleterious circumstances effectively intervene in brain functions. In essence, neurotechnology bridges one of the final technological barriers—specifically, our ability to directly interface with the mind. Furthermore, unlike other ongoing technology trends such as microelectronics and nanotechnology, neurotechnology has a relatively low cost to entry for anyone wishing to explore the possibilities, enabling opportunities for rapid innovation.

Almost a decade has passed since these assertions, and while neurotechnology remains unfamiliar to most people, the initial hints of an impending wave of new technology can be found. These can be seen in the substantial investments in research and development by the US Department of Defense. Low-cost, consumer-grade brain monitoring equipment is now readily available (e.g., Emotiv Epoch). With the increasing acceptance of physiological self-monitoring in personal health, a market has emerged for personal biometrics. Recently, there was a second meeting (NeuroGaming Conference) of industry leaders from the video game industry was held to share perspectives on the prospects for the integration of neurotechnologies, with the gaming industry recognized as fertile territory for the earliest wide-scale adoption of neurotechnologies. Perhaps, most significantly, there has been growing interest in brain science across domains extending beyond health to include education, marketing, engineering, and entertainment.

Neurotechnology to Augment, Train, Preserve, or Repair Cognitive Skills

Augmentation

Advances under the umbrella of *augmented cognition* have involved adaptive systems where physiological data from human operators allow systems to automatically adjust to the cognitive load and other ongoing cognitive demands (Forsythe et al., 2005). Within the systems that have been demonstrated to date, the system adaptations have taken several forms:

- *Task Scheduling*: the detection of high levels of cognitive demand prompted the delay of nonurgent tasks, with tasks held in a buffer until cognitive demands had subsided.
- *Task Switching:* where multiple operators were capable of performing a task, the detection of high levels of cognitive demand on one operator prompted the transfer of tasks to another operator, for whom there was a lower level of demand.
- *Adaptive Automation*: the detection of high levels of cognitive demand prompted the allocation of tasks for system automation.
- *Modality Switching*: the recognition that task demands consumed the resources associated with one sensory modality prompted the system to switch the mode of information transmission to another sensory modality (e.g., if consumed with a visual task, information would be transmitted via the auditory modality).
- *Adaptive Interfaces*: the recognition that an operator's attention was focused on a given region of an interface prompted the system to display other urgent information within that same region.
- *Contextual and Other Cues for Task Support*: the detection of high levels of cognitive demand prompted the system to provide users with mechanisms to support memory retention, context switching, and related cognitive functions.

Training

Advances under the umbrella of *brain training* emphasize activities (e.g., video games) that exercise specific brain functions. These activities are touted to provide a cognitive advantage, are highly accessible to anyone seeking them, require no special equipment other than a personal computer or gaming device, and have been designed to be engaging and entertaining, while offering personalized measures to track one's progress and achievements over time. A significant amount of research in this area has explored the cognitive effects of video games (Bavelier et al., 2011), with some researchers touting the positive effects that certain games have on the low-level vision, visual attention, and information-processing speed of the players who play them (Green and Bavelier, 2006).

A more recent trend in research on brain training involves various Internet sites such as Lumosity (Hardy and Scanlon, 2009) or MyBrainSolutions (Connole, 2011), which provide games that are designed to train diverse aspects of cognition (e.g., working memory capacity, visuospatial reasoning). While the effectiveness of these sites is a subject of debate (Slagter, 2012;

Redick et al., 2012; Kpolovie, 2012; Gordon et al., 2013), the sheer number of users (i.e., tens of millions of users) signals the demand for this kind of service.

Preservation and Repair

The preservation and repair of cognitive skills can be seen as an extension of the neurotechnology that falls under the umbrella of brain training. The motivation of the users of these systems, however, is to stave off age-related cognitive decline or to help rehabilitate physical and psychological maladies. A popular noninvasive approach involves the use of video games to prevent cognitive decline in older adults (Lange et al., 2010; Whitlock et al., 2010, 2012; Trujillo et al., 2011). More invasive approaches include transcranial magnetic stimulation (TMS), transcranial direct current stimulation (tDCS), deep brain stimulation (DBS), and vagus nerve stimulation (VNS) (Malhi and Sachdev, 2002). There has similarly been research on the use of neurosurgical implants that are designed to serve as a substitute for biological neuronal tissue (Berger et al., 2008).

Neurotechnology as a Tool to Design or Adapt Human–Computer Interaction

Other conceptions of neurotechnology have come from the field of human–computer interaction (HCI). Opportunities exist to leverage insights regarding the functioning of the brain and the central nervous system as a motivation for the design of computer systems intended for human use. For example, Causse et al. (2012) based their design of a system for aircraft terrain avoidance on insights gained from the brain's mirror neurons. Using an avatar to demonstrate the desired actions, they found superior performance as compared with traditional warnings. With product development and testing, measurement has generally involved behavioral assessments of performance in combination with a variety of techniques that elicit responses of varying degrees of subjectivity. Recently, researchers have begun to use neurophysiological measurements as a means of supplementing traditional assessments of usability (Hirshfield et al., 2009).

Neurotechnology provides a basis for inferring information about users that they might not willingly divulge, but is helpful in conceptualizing and engineering HCIs. When humans interact with computing systems, the exchange can be thought of as purposeful; users have an explicit purpose when they interact with the system, and use the information available to them (the system's status, the software's user interface, etc.) to achieve their goals. Unfortunately, the computer has disproportionately less information on which to operate, as it only knows what is communicated through its input devices (traditionally, a mouse and keyboard). Advances in HCI under the umbrella of *physiological computing* (Fairclough, 2009) have attempted to bridge that information gap by furnishing the computer with information concerning a user's psychological state, including the user's focus of attention, intentions, and motivations. These advances introduce an "improvisatory element" to the HCI and bring HCI closer to a "true dialogue with the user" (Norman, 2009), interpreting the user's behavioral cues and reacting to them dynamically. Examples within this field include the following:

- *Management of Affective State*: managing the trade-off between cognitive and affective student outcomes in intelligent tutoring systems (Boyer et al., 2008).
- *Detecting Motivational State*: activating context-specific help if a user is frustrated with a user interface or system (Scheirer et al., 2002).
- *Mediating Individual Engagement and Entertainment*: adapting an interactive experience to a user's sense of engagement (El-Nasr et al., 2010).
- *Distinguishing Classes of Users*: classifying students by their proficiency through measurements of the heart-rate variability (Zotov et al., 2011).
- *Assessing Group Engagement*: assessing the extent to which team members are mutually engaged in a task via the electroencephalogram (EEG)-based profiles of team members (Dodel et al., 2011).

Neurotechnology as a New Modality through Which Systems Are Controlled

Brain–computer interfaces (alternatively, *brain–machine interfaces* [BMI]) have been a topic of interest for many years (Vidal, 1973). The distinguishing feature of these systems is that the primary mode of interaction is via an externally derived neural command source, captured through a direct and invasive or indirect and noninvasive BMI. There has been a resurgence of interest in the use of neural interfaces to establish a communication channel between humans and machines (Donoghue, 2002). The communication channel is two way, creating two broad classes of BMIs. One class of BMI, known as "output BMI," focuses on control of external devices. Initial demonstrations of output BMIs used an EEG and allowed a user to control a cursor or other objects on a screen by producing specific patterns of brain activity (e.g., Wolpaw et al., 1991).

However, recent interest has turned to direct interfaces in which sensors are embedded within an individual's brain and input from the system comes through a low-impedance transduction of neural signals. For example, using monkeys, researchers have demonstrated the direct control of a prosthetic limb through signals emanating from the motor cortex (Velliste et al., 2008) and the control of two virtual arms through signals emanating from neurons in several frontal and parietal cortical areas (Ifft et al., 2013). In humans, direct neural control has been used to manipulate computer functions (e.g., open emails), as well as to control electronic devices such as a television (Hochberg et al., 2006).

The other class of BMI, known as input BMI, focuses on efforts to provide the brain with direct feedback from a computer device. This research is exemplified by work that is focused on enabling the blind to see through camera devices that transfer image signals directly to the visual cortex (e.g., Dobelle, 2000).

Neurophysiological Measurement

An essential component that all neurotechnology systems have in common is a mechanism for sensing some facet of a person's physiological state, with this generally occurring in real time. While brain-based measurement has been the most common basis for physiological recordings, other data sources have also been explored (e.g., heart-rate variability, pupillometry, and posture) Additionally, with many systems, mechanisms have been employed that use various system and sensor data as a means of establishing the ongoing situational context, with contextual information providing a reference for enhancing the interpretation of physiological data. For example, in automotive applications, data generated by various vehicle systems (e.g., steering rate, pressure applied to the accelerator, wheel speed) provide the basis for inferring the ongoing driving context (e.g., entering a high-speed roadway) and estimating the associated level of cognitive load that is experienced by the driver (Dixon et al., 2005).

Strengths and Challenges

Unfortunately, there is no direct indicator of cognitive function. Here, "cognitive function" is used to denote either a cognitive process or a cognitive state. The techniques outlined in Chapter 2 are indirect indicators, which measure brain activity as a function of the brain's electrical signals (i.e., EEG or magnetoencephalography [MEG]), or as a function of the brain's blood flow and blood oxygenation levels (i.e., positron emission tomography [PET] and magnetic resonance imagery [fMRI]). Because we have no way of directly measuring cognitive function or state, we must posit and then measure indirect brain activity indicators, which we have good reason to believe

are somehow correlated with the cognitive function or state we are interested in measuring. However, this methodological challenge is not unlike
that faced by physicists who study subatomic particles through interactions
in particle colliders. Thus, the nature of the problem is not one of indirect
measures, but more that we know very little about how what we measure
(e.g., electrical activity, blood flow) signifies what we want to characterize
(i.e., cognitive function or state).

Desiderata for Design in Neurotechnology

Being cognizant of the shortcomings of neurophysiology allows us to be
critical in the design of systems that intend to use neurotechnology. Despite
the shortcomings, neurotechnology is a resource of valuable information,
and if we take care to design around the shortcomings, we can still make
significant progress; such was the route taken by Petersen et al. (1988) in
their landmark article on the use PET to study word processing. Their use
of PET, however, was combined with a clever use of experimental protocols
that allowed them to assess brain activity incrementally (through a "subtrac-
tion paradigm"), such that the brain activity that they recorded showed only
the activity that they wanted to characterize.

What follows is a tripartite desiderata for design considerations in the
deployment of neurotechnological solutions. These considerations are
adapted from Fairclough (2009) and Cacioppo et al. (2000).

Desideratum 1: What Is the Relationship between the Neurophysiological Measures and the Psychological Measurement of Interest?

As mentioned, we must often tacitly assume that what we intend to measure
correlates in some way to the cognitive function of interest. There are several
ways to analyze the relationship between measures and cognitive functions
or states. In designing systems, each of the following questions should be
considered:

What Is the Assumed Mapping between the Measure and the Function?

Cognitive function is associated with some measure of activation at the neural level, but for any given function's activation, the same (or similar) activations may appear for similar or dissimilar cognitive functions. Cacioppo
et al. (2000) outlined a taxonomy of potential mappings between measures
and cognitive functions:

1. One-to-one: a measure has an isomorphic relationship with a function (the ideal case).
2. Many-to-one: several measures are associated with a function.
3. One-to-many: a measure is concordant to several functions.
4. Many-to-many: several sets of measures are concordant to several functions.

What Is the Diagnosticity of the Measure?

Diagnosticity refers to the ability of a measure to target a specific function and to remain invariant in the presence of potentially spurious influences (O'Donnell and Eggemeier, 1986). Establishing the absence of spurious influences is key to ensuring that a measure is useful.

What Is the Sensitivity of the Cognitive Function to the Measure?

Sensitivity refers to the degree to which a measure maps the fluctuation of the cognitive function of interest (O'Donnell and Eggemeier, 1986). In the design of neurotechnology systems, it is paramount to specify the expected range of the measure and whether or not this range is sufficient to distinguish between different cognitive processes. For example, if we were to use blood oxygenation levels as a proxy for a problem-solving activity, we should be able to state what our fMRI scans could reasonably pick up and, in addition, we should be able to state whether or not these scans could distinguish between high or low levels of problem-solving activity.

What Is the Reliability of the Inference?

Reliability refers to the ability of the measure to perform consistently across sessions with a given individual and across different individuals (O'Donnell and Eggemeier, 1986).

Desideratum 2: How Valid Are Inferences Concerning Cognitive Function from the Neurophysiological Measures?

Beyond establishing a precedent for the use of specific measures as proxies for specific functions (as outlined for the first desideratum), practitioners should also demonstrate that the specific measure is capable of predicting the function of interest in the respective domain-specific context. Neurotechnology designers should establish validity across a variety of representative conditions and environments, and with representative subject populations.

Validation through Laboratory Tasks

Borrowing from experimental psychology, this type of validation involves the use of standardized tasks such as mental rotation (Shepard and Metzler, 1971) or problem-solving tasks (Baker et al., 1996), for which there are known correlations between measures and functions. Validation through laboratory tasks requires that there exist a strong relation between the task and the target psychological construct. Given that relation, we can verify that a specific neurophysiological measure captures brain activity in the context of the task of interest. Ideally, multiple experimental contexts involving the cognitive function of interest are available, such that we can assess the range of potential neurophysiological responses.

Validation through Subjective Measures

Subjective self-reports are useful in the design of neurotechnological systems since they represent the experience of individual users. Invariably, there will be individual differences across users who use neurotechnology applications, and subjective measures can help fine-tune the experience for an individual user.

Desideratum 3: How Are We Representing the User?

A third important concern is how users of the neurotechnological application are represented by the system. Neurotechnology systems, based on neurophysiological measures, will typically represent the user in terms of cognitive functions. For example, a system could characterize a user engaged in problem-solving tasks in terms of his or her estimated task engagement and distress (Matthews et al., 2002). These composite measures might be derived from the neurophysiological measures. To represent the user, designers will typically need to decide two things.

What Is the Dimensionality of the Representation?

The dimensionality refers to the number of variables that the system will compute as a function of the neurophysiological measures. Designers must decide on a representation that is rich enough to afford meaningful interaction for the user and is constrained enough in scope so that the computations needed to assess the user are tractable. As seen in Fairclough (2009), the dimensionality of neurotechnology applications often does not exceed two dimensions (e.g., tracking engagement and distress) due to the combinatorial explosions that can result from tracking more variables. Typical representations are:

1. One-dimensional continuum
2. One-dimensional discrete

3. Two-dimensional continuum

4. Two-dimensional discrete

What Is the Modality of the Representation?

Beyond considering issues of dimensionality, designers may want to consider combining neurophysiological data with context-specific data (e.g., task progression, time spent in an estimated psychological state), to give computational systems greater information than the moment-to-moment calculations of the psychological state.

Future Directions

Neurogaming

Perhaps the first domain in which there will be broad acceptance of neurotechnology is gaming, with neurogaming now recognized as an emerging field within the gaming industry. Today, gaming is a greater than $20 billion industry (Entertainment Software Association, 2012) in which manufacturers are constantly seeking opportunities to differentiate themselves from their competition and users are generally accepting of new technologies. Relatively low-cost, reliable, and easy-to-use headsets that measure brain activity are now available from various companies. However, neurotechnology is only starting to impact gaming. This is most likely attributable to the newness of the technology and that a compelling application has not yet been identified. Yet, recently, titles such as Son of Nor (Stillalive Studios, 2013) have appeared where the player can move and explode objects by producing specific patterns of brain activity, effectively giving the player telekinetic powers. Moreover, there are several aspects of neurogaming that have the potential to be transformative.

Multiplayer Neurogaming

Multiplayer gaming is enormously popular, with players able to meet within a virtual space and simultaneously conduct activities in unison or in opposition to one another. When a given player takes an action, he or she can observe behaviorally how that action has affected other players, which is the same experience we have within the real world. However, if players are each wearing headsets and their respective brain activity is being monitored and displayed to other players, a given individual can not only see how his or her actions have affected other players behaviorally, but also physiologically and, by inference, psychologically. This has the potential to be transformative in that this is an experience that is readily achievable within a gaming environment, yet it is not possible in real life. Thus, within gaming environments, there is an opportunity to attain a level of interpersonal awareness for which it is difficult to anticipate its ramifications. Furthermore, if such a capability arises and flourishes within gaming environments, it is likely that analogs will soon emerge within nongaming environments, promoted by the growing integration of gaming and everyday, nongaming devices through the spread of increasingly powerful go-anywhere mobile electronics.

Neurocognitive Approaches to Interactive Narratives

Game environments increasingly rely on narrative structures to guide players toward the completion of specific in-game tasks. While playing games that provide an interactive narrative experience, players' story comprehension faculties are engaged as they project a fictional world (Gerrig and Bernardo, 1994; Sengers, 1998; Ryan, 1999; Gerrig, 2013), such that players project themselves as the avatars under their control, and that the story context in which they are embedded plays a key role in how they perceive their potential actions. Designers of interactive narrative experiences would do well to go beyond ensuring that game story structures are logically coherent, and should take care to account for how the player experiences the narrative (Szilas, 2010). Indeed, efforts are underway to study the effect that games and narratives have on players at a cognitive level (Cardona-Rivera et al., 2012; Cardona-Rivera and Young, 2013). These efforts stand to be enhanced through the incorporation of insights gained through advances in the study of the neuropsychology of narrative (Mar, 2004), as well as an understanding of the neuroscientific underpinnings of play.

Acknowledgments

Sandia National Laboratories is a multiprogram laboratory managed and operated by Sandia Corporation, a wholly owned subsidiary of Lockheed Martin Corporation, for the US Department of Energy's National Nuclear Security Administration under contract DE-AC04-94AL85000. This chapter was supported in part by a Department of Energy Computational Science Graduate Fellowship, Grant No. DE-FG02-97ER25308.

References

Baker, S.C., Rogers, R.D., Owen, A.M., Frith, C.D., Dolan, R.J., Frackowiak, R.S. and Robbins, T.W. (1996). Neural systems engaged by planning: A PET study of the Tower of London task. *Neuropsychologia*, 34(6), 515–526.

Bavelier, D., Green, C.S., Hyun Han, D., Renshaw, P.F., Merzenich, M.M. and Gentile, D.A. (2011). Brains on video games. *Nature Reviews Neuroscience*, 12(12), 763–768.

Berger, T.W., Gerhardt, G., Liker, M.A. and Soussou, W. (2008). The impact of neuro-technology on rehabilitation. *IEEE Reviews in Biomedical Engineering*, 1, 157–197.

Boyer, K.E., Phillips, R., Wallis, M., Vouk, M. and Lester, J. (2008). Balancing cognitive and motivational scaffolding in tutorial dialogue. In B.P. Woolf, E. Aimeur, R. Nkambou and S. Lajoie (eds), *Proceedings of the 9th International Conference on Intelligent Tutoring Systems*, pp. 239–249. Heidelberg: Springer.

Cacioppo, J.T., Tassinary, L.G. and Berntson, G. G. (2000). Psychophysiological science. In J.T. Cacioppo, L.G. Tassinary and G.G. Berntson (eds), *Handbook of Psychophysiology*, pp. 3–26. Cambridge: Cambridge University Press.

Cardona-Rivera, R.E. and Young, R.M. (2013). A cognitivist theory of affordances for games. In *Proceedings of the Digital Games Research Conference: DeFragging Game Studies*. August 26–29, Atlanta, GA.

Cardona-Rivera, R.E., Cassell, B.A., Ware, S.G. and Young, R.M. (2012). Indexter: A computational model of the event-indexing situation model for characterizing narratives. In *Proceedings of the Working Notes of the Workshop on Computational Models of Narrative at the Language Resources and Evaluation Conference*, pp. 32–41. May 26–27, Istanbul, Turkey.

Causse, M., Phan, J., Segonzac, T. and Dehais, F. (2012). Mirror neuron based alerts for control flight into terrain avoidance. *Advances in Cognitive Engineering and Neuroergonomics*, 16, 157–166.

Connole, I. (2011). MyBrainSolutions. *Journal of Sport Psychology in Action*, 2(3), 197.

Dixon, K.R., Lippitt, C.E. and Forsythe, J.C. (2005). Supervised machine learning for modeling human recognition of vehicle-driving situations. In *Proceedings of International Conference on Intelligent Robots and Systems*, pp. 604–609. Edmonton, AB: IEEE.

Dobelle, W.H. (2000). Artificial vision for the blind by connecting a television camera to the visual cortex. *ASAIO Journal*, 46(1), 3–9.

Dodel, S., Cohn, J., Mersmann, J., Luu, P., Forsythe, J.C. and Jirsa, V. (2011). Brain signatures of team performance. In *Proceedings of the 6th International Conference on Foundations of Augmented Cognition: Directing the Future of Adaptive Systems*, pp. 288–297. July 9–14, Orlando FL.

Donoghue, J.P. (2002). Connecting cortex to machines: Recent advances in brain interfaces. *Nature Neuroscience*, 5, 1085–1088.

El-Nasr, M.S., Morie, J.F. and Drachen, A. (2010). A scientific look at the design of aesthetically and emotionally engaging interactive entertainment experiences. In D. Gökçay and G. Yildirim (eds), *Affective Computing and Interaction: Psychological, Cognitive, and Neuroscientific Perspectives*, pp. 281–307. Hershey, PA: IGI Global.

Entertainment Software Association. (2012). *The Entertainment Software Association—Industry Facts*. Retrieved December 3, 2013, http://www.theesa.com/facts/index.asp.

Fairclough, S.H. (2009). Fundamentals of physiological computing. *Interacting with Computers*, 21(1), 133–145.

Forsythe, J.C., Kruse, A. and Schmorrow, D. (2005). Augmented cognition. In J.C. Forsythe, M.L. Bernard and T.E. Goldsmith (eds), *Cognitive Systems: Human Cognitive Models in Systems Design*, pp. 99–135. Mahwah, NJ: Lawrence Erlbaum.

Gerrig, R.J. (2013). *A Participatory Perspective on the Experience of Narrative Worlds*. New York: Stony Brook University.

Gerrig, R.J. and Bernardo, A.B. (1994). Readers as problem-solvers in the experience of suspense. *Poetics*, 22(6), 459–472.

Gordon, E., Palmer, D.M., Liu, H., Rekshan, W. and DeVarney, S. (2013). Online cognitive brain training associated with measurable improvements in cognition and emotional well-being. *Technology and Innovation*, 15, 53–62.

Green, C.S. and Bavelier, D. (2006). The cognitive neuroscience of video games. In P. Messaris and L. Humphreys (eds), *Digital Media: Transformations in Human Communication*, pp. 211–223. New York: Peter Lang International Academic Publishers.

Hardy, J. and Scanlon, M. (2009). The science behind lumosity. www.lumosity.com/documents/the_science_behind_lumosity.pdf. Retrieved May 30, 2014.

Hirshfield, L.M., Solovey, E.T., Girouard, A., Kebinger, J., Jacob, R.J., Sassaroli, A. and Fantini, S. (2009). Brain measurement for usability testing and adaptive interfaces: An example of uncovering syntactic workload with functional near infrared spectroscopy. In *Proceedings of the SIGCHI Conference on Human Factors in Computing Systems*, pp. 2185–2194. New York: ACM.

Hochberg, L.R., Serruya, M.D., Friehs, G.M., Mukand, J.A., Saleh, M., Caplan, A.H., Branner, A., Chen, D., Penn, R.D. and Donoghue, J.P. (2006). Neuronal ensemble control of prosthetic devices by a human with tetraplegia. *Nature*, 442, 164–171.

Ifft, P.J., Sokur, S., Li, Z., Lebedev, M.A. and Nicolelis, M.A. (2013). A brain-machine interface enables bimanual arm movements in monkeys. *Science Translational Medicine*, 5, 210.

Kpolovie, P.J. (2012). Luminosity training and brain-boosting food effects on learning. *Educational Research Journals*, 2(6), 217–230.

Lange, B.S., Requejo, P., Flynn, S.M., Rizzo, A.A., Valero-Cuevas, F.J., Baker, L. and Winstein, C. (2010). The potential of virtual reality and gaming to assist successful aging with disability. *Physical Medicine and Rehabilitation Clinics of North America*, 21(2), 339–356.

Malhi, G.S. and Sachdev, P. (2002). Novel physical treatments for the management of neurpsychiatric disorders. *Journal of Psychosomatic Research*, 53, 709–719.

Mar, R.A. (2004). The neuropsychology of narrative: Story comprehension, story, production and their interrelation. *Neuropsychologia*, 42(10), 1414–1434.

Matthews, G., Campbell, S.E., Falconer, S., Joyner, L.A., Huggins, J., Gilliland, K., Grier, R. and Warm, J.S. (2002). Fundamental dimensions of subjective state in performance settings: Task engagement, distress, and worry. *Emotion*, 2(4), 315–340.

McBride, D. (2007). *Neurotechnology Futures Study*. Arlington, VA: Potomac Institute for Policy Studies, Potomac Institute Press.

Norman, D.A. (2009). *The Design of Future Things*. New York: Basic Books.

O'Donnell, R.D. and Eggemeier, F.T. (1986). Workload assessment methodology. In K. Boff, L. Kaufman and J. Thomas (eds), *Handbook of Human Perception and Performance*, vol. 2, pp. 42.1–42.49. New York: Wiley.

Petersen, S.E., Fox, P.T., Posner, M.I., Mintun, M. and Raichle, M.E. (1988). Positron emission tomographic studies of the cortical anatomy of single-word processing. *Nature*, 331(6157), 585–589.

Redick, T.S., Shipstead, Z., Harrison, T.L., Hicks, K.L., Fried, D.E., Hambrick, D.Z., Kane, M.J. and Engle, R.W. (2012). No evidence of intelligence improvement after working memory training: A randomized, placebo-controlled study. *Journal of Experimental Psychology: General*, 142(2), 359–380.

Ryan, M.-L. (1999). Immersion vs. interactivity: Virtual reality and literary theory. Technical report, Department of English, Colorado State University, Fort Collins, CO.

Scheirer, J., Fernandez, R., Klein, J. and Picard, R.W. (2002). Frustrating the user on purpose: A step toward building an affective computer. *Interacting with Computers, 14*(2), 93–118.

Sengers, P. (1998). Narrative intelligence. Technical report, Institute for Visual Media, Center for Art and Media Technology (ZKM), Karlruhe, Germany.

Shepard, R.N. and Metzler, J. (1971). Mental rotation of three-dimensional objects. *Science, 171*(3972), 701–703.

Slagter, H.A. (2012). Conventional working memory training may not improve intelligence. *Trends in Cognitive Sciences, 16*(12), 582–583.

Stillalive Studios. (2013). Son of Nor. Stillalive Studios, Innsbruck.

Szilas, N. (2010). Requirements for computational models of interactive narrative. In *Proceedings of the AAAI Fall Symposium on Computational Models of Narrative*, pp. 62–68. November 11–13, Arlington, VA.

Trujillo, A.K., Whitlock, L.A., Patterson, T., McLaughlin, A.C., Allaire, J.C. and Gandy, M. (2011). Benefits of playing a complex spatially challenging video game on cognitive functioning in older adults. *Gerontologist, 51*, 278.

Velliste, M., Perel, S., Spalding, C., Whitford, A.S. and Schwartz, A.B. (2008). Cortical control of a prosthetic arm for self-feeding. *Nature, 453*(7198), 1098–1101.

Vidal, J.-J. (1973). Toward direct brain-computer communication. *Annual Review of Biophysics and Bioengineering, 2*(1), 157–180.

Whitlock, L.A., McLaughlin, A.C. and Allaire, J.C. (2010). Training requirements of a video game-based cognitive intervention for older adults: Lessons learned. *Proceedings of the Human Factors and Ergonomics Annual Meeting, 54*, 2343–2346.

Whitlock, L.A., McLaughlin, A.C. and Allaire, J.C. (2012). Individual differences in response to cognitive training: Using a multi-modal, attentionally demanding game-based intervention for older adults. *Computers in Human Behavior, 28*, 1091–1096.

Wolpaw, J.R., McFarland, D.J., Neat, G.W. and Forneris, C.A. (1991). An EEG-based brain-computer interface for cursor control. *Electroencephalography and Clinical Neurophysiology, 78*(3), 252–259.

Zotov, M., Forsythe, C., Voyt, A., Akhmedova, I. and Petrukovich, V. (2011). A dynamic approach to the physiological-based assessment of resilience to stressful conditions. In D. Schmorrow and C.M. Fidopiastis (eds), *Foundations of Augmented Cognition: Directing the Future of Adaptive Systems*, pp. 657–666. Berlin: Springer-Verlag.

Index

Printed and bound by CPI Group (UK) Ltd, Croydon, CR0 4YY

18/10/2024

01776271-0007